Y0-BJM-535

Research Design
In Speech Pathology
And Audiology

*asking and
answering questions*

FRANKLIN H. SILVERMAN

Marquette University

Research Design In Speech Pathology And Audiology

asking and answering questions

Prentice-Hall, Inc., Englewood Cliffs, New Jersey   07632

Library of Congress Cataloging in Publication Data

SILVERMAN, FRANKLIN H (Date)
   Research design in speech pathology and audiology.

   Includes bibliographies and index.
   1. Speech, Disorders of—Research. 2. Audiology
—Research. I. Title. [DNLM: 1. Speech disorders.
2. Hearing disorders. 3. Research. WM475 S587r]
RC423. S52   616. 8'55'00184   76-45471
ISBN 0-13-774117-0

© 1977 by Prentice-Hall, Inc., Englewood Cliffs, New Jersey 07632

*All rights reserved. No part of this book may
be reproduced in any form or by any means without
permission in writing from the publisher.*

Printed in the United States of America

10 9 8 7 6 5

Prentice-Hall International, Inc., *London*
Prentice-Hall of Australia Pty. Limited, *Sydney*
Prentice-Hall of Canada, Ltd., *Toronto*
Prentice-Hall of India Private Limited, *New Delhi*
Prentice-Hall of Japan, Inc., *Tokyo*
Prentice-Hall of Southeast Asia Pte. Ltd., *Singapore*
Whitehall Books Limited, *Wellington, New Zealand*

*To my wife Ellen-Marie and my daughter Catherine,
for establishing an environment of love
that made it possible for this book to be written*

CONTENTS

PREFACE *xiii*

part I
Introduction 1

ONE
NEED FOR RESEARCH IN
SPEECH PATHOLOGY AND AUDIOLOGY *3*

    Questioning and Clinical Effectiveness *4*
    Need for Systematic Observation in Answering Questions *5*
    Satisfying the Need for Systematic Observation *7*
    Questions and Answers *8*
    Has the Need Been Met? *11*
    References *11*

TWO
RESEARCH AND THE CLINICIAN *13*

Why be a Clinician-Investigator? *14*
Who Can be a Clinician-Investigator? *20*
References *25*

THREE
RESEARCH AS A PROCESS
OF ASKING AND ANSWERING QUESTIONS *27*

What is the Scientific Method? *29*
The Scientific Method as a Set of Rules
   for Asking and Answering Questions *43*
References *44*

part II
Asking and Answering Questions 47

FOUR
ASKING QUESTIONS
THAT ARE BOTH RELEVANT AND ANSWERABLE *49*

Generating Relevant Questions for Research *51*
Structuring Research Questions to Make Them Answerable *62*
References *64*

FIVE
SELECTING THE APPROPRIATE DESIGN
FOR ANSWERING SPECIFIC QUESTIONS *65*

Differences Between Individual Subject
   and Typical Subject Designs *67*
Advantages and Disadvantages of Each Design *72*

Variations Possible Within Each Category of Design *75*
Which Type of Design Should You Use? *87*
References *87*

SIX
TYPES OF DATA *89*

What are Data? *89*
Types of Data *92*
Measurement–Related Properties of Quantitative Data *97*
References *107*

SEVEN
APPROACHES TO GENERATING QUANTITATIVE DATA *109*

Role of the Observer in the Measurement Process *109*
Measurement Schemes Which Utilize an Instrument
  to Supplement Observer Judgment *113*
Measurement Schemes That Rely Primarily Upon Observer
  Judgment: Psychological Scaling Methods *130*
References *161*

EIGHT
ORGANIZING DATA FOR ANSWERING QUESTIONS *165*

Strategies for Organizing Qualitative Data
  for Answering Questions *166*
Strategies for Organizing Quantitative Data
  for Answering Questions *170*
References *215*

NINE
CONSIDERATIONS IN INTERPRETING ANSWERS
TO QUESTIONS *216*

Dimensions to Consider When Evaluating Answers *217*
Criteria for Evaluating Reliability, Validity, and Generality *222*
References *227*

TEN
COMMUNICATING
QUESTIONS AND ANSWERS *228*

    Modes for Disseminating Research Findings *228*
    Objectives of Scientific Communication *231*
    Organization of Written Reports *233*
    Organization of Oral Presentations *238*
    Preparation of Written and Oral Reports *239*
    Locating Outlets for Speech Pathology and Audiology Research *240*
    Editorial Processing of Manuscripts *241*
    References *243*

part III
Clinical Research Considerations 245

ELEVEN
ASSESSING
THE EFFECTS OF THERAPIES *247*

    Choice of Presumption *247*
    Questions to Consider When Evaluating a Therapy *250*
    Research Design Considerations
       for Assessing the Effects of Therapies *252*
    References *269*

TWELVE
ESTABLISHING A COMMUNICATIVE DISORDERS
RESEARCH PROGRAM IN A CLINICAL SETTING *270*

    Achieving Administrative Support *270*
    Preparing a Research Proposal *271*
    Research Funding *274*
    Use of Consultants *275*
    References *276*

Appendices 277

A

COMPUTATIONAL FORMULAS, WORKED EXAMPLES, AND EXERCISES FOR SELECTED DESCRIPTIVE AND INFERENTIAL STATISTICS THAT ARE PRACTICAL TO COMPUTE WITH A DESK OR SLIDE RULE CALCULATOR *279*

Contents *279*
References *326*

B

TABLE OF RANDOM NUMBERS *327*

GLOSSARY *336*

AUTHOR INDEX *343*
SUBJECT INDEX *346*

PREFACE

With the present emphasis on "accountability," speech pathologists and audiologists are finding it increasingly advantageous to be able to demonstrate "scientifically" the impacts of their clinical programs—both diagnostic and therapeutic—on their clients. Providing such a demonstration involves the asking and answering of certain questions. This book deals with the methodologies involved in identifying, formulating, and answering these questions as well as those related to the symptomatology (phenomenology) and etiology of communicative disorders. It is intended to acquaint the advanced undergraduate and masters level graduate student as well as the professional speech pathologist and audiologist and professionals in related fields (such as the language pathologist and learning disabilities specialist) with the meaningfulness of research findings to the clinician and to help them understand on an "intuitive" level the process of designing clinically-relevant research. Its main purpose is to provide clinicians with the essential information they need to function as investigators (i.e., *clinician-investigators*) if they so choose.

The book is divided into three parts. In the first, or introductory, part (which consists of the first three chapters) I indicate the relevance of research to the clinician; why he or she probably would find it advantageous to do clinical research (i.e., function as a clinician-investigator); and the nature of the scientific method which underlies the research process—i.e., the asking and answering of questions.

In the second part of the book (which includes chapters four through 10) I describe a process for asking and answering questions based on the scientific method. I begin with that for asking questions, particularly the process by which questions are generated for research that both are relevant and "answerable." I then deal with that for answering questions including selection of an appropriate design for making the necessary observations, describing the observations made (quantitatively and/or qualitatively), and organizing and summarizing (numerical and verbal) descriptions of observations so they can be used to answer questions. Next, some factors that must be considered when interpreting answers to questions are described. The dissemination of research findings, with particular emphasis on the preparation of written reports and oral presentations, follows.

In the third part of the book (which includes chapters 11 and 12) I discuss two topics that are relevant to functioning as a clinician-investigator. The first deals with assessing the effects of therapies with particular emphasis on seven questions it would be desirable to answer when assessing the impact of any therapy on a person who has a communicative disorder. The second presents some considerations when attempting to establish a communicative disorders research program in a clinical setting.

It is impossible to give credit to the many sources from which the concepts presented in this book have been drawn. This book is the result of years of reading and thousands of hours of conversation with students and colleagues in the areas of communicative disorders and research methodology. Thus, I cannot credit this or that concept to a specific person, but I can say "thank you" to all who have helped, particularly my graduate students at Marquette University and the University of Illinois at Urbana-Champaign whose questions and criticisms through the years have helped me to clarify my own ideas.

Some special thanks are due to Dr. Dorothy Sherman of the University of Iowa—pioneer research methodologist in the field of communicative disorders—for introducing me to the "intuitive" approach to research methodology and psychological scaling. Special thanks also are due to Dr. David Lilly of the University of Iowa for introducing me to instrumentation schemes for measurement and to Dean Alfred J. Sokolnicki of the Marquette University College of Speech for reducing my teaching load several semesters to facilitate the writing of this book. And last, but certainly not least, I wish to thank my wife Ellen-Marie for her many questions, criticisms, and suggestions which helped me to clarify many of the concepts presented here.

FRANKLIN H. SILVERMAN

part I

Introduction

ONE

NEED FOR RESEARCH IN SPEECH PATHOLOGY AND AUDIOLOGY

The objective of this chapter is to demonstrate the relevance of pure and applied research to evaluation and therapy (clinical process) in speech pathology and audiology. *Pure research* means research that implicitly or explicitly is intended to increase our understanding of the etiology (that is, the predisposing, precipitating, and maintaining causes) of communicative disorders. *Applied research* means research that implicitly or explicitly is intended to increase our understanding of how to prevent the development of, or modify behaviors contributing to, communicative disorders. Some research serves both functions: it provides data relevant to the etiology of communicative disorders as well as to their prevention or treatment.

The term *research* in this book refers to the processes underlying the *asking* and *answering* of questions as well as to the "answers" that can be abstracted from the observations provided by such processes. In a sense, the overall objective of this book is to clarify and elaborate upon this definition of research as it applies to clinical process in speech pathology and audiology.

You, the readers of this book, must have as strong a belief as possible in the relevance of research to your activities before deciding how much to invest in acquiring a knowledge of research methodology. The amount you are willing to invest to attain a goal is at least partially a function of the return you anticipate from the investment. If you expect a substantial return, you will usually invest more than if you anticipate little, if any, return. The stronger your belief that learning certain material will directly influence your activities, the more time and energy you will probably devote to learning that material. Also, the stronger your belief that learning certain material will directly influence your activities, the more willing you would probably be to tackle material you expect to be difficult, such as statistical and research design concepts. And the more willing you are to tackle such material and the more time and energy you devote to mastering it, the more likely you are to be successful in mastering it. Many people who have difficulty understanding statistical and research design concepts appear to experience difficulty *not* because of lack of ability, but because they are not convinced of the relevance of such concepts to their activities and, therefore, do not invest the time and energy necessary to understand them. The goal of this chapter is to strengthen your belief in the relevance of research to your activities.

QUESTIONING AND CLINICAL EFFECTIVENESS

We will begin our discussion of the relevance of research to clinical process in speech pathology and audiology with the following premise: To be even minimally effective, a clinician must be able to answer at least partially certain questions. These questions include:

1. Is the communicative behavior of the child or adult whom I am evaluating "within normal limits?"
2. If his communicative behavior is not "within normal limits," what is the reason?
3. How can his communicative behavior be modified to bring it "within normal limits," or as close as possible to this goal?

If we are not aware of "normal limits" for such dimensions as articulation, fluency, syntax, and language comprehension, we will be unable to determine reliably whether a child or adult (particularly a child) has a communicative disorder. We will tend to make one or both of the following errors more often than we should: (1) classifying a person whose communicative behavior is "within normal limits" as having a communicative disorder, or (2) classifying a person who has a communicative disorder as having communicative behavior "within normal limits." We may, for example, classify a four-year-old who has an IQ of approximately 100 and consistently substitutes /d/ for /ð/ as not having articulation "within normal limits." Also, we might classify a four-year-old who is "effortlessly" repeating some words as beginning to stutter. To answer questions concerning the normality of a four-year-old's communicative behavior, we must have information concerning the communicative behavior of "normal" four-year-olds. That is, we must have access to relevant normative data.

If the answer to the first question is *no* (that is, if we do not judge the person's communicative behavior to be "within normal limits"), we then attempt to answer the second, or "why," question. To answer this question, we have to be able to specify the possible causes for the deviation or deviations we have observed. We need this information to perform a differential diagnosis—to rule in and rule out possible causes systematically. We also need this information to plan therapy. For a therapy strategy to have maximum probability of success, it should be based upon, or derived from, our assumption or assumptions about why a client's communicative behavior is not "within normal limits."[1]

Once we have at least partially established the reason or reasons for a client's communicative behavior not being "within normal limits," we then plan a therapy strategy that will hopefully either bring it "within normal limits" or as close as possible to this goal. To plan such a strategy, or to answer the "how" question, we need information concerning the relative effectiveness of the various strategies that could be used. For each possible strategy, we also need related information, including negative side effects and susceptibility to relapse. Such information provides guidelines for answering the "how" question and thereby helps to maximize the probability of achieving the therapy goal or goals.

NEED FOR SYSTEMATIC OBSERVATION IN ANSWERING QUESTIONS

How do we go about answering questions such as the three previously discussed so that the probability of a correct answer is maximized? Answering questions in this manner requires the type of data that results from systematic observation. The term *data* as used here refers to numerical and verbal descriptions of attributes of events. Attributes of the event "speech," for example, would include "accuracy of articulation" and "amount of word repetition." And attributes of the event "listening" would include "sound discrimination ability" and "level of comprehension." Numerical descriptions of attributes of events are referred to as *quantitative* and verbal as *qualitative*.

Systematic observation is a process that permits us to describe individual attributes of events. We decide in advance which attributes of which events we wish to describe and then for each attribute devise a "filter" that

[1]See Williams (1968) for a discussion of the role of such assumptions in planning stuttering therapy.

will permit us to make the desired observations. The filter makes each target attribute—each attribute we seek to describe—stand out sufficiently from the others so that it can be described reliably. The filter, then, enhances the figure-background relationship (the target attribute being the figure and the other attributes the background). The filter may include instrumentation to enhance the observer's ability to restrict his observational processes, or it may consist solely of a "set" the observer gives himself to restrict his observational processes. Speech pathologists usually give themselves such a set during the administration of a picture articulation test, since they pay most attention to the particular speech sound each picture was included to elicit. This sound would be the figure (i.e., the target attribute), the other sounds in the word would be the background. Instrumentation used by speech pathologists and audiologists for this purpose is described in Chapter 7.

Systematic observation maximizes the probability that the data used to answer questions will yield correct answers by maximizing the probability that they will possess adequate validity and reliability for the purpose. By adequate *validity* in this context, we mean that the filter used to observe and describe a particular attribute of a particular event actually permits us to observe and describe that attribute of that event. If we wished, for example, to determine how frequently a child produced a lateral /s/ (attribute) during conversational speech (event), having observers listen to tape recordings of the child's conversational speech and identifying instances of lateral /s/ on typescripts of the recordings should yield data which possess adequate validity for this purpose. Also, if one wished to estimate how much an adult understands when he listens to someone speak (event), his ability to understand single words (attribute)—e.g., a PB-50 world list (Egan, 1948)—would probably possess adequate validity for the purpose.

By maximizing the probability that the data used to answer a question will possess adequate *reliability*, we mean that the filter used to observe and describe an attribute of an event permits this to be done with a *sufficient level of accuracy*—that is, a level that permits the minimum desired degree of confidence in the correctness of the answer. The less distortion (or error) introduced by the filter, the more reliable will be the resulting data. As indicated in the previous paragraph, a valid method for estimating how frequently a child produced a lateral /s/ probably would be to tape record his conversational speech and have trained listeners indicate instances of lateral /s/ on a typescript of the recording. For this methodology to be adequately reliable as well as valid, the tape recordings would have to be of sufficiently high quality that instances of lateral /s/ could be identified from them with minimal error. Similarly, for estimates of an adult's ability to understand single words to be adequately reliable as well as valid, the environment in which the words are presented would have to be sufficiently noise-free.

Systematic observation, in addition to maximizing the probability that the data used to answer a question will possess adequate levels of validity and reliability for the purpose, also provides a methodology for determining whether this goal has been achieved. In fact, this methodology permits us to estimate the validity and reliability levels of a set of data. These constructs will be discussed further in Chapter 9.

SATISFYING THE NEED FOR SYSTEMATIC OBSERVATION

The preceding section discussed why systematic observation could be expected to result in the type of data which maximizes the probability of correct answers to questions. We will now consider how pure and applied research can satisfy, at least partially, the need for systematic observation.

Systematic observation is used in both pure and applied research. It is, in fact, a component (as will be shown in Chapter 3) of the scientific method that underlies almost all research. For this reason, data yielded by both types of research can be used by speech pathologists and audiologists to answer questions of professional interest, including those on clinical process.

The previous section discussed three questions that a clinician needs to be able to answer to function effectively. *How can data from pure and applied research help to maximize the probability of a correct answer to each question?*

The first of these questions was: Is the communicative behavior of the child or adult whom I am evaluating "within normal limits?" To maximize the probability of a correct answer, a clinician needs *normative data*—data that help to define "normal limits" for each attribute of communicative behavior being evaluated. Such data have been reported for a number of attributes of communicative behavior in research papers appearing in such journals as the *Journal of Speech and Hearing Disorders* and the *Journal of Speech and Hearing Research*. Attributes of communicative behavior for which normative research-based data have been reported include speech fluency (Johnson, 1959, 1961), speech articulation (Templin, 1957), and ability to comprehend words (Dunn, 1959).

The second question was: If the client's communicative behavior is not "within normal limits," what is the reason? To answer this question, we need to know the possible causes for each deviation from "normal limits" a client exhibits. Considerable relevant research-based information has appeared in the *Journal of Speech and Hearing Disorders* and the *Journal of Speech and Hearing Research*. Such research-based information, incidently, is the source of lists of possible causes of articulation disorders, voice disorders, stuttering, delayed speech and language development, hearing loss, and other communicative disorders which appear in speech pathology and audiology textbooks.

The final question was: How can the client's communicative behavior be modified to bring it within "normal limits," or as close as possible to this goal? To answer this question, we need information concerning the possible impacts of each therapy strategy we are considering, on the client in general and his communicative behavior in particular. We are not only interested in information about the possible positive effects of a therapy strategy on a client's communicative disorder, but also in information about possible negative side effects and the permanence of the change in a client's communicative behavior resulting from its use. Relevant data for some therapy approaches used to treat communicative disorders have been reported in such journals as the *Journal of Speech and Hearing Disorders*. There is a need for considerably more therapy outcome research; some therapy approaches have not been evaluated systematically, and most others show incomplete data. This need will be further explored in Chapters 2 and 11.

QUESTIONS AND ANSWERS

To demonstrate the relevance of research to clinical decision making in speech pathology and audiology, we have argued that a clinician has to be able to answer certain questions to be even minimally effective. In this section we will indicate more specifically how research can provide the data needed to maximize the probability of correct answers to questions concerning evaluation and therapy. We will pose five questions a clinician might need to answer and indicate how data published in several *randomly* selected issues of the *Journal of Speech and Hearing Research* could provide at least a partial answer to each question. The format used for each question will be: (1) a statement of the question, (2) a reference for the data, (3) a description of the observational procedures, (4) a summary of the observations made (i.e., data) that are relevant to answering the question, and (5) a tentative answer to the question. In addition to demonstrating the relevance of research to clinical decision making, this presentation is also intended as an informal introduction to the structure of a research report.

1. ARE THE EARPHONES I USE FOR MY CLINICAL AUDIOLOGICAL EVALUATIONS LIKELY ENOUGH TO BECOME CONTAMINATED TO WARRANT THE EXPENSE OF ROUTINE DECONTAMINATION?

Data Source. Talbott, R. E., Bacteriology of earphone contamination. *Journal of Speech and Hearing Research*, 12, 326–329 (1969).

Observational Procedure. Bacterial samples of earphone earcushions used for clinical audiological evaluations in a hospital setting were examined for the presence of three pathogenic microorganisms that have been associated with otitis media and otitis externa.

Observations Made. Staphylococcus aureus, a pathogenic microorganism, was recovered "in great quantities" from all earcushions sampled.

Tentative Answer to Question. Earphones used for clinical audiological evaluations appear likely enough to become contaminated by pathogenic microorganisms to warrant the expense of routine decontamination.

Remarks. A clinician also could obtain data to answer this question through systematic observation of his own earphones.

2. WHAT ATTRIBUTES OF SPEECH AND VOICE WOULD IT BE PARTICULARLY IMPORTANT TO CHECK WHEN EVALUATING A PATIENT WHO HAS DIAGNOSED DYSTONIA?

Data Source. Darley, F. L., Aronson, A. E., and Brown, J. R., Differential diagnostic patterns of dysarthria. *Journal of Speech and Hearing Research,* 12, 246–269 (1969).

Observational Procedure. Three judges independently rated thirty-second speech samples from each of 30 patients unequivocally diagnosed as having dystonia on each of 38 attributes of speech and voice using a seven-point scale of severity.

Observations Made. The attributes of speech and voice judged most characteristic of the patients in this group were imprecise consonants, vowels distorted, harsh voice, irregular articulatory breakdown, strained-strangled voice, monopitch, and monoloudness.

Tentative Answer to Question. When evaluating a patient with dystonia, it would be important to check on both consonant and vowel production as well as pitch and loudness variation and voice quality.

3. SHOULD I ROUTINELY EVALUATE CHILDREN WHO HAVE RELATIVELY SEVERE ARTICULATION PROBLEMS FOR THE POSSIBILITY THAT THEY ARE AVOIDING TALKING?

Data Source. Shriner, T. H., Holloway, M. S., and Daniloff, R. G., The relationship between articulation defects and syntax in speech defective children. *Journal of Speech and Hearing Research,* 12, 319–325 (1969).

Observational Procedure. Each of 30 first- through third-grade children diagnosed by a speech clinician as having "severe problems with articulation" and 30 matched controls who had no speech problems told a story about a picture. Average sentence length (i.e., total number of words per response) was computed for each child.

Observations Made. The mean number of words per response was lower for the speech defective children.

Tentative Answer to Question. Since these data suggest that at least some children who have relatively severe articulation problems are apt to talk less than their peers, such children should be routinely evaluated for the possibility that they are avoiding talking.

4. IS IT LIKELY TO MAKE A DIFFERENCE IN AN APHASIC'S LANGUAGE PERFORMANCE IF I SCHEDULE HIM FOR SPEECH THERAPY AFTER HE HAS HAD PHYSICAL THERAPY?

Data Source. Marshall, R. C., and King, P. S., Effects of fatigue produced by isokinetic exercise on the communication ability of adult aphasics. *Journal of Speech and Hearing Research*, 16, 222–230 (1973).

Observational Procedure. The Porch Index of Communicative Ability (PICA) was administered to 16 adult aphasics twice—once following a period of isokinetic exercise and once immediately following a rest period.

Observations Made. Fourteen of the 16 subjects had lower PICA mean scores when testing followed exercise than when testing followed a period of rest.

Tentative Answer to Question. Since exercise of the type encountered in physical therapy appears likely to influence adversely an aphasic's language performance, such patients should not be scheduled for speech therapy following a period of physical therapy if it is avoidable.

5. IS IT SAFE TO ASSUME THAT HAVING A STUTTERER REPEATEDLY ENTER A SPEAKING SITUATION (E.G., SPEAKING ON THE TELEPHONE) WILL NOT RESULT IN A SYSTEMATIC INCREASE IN HIS FREQUENCY OF STUTTERING IN THAT SITUATION?

Data Source. Bloom, C., and Silverman, F. H., Do all stutterers adapt? *Journal of Speech and Hearing Research*, 16, 518–521 (1973).

Observational Procedure. An adult stutterer made five consecutive four-minute telephone calls to the same person on each of three consecutive days. On the fourth day, she telephoned a different person five times one after the other. Several weeks later, she also made 10 consecutive four-minute phone calls to the same person she had spoken to the first three days. All telephone calls were tape-recorded, and each day she spoke about the same topic during all calls. Her total frequency of disfluency per 100 words was computed for each telephone call on each day.

Observations Made. The subject's frequency of disfluency on the last call of each day was higher than on the first. On four of the five days, her frequency of disfluency on the first call was lower than on any of the subsequent calls. Her performance on this task, incidently, differed from that of 13 other adult stutterers.

Tentative Answer to Question. Judging by the consistency of the subject's performance, it does not appear safe to assume that having a stutterer repeatedly enter a speaking situation will not result in a systematic increase in his frequency of stuttering in that situation.

If you would like an additional demonstration of how research can provide the data needed to answer questions concerning clinical process, I would recommend that you read two papers (Jerger and Speaks, 1967; Lilly, Sherman, Compton, Fisher, and Carney, 1968) in which the authors attempted to indicate the clinical relevance of the data reported in two volumes of the *Journal of Speech and Hearing Research.*

HAS THE NEED BEEN MET?

This chapter has placed considerable emphasis on the fact that existing research can provide data helpful in answering questions concerning clinical process. This emphasis was not meant to imply that the need for such data has been met. To the contrary, more data are needed (*Human Communication and its Disorders: An Overview,* 1969; Morley, 1962; Public school speech and hearing services, 1961; Research needs in speech pathology and audiology, 1959; Templin, 1953). This need is, incidently, one of the main reasons for arguing in the next chapter that clinicians should be producers as well as consumers of research.

REFERENCES

BLOOM, C., and SILVERMAN, F. H., Do all stutterers adapt? *Journal of Speech and Hearing Research,* 16, 518–521 (1973).

DARLEY, F. L., ARONSON, A. E., and BROWN, J. R., Differential diagnostic patterns of dysarthria. *Journal of Speech and Hearing Research,* 12, 246–269 (1969).

DUNN, L. M., *Peabody Picture Vocabulary Test.* Minneapolis, Minn.: American Guidance Service, Inc. (1959).

EGAN, J. P., Articulation testing methods. *Laryngoscope,* 58, 955–991 (1948).

Human Communication and its Disorders—An Overview. National Institute of Neurological Diseases and Stroke (1969).

JERGER, J., and SPEAKS, C., Annual review of JSHR research, 1966. *Journal of Speech and Hearing Disorders,* 32, 197–211 (1967).

JOHNSON, W., Measurement of oral reading and speaking rate and disfluency of adult male and female stutterers and nonstutterers. *Journal of Speech and Hearing Disorders,* Monograph Supplement 7, 1–20 (1961).

Johnson, W., and Associates, *The Onset of Stuttering*. Minneapolis, Minn.: University of Minnesota Press (1959).

Lilly, D. J., Sherman, D., Compton, A. J., Fisher, C. G., and Carney, P. J., Annual review of JSHR research, 1967. *Journal of Speech and Hearing Disorders*, 33, 303–317 (1968).

Marshall, R. C., and King, P. S., Effects of fatigue produced by isokinetic exercise on the communication ability of adult aphasics. *Journal of Speech and Hearing Research*, 16, 222–230 (1973).

Morley, D. E., Research needs in communication problems of the aging. *Asha*, 4, 345–347 (1962).

Public school speech and hearing services. *Journal of Speech and Hearing Disorders*, Monograph Supplement 8, 114–123 (1961).

Research needs in speech pathology and audiology. *Journal of Speech and Hearing Disorders*, Monograph Supplement 5, 1–78 (1959).

Shriner, T. H., Holloway, M. S., and Daniloff, R. G., The relationship between articulation defects and syntax in speech defective children. *Journal of Speech and Hearing Research*, 12, 319–325 (1969).

Talbott, R. E., Bacteriology of earphone contamination. *Journal of Speech and Hearing Research*, 12, 326–329 (1969).

Templin, M. C., *Certain Language Skills in Children* (*Institute of Child Welfare Monograph Series*, No. 26). Minneapolis, Minn.: University of Minnesota Press (1957).

Templin, M. C., Possibilities of research for public school speech therapists. *Journal of Speech and Hearing Disorders*, 18, 355–359 (1953).

Williams, D. E., Stuttering therapy: An overview. In Hugo Gregory (Ed.), *Learning Theory and Stuttering Therapy*, Evanston, Ill.: Northwestern University Press, 52–66 (1968).

TWO

RESEARCH AND THE CLINICIAN

The previous chapter dealt with the need for research in speech pathology and audiology to answer questions concerning clinical process. This chapter will discuss *the need for clinicians to undertake such research*. Specifically, we will argue that it is desirable for clinicians to function as producers as well as consumers of research, that is, to function as researchers or investigators.

The term *clinician-investigator* will be used in this book to designate a speech pathologist or audiologist who functions both as a clinician and a clinical investigator, or researcher. A hyphen was inserted between "clinician" and "investigator" to indicate that the two roles are not independent but interdependent. Thus, being a clinician would probably influence the kinds of research questions an investigator would ask, and being an investigator would probably influence a clinician's approach to problem-solving in diagnosis and therapy. Also, a speech pathologist or audiologist might perform both functions simultaneously. That is, he might gather clinical research data while performing clinical functions (diagnosis and therapy). The individual clinical case study that utilizes data gathered as part of diagnosis or therapy, or both, illustrates this combined function. The term "clinician-investigator," incidently, was derived from "teacher-investigator," a term used in some colleges and universities to designate the dual interrelated roles of a professor —teaching and research.

WHY BE A CLINICIAN-INVESTIGATOR?

What benefits would a clinician derive from functioning as a clinician-investigator? The following discussion suggests several benefits. However, the order in which they are discussed is not intended to reflect their relative importance.

First of all, functioning as a clinician-investigator would probably make one's job more stimulating, less routine, and would probably increase the possibilities for positive reinforcement. In addition to feeling successful at clinical activities, the clinician-investigator would have a second potential source of reinforcement—his research activities. This reinforcement could arise from any of the following factors: the feeling of accomplishment that comes from formulating a research question (or questions) and making the necessary observations to answer it (or them) at least partially; reporting the results of research to professional colleagues on the program of a professional meeting (for example, a state speech and hearing association or the American Speech and Hearing Association), or in a professional journal; and knowing that your professional efforts can help not only your own clients, but also those of other speech pathologists and audiologists. Thus, communicating your clinical knowledge and experience of the communicatively handicapped can spread the benefits to others.

Next, functioning as a clinician-investigator could probably help you become a more effective clinician, for several reasons. First, the dual role could provide answers to questions relevant to managing your own caseload. For example, it could help you to determine whether a therapy approach you are using is effective and whether, therefore, you should continue to use it. Or it could help you to determine whether a newer therapy approach is more effective than one you are currently using and, therefore, whether you should adopt the newer approach. It could also help you to establish whether your diagnostic procedures are adequately reliable and to provide normative data for diagnostic procedures you use that are not standardized on the specific populations in your caseload. Finally, it could provide information about the effectiveness of new clinical programs that could be useful when you are deciding whether to continue them.

Functioning as a clinician-investigator could improve effectiveness by helping to develop a more "scientific" approach to clinical decision making. The problem-solving approach based on the scientific method that is essential for functioning as an investigator is also desirable for functioning as a clinician. This approach has several aspects, including: (1) stating goals, or objectives, clearly; (2) asking questions that are "answerable" and stating hypotheses that are "testable"; (3) being systematic in making observations to answer questions and test hypotheses; and (4) being aware of the *tentative* nature of answers and hypotheses.

The need for clinical goals and objectives to be stated clearly has been discussed by a number of authors (e.g., Williams, 1968; Johnson, 1946). Obviously, if a clinical objective or goal were not clearly stated, a clinician could never be reasonably certain whether or not it had been achieved. This situation probably would not be positively reinforcing for either client or clinician.

Another clinically relevant aspect of this approach is asking questions that are "answerable" and stating hypotheses that are "testable." Rather than asking, for example, whether a given therapy approach has been effective, you would ask whether it resulted in certain behavioral changes. (The reason why the second question would be more "answerable" than the first will be discussed in Chapter 4.) Also, rather than hypothesizing that a child is slow in learning to talk because he is "emotionally disturbed," you would define operationally what you meant by being emotionally disturbed. This definition would suggest the diagnostic procedures you would need to test your hypothesis.

A third aspect is being systematic in making observations to answer questions and test hypotheses. The considerations described in Chapter 11 for designing research to evaluate the effects of therapies, for example, are relevant *clinically* for making observations to evaluate the effects of therapies you are using with clients. That is, the approaches used to answer systematically clinical questions for both clinical and research purposes are identical. The approaches used for making observations to "test" clinically relevant hypotheses also are identical. There should be no difference, therefore, in the way you would go about answering clinically relevant questions or testing clinically relevant hypotheses for clinical and research purposes. This similarity in approach is not surprising since no sharp line of demarcation exists between clinical work and clinical research. Overlap is particularly evident with regard to the individual case study and other single subject (i.e., $N = 1$) clinical research (Gottman, 1973).

The final aspect of the scientific approach, being aware of the *tentative* nature of answers and hypotheses, is one of the most important, because it indicates that no answer to a question or test of a hypothesis is *final*. As new information becomes available, the answers to questions may change. Also as new information becomes available, hypotheses that appeared viable may no longer appear so. The answer to every question and the viability of every hypothesis must therefore be regarded as tentative. Both have implicit qualifiers attached. For answers to questions, the implicit qualifier would be: "With the information I currently have available, the answer to the question is...." And for statements concerning the viability of hypotheses, the implicit qualifier would be: "Judging by the information I currently have available, the hypothesis seems viable."

The tentative nature of answers and hypotheses is due at least partially to the fact that observations are never complete. In other words, "the data are never all in." It is more appropriate to conclude, therefore, that available research data *suggest* a therapy is effective, rather than available data *prove* a therapy is effective. This concept will be further discussed in Chapter 3.

If clinicians functioned as clinician-investigators, furthermore, another important benefit would be to help provide data needed to answer questions on diagnosis and therapy for persons who have a communicative disorder. The answers to many questions sought by clinicians require observations that are as validly and efficiently (or more validly and efficiently) made in the clinic as in the laboratory. That is, they can at least as validly and efficiently be made in a "real" clinic environment as in a laboratory. If you wished to evaluate, for example, a therapy approach intended for use in a school setting, it probably would make most sense for you to evaluate it in a school setting. One reason is that the setting in which therapy is done may place constraints upon what can be done. Thus, a therapy approach might be quite effective if a child can be seen five days a week for an hour a day, but this time investment might not be possible in the typical school setting. Also, data on the long-term effects of therapies probably can be gathered as validly, and more efficiently, in a clinical than it can in a laboratory setting. Additionally, the populations that must be observed to answer certain clinical questions may be more available to an investigator who works in a setting where such cases are seen for therapy than to one who is not employed in such a setting.

Finally, the data necessary to answer many clinically relevant questions can be gathered over a period of time as a part of diagnosis and therapy. Some of the best data we have on the symptomatology, etiology, diagnosis, and treatment of communicative disorders have come from this source. Several examples are the data on aphasia gathered at the Minneapolis Veterans' Administration Hospital (Schuell, Jenkins, and Jiménez-Pabón, 1964), the data on dysarthria gathered at the Mayo Clinic (e.g., Darley, Aronson, and Brown, 1969), the data on voice disorders gathered at the Jewish Hospital in St. Louis (Wilson, 1971), and the data on public school speech and hearing therapy gathered at the Oakland Schools (Freeman, 1971; Baynes, 1966).

A clinician often is in a better position to make the observations needed to answer questions of clinical interest than is an investigator not actively engaged in clinical work. As previously mentioned, a clinician sometimes can make and record such observations within the context of his clinical work. In fact, the observations a clinician makes and records during diagnosis and therapy may be used to answer clinically relevant questions. It is necessary, though, that these observations be made in such a way that they possess relatively high levels of validity and reliability. This, incidently, would also be a requirement for making such observations for clinical purposes. Observations that are not adequately reliable and valid would not be particularly useful for these purposes, either.

A clinician may also be able to make the observations needed to answer certain questions more reliably than an investigator not actively engaged in clinical work, because of his clinical background and experience. This would be especially likely, for example, if the observations were of performance on clinical diagnostic tests and procedures. An experienced administrator's and interpreter's observations of performance on a diagnostic test probably would be more reliable than those of an investigator who is not experienced with the test, particularly one who has not administered or interpreted it prior to doing so for a research project.

A clinician-investigator would also probably be better able both to evaluate therapies and to design research for this purpose than an investigator not actively engaged in clinical work would. This is especially true if the research involves experimental therapy and the design calls for the investigator to serve as clinician. An experienced clinician probably would do a better job administering an experimental therapy than an inexperienced one would. Additionally, an experienced clinician would probably be more aware of the "reality" factors which have to be considered when designing clinical research, particularly those introduced by the environment in which the data are being gathered. It may not be realistic, for example, to expect a classroom teacher to consistently reinforce "target" behaviors in a specified manner. It also may be unrealistic to expect a child's parents to reinforce "target" behaviors as instructed. Such factors probably would be taken into consideration by an experienced clinician when planning therapy outcome research.

Thus far we have argued that: (1) many questions to which clinicians seek answers require observations that are at least as validly made in the clinic as in the laboratory, and (2) a clinician may be in a better position to make the observations necessary to answer such questions than an investigator not actively engaged in clinical work. Hopefully, we have demonstrated why a speech pathologist or audiologist would have the *possibility* of functioning as a clinician-investigator. Is there a *need*, however, for speech pathologists and audiologists to function in this manner? We believe such a need exists for several reasons, including the following:

1. He may be in the best position to make the observations necessary to answer clinically relevant questions, particularly those related to diagnosis and therapy. There are several reasons why the clinician-investigator

might be in an advantageous position to answer such questions, including: (a) the setting in which he or she works, (b) the populations in his caseload, (c) his or her background and experience, (d) the availability of equipment and facilities for making the necessary observations, (e) the availability of collaborators from other disciplines, (f) the availability of an existing research program as a part of which the desired observations could be made, and (g) the availability of consultants and other supportive research personnel. The first three reasons were discussed earlier in the chapter; let us briefly examine the others here.

A speech pathologist or audiologist may be in an excellent position to make the observations necessary to answer certain questions of clinical interest because of available facilities, equipment, or both. This is particularly true if he has certain instruments or facilities that are unique or not generally available. An audiologist, for example, may have testing instrumentation or facilities that are unavailable in most audiological settings because of their cost or relatively limited usefulness. A speech pathologist may have one or more instruments for behavior modification, programmed learning, biofeedback, or diagnostic testing that are not available in most speech clinics. If a speech pathologist or audiologist is able to exploit such facilities or instrumentation, he may be in a unique position to gather data necessary to answer questions of clinical importance.

A speech pathologist or audiologist may also have the opportunity to collaborate with investigators in other disciplines. A speech pathologist might collaborate with an otolaryngologist to assess the effects of a therapy on vocal nodules, or with a reading specialist to determine the effect of articulation errors on reading ability. An audiologist might collaborate with a microbiologist to determine if audiometer earphones are likely to contain pathogenic microorganisms. Again, if a speech pathologist or audiologist "exploits" opportunities for interdisciplinary research, he may be able to make the observations necessary to answer at least partially questions of clinical significance.

Another opportunity for a speech pathologist or audiologist to gather clinically relevant data is to become involved with an ongoing research program, especially an interdisciplinary one. If a clinician is working in a setting where research is being conducted in a related area such as psychology, learning disabilities, physical therapy, occupational therapy, rehabilitation counseling, social work, medicine, or dentistry, he may be able to gather clinically relevant data on communicative disorders by participating in the research program. In fact, by becoming involved when such a program is being planned, the clinician may be able to arrange for relevant data on communicative disorders to be gathered at the same time subjects are being seen by the other discipline or disciplines involved. To illustrate how this combining of interests can be accomplished, in the late 1950s a group of audiologists at a Veterans' Administration Outpatient Center were able to gather data on the hearing of men well past the age of seventy by arranging to do an audiometric evaluation on each of a group of Spanish-American War veterans being seen at the Center for other reasons. In this way speech pathologists and audiologists can take advantage of available opportunities to gather the data they need to answer clinically relevant questions.

The final factor to consider is the availability of consultants and supportive research personnel. Included here would be persons with expertise in statistics and research design, computer programming, electronics, manuscript editing, and grant writing for research. If such persons are available, a clinician with clinically relevant questions to be answered who is relatively unsophisticated in research methodology can, with their help, make the observations necessary to answer the questions.

2. Much of the needed clinical research probably will not be done unless more clinicians are willing to function as clinician-investigators. In the first place, investigators who are not actively involved in clinical work are unlikely to be as *aware* as clinician-investigators are of at least some clinically relevant questions that need to be answered. This is particularly true of practical questions of clinical program procedure. Such questions might deal with the effectiveness of paraprofessionals in various roles in speech and hearing habilitation and rehabilitation, or with the efficacy of teacher referral for identifying children with various communicative disorders.

Second, investigators who are not clinicians are unlikely to be as *interested* as clinician-investigators are in answering many questions of clinical interest, particularly those on clinical program procedure and therapy outcome. Such investigators may view questions on clinical program procedure as having limited theoretical significance. They may also be less interested in questions on therapy outcome for one or more of the following reasons: (a) the effects of extraneous variables are more difficult to control than in much laboratory research; (b) the time it takes to collect data may be longer than for many types of laboratory research; and (c) the likelihood of a publishable result may not be as high in outcome research as in many types of laboratory research.

Third, investigators who are not clinicians might lack the *opportunity* to make the observations needed to answer many clinically relevant questions even if they were interested in doing so. Possible reasons for this lack of opportunity have already been discussed.

3. More clinicians functioning as clinician-investigators would probably help break down the clinician-researcher dichotomy that exists to some extent in speech pathology and audiology (Goldstein, 1972; Hamre, 1972; Jerger, 1963a, 1963b, 1964; Powers, 1955; Ringel, 1972; Schultz, Roberts, and Yairi, 1972). While this is certainly not the primary reason speech pathologists and audiologists should function as clinician-investigators, it

nevertheless is an important one, since (for reasons previously discussed) it seems reasonable to conclude that clinical research and clinical practice are interdependent activities.

WHO CAN BE A CLINICIAN-INVESTIGATOR?

The previous section attempted partially to answer the question, "What benefits would a clinician derive from functioning as a clinician-investigator?" The word "partially" was inserted here to indicate that the reasons discussed are not the only possible ones. As general semanticists (e.g., Johnson, 1946) and others have pointed out, it is quite doubtful that any question can be completely answered, or, for that matter, that everything can be said about anything.

This section will attempt partially to answer the question: *What attributes and competencies are necessary for a clinician to function successfully as a clinician-investigator, and how do these differ from those necessary to function successfully solely as a clinician?* It also will attempt to answer the related question: *What attitudes and competencies are not essential for a clinician to function successfully as a clinician-investigator that might be regarded as necessary for him to function successfully in this role?* More broadly, this section will attempt to develop in the reader an objective attitude toward research.

Why is it necessary to be concerned about developing an objective attitude toward research? The term "objective attitude" is used here to indicate that your attitude toward research and your ability to function as a researcher should be as rational, or reality-oriented, as possible. If you were to view research as an activity possible for Ph.D.s in universities but not for clinicians who have masters' degrees, your attitude would not be objective. Speech pathologists and audiologists employed in clinical settings who are not Ph.D.s both have done and continue to do research. Viewing research as an activity that requires extensive training in statistics and research methodology or considerable expenditure of time is likewise not an objective attitude, because neither is absolutely essential for at least some clinical research.

The more objective a clinician's attitude toward research, the higher the probability he will consider functioning as a clinician-investigator. And the more certain the clinician is that this is a possibility, the more likely it is that he would attempt to function in this role. Some clinicians do not function as clinician-investigators because their attitudes toward research are not objective, not because their interest is lacking. They may assume, for example, that to do clinical research, a speech pathologist or audiologist must have a doctoral degree, or advanced training in statistics or research design, or considerable time available, or certain personal attributes that are not generally regarded as essential for clinicians. While these are not the only such assumptions made by clinicians, they appear to be among the most frequent, judging by the results of a survey of speech clinicians in Wisconsin (Silverman, Halback, and Palmer, unpublished data). For this reason, the validity of each assumption will be considered here.

Neither a Ph.D. degree nor extensive training in statistics are essential for a speech pathologist or audiologist to make many (but not necessarily all) of the observations needed to answer clinical questions and report the answers in oral convention presentations or journal articles. While training on a doctoral level is desirable for an investigator because it is usually in large part research training, it is not a prerequisite. The investigator responsible for the scientific exhibit that won First Prize for Scientific Excellence at the 1972 Annual Convention of the American Speech and Hearing Association was a high school student. His competition, incidently, consisted of 19 exhibits by speech pathologists, audiologists, and speech and hearing scientists with doctoral degrees (including the author). Perhaps the strongest evidence that a Ph.D is not a prerequisite for at least some clinical research is the fact that clinical research done by speech pathologists and audiologists with masters' degrees has been reported at annual conventions of the American Speech and Hearing Association as well as in the clinical journals published by the American Speech and Hearing Association—the *Journal of Speech and Hearing Disorders* and *Language, Speech, and Hearing Services in Schools*. A dozen representative clinical research studies reported in the *Journal of Speech and Hearing Disorders* by speech pathologists and audiologists who did not have a Ph.D degree and were employed in a clinical setting when the study was done are listed in Table 2.1. These are not the only such studies reported in this journal nor is this the only journal where such studies have been reported. They have been reported in a number of national organization journals and convention programs as well as in state speech and hearing association journals and convention programs.

Extensive knowledge of statistics and research methodology, like doctoral level training, though desirable for a speech pathologist or audiologist who wishes to function as a clinician-investigator, is not essential. The information presented in this book will suffice to formulate a plan for making the observations necessary to answer some questions. To answer others, the clinician-investigator may have to consult with persons who are knowledgeable in statistics and research design. Such consultants are available in many school systems, hospitals, rehabilitation centers, and other clinical settings. In addition, faculty members at nearby colleges and universities with expertise in statistics and research methodology, or statisticians employed by local companies, might be willing to consult on research design problems. One approach to identifying possible local consultants, incidently, is to consult the geographical listing in *Statisticians and Others in Allied Professions* published by the American Statistical Association, 806 15th Street, N.W., Washington, D.C 20005.

TABLE 2.1. Representative clinical research studies reported in the *Journal of Speech and Hearing Disorders* (JSHD) by speech pathologists and audiologists who did not have a Ph.D. degree and were employed in a clinical setting when the study was done.

Author	Highest Degree[1]	Place of Employment[2]	Title of Study	Reference
Jerry Summers	M.A.	LaCrosse Lutheran Hospital, LaCrosse, Wisconsin	The use of the electrolarynx in patients with temporary tracheostomies	JSHD, 38, 335–338 (1973)
Zane E. LaCroix	M.S.	Enid State School, Enid, Oklahoma	Management of disfluent speech through self-recording procedures	JSHD, 38, 272–274 (1973)
Edmund Lauder	M.A.	American Cancer Society, San Antonio, Texas	The laryngectomee and the artificial larynx—A second look	JSHD, 35, 62–65 (1970)
Margery Wessell	M.A.	Speech Correction Center, Shreveport, Louisiana	A language development program for a blind language-disordered preschool girl: A case report	JSHD, 34, 267–274 (1969)
Julia Adams	M.A.	Iowa State Services for Crippled Children, Iowa City, Iowa	Delayed language development	JSHD, 34, 169–171 (1969)
Ethel Slipakoff	M.A.	Houston Public Schools, Houston, Texas	An approach to the correction of the defective /r/	JSHD, 32, 71–75 (1967)
Marjorie Burkland	M.A.	Evanston Township High School, Evanston, Illinois	Use of television to study articulation problems	JSHD, 32, 80–81 (1967)
Robert C. Cody	M.A.	Siouxland Rehabilitation Center, Sioux City, Iowa	Instrumentation: SAL technique with a Grason-Stadler Speech Audiometer	JSHD, 31, 257–258 (1966)
Robert A. Baynes	M.A.	Oakland Schools Speech and Hearing Clinic, Pontiac, Michigan	An incidence study of chronic hoarseness among children	JSHD, 31, 172–176 (1966)
Duane Anderson	M.S.	Hearing Conservation Program, Oregon State Board of Health, Portland, Oregon	The effect of climate on the incidence of hearing loss	JSHD, 30, 66–70 (1965)
Irwin Shore Joan C. Kramer	M.A. M.S.	Central Institute for the Deaf, St. Louis, Missouri	A comparison of two procedures for hearing-aid evaluation	JSHD, 28, 159–170 (1963)
Venus E. Tretsven	M.A.	Cleft Lip and Palate Program, Montana State Board of Health, Helena, Montana	Incidence of cleft lip and palate in Montana Indians	JSHD, 28, 52–57 (1963)

[1]Degree information was from the *1973 American Speech and Hearing Association Membership Directory* or the article.
[2]Place of employment was from the article.

Another potentially unobjective attitude is that clinical research requires more time than a speech pathologist or audiologist would have available for the purpose. This reason was one of the most frequently mentioned for not doing research in the survey of Wisconsin speech clinicians cited previously. The objectivity of this attitude is a function of the question, or questions, the clinician seeks to answer. If these questions require observations that *the clinician has to make as part of his routine clinical responsibilities* (or observations he would not routinely make but could make within the context of his clinical responsibilities), this attitude would probably not be objective. Such questions might deal with the effectiveness of therapies being used with clients in the clinician's caseload. It seems reasonable to assume that the clinician would make some observations to evaluate the effectiveness of the therapies being used to improve clinical effectiveness. If these observations were reasonably reliable and valid (which also would be necessary to make them useful for clinical purposes), they could be used to answer questions for clinical research. Such research, furthermore, probably would not be particularly time-consuming.

Other research likely to place minimal demands upon a clinician's time is that which utilizes client folder data—i.e., the diagnostic and therapy data recorded in clients' folders. For such data to be useable for this purpose, they must be reasonably complete, reliable, and valid. They also must be easily retrievable: that is, the files must be organized so that the folders of clients in the "population" to be studied can be located fairly easily. A variety of clinically relevant questions can be answered, at least partially, through the use of such data. These would include those pertaining to: (1) factors influencing the prognosis for various communicative disorders, (2) interrelationships between test results (e.g., audiometric test results) for specific clinical "populations," (3) negative side-effects of specific therapies, (4) positive effects of specific therapies upon specific communicative disorders, and (5) factors that influence the probability a client will terminate therapy before his clinician feels he is ready.

A final misconceived attitude is that clinicians, to do research, need to have more of certain personal attributes than are strictly necessary in their present role. The attribute most frequently mentioned by speech clinicians in the Wisconsin survey was "intelligence." More than a third of the clinicians surveyed indicated that they did not consider themselves sufficiently intelligent to do clinical research. Several assumptions appear to underlie this attitude. One is that clinical research is relatively homogeneous in the demands it places on an investigator's intelligence, that is, that the level of intelligence required to answer most questions of clinical interest is approximately the same. A second, related assumption implicit here is that the level of intelligence required to answer clinically relevant questions for research purposes exceeds that required to answer such questions for clinical purposes. (We are assuming here that a clinician would regard his level of intelligence as adequate for answering clinically relevant questions for clinical purposes.)

While clinical research may possibly be relatively homogeneous in the demands it places on an investigator's intelligence, this still seems quite unlikely, for several reasons. First, this assumption would violate the principle posited by general semanticists (e.g., Johnson, 1946) and others that the members of a "class of events" (clinical research studies would constitute such a class) are not identical in any attribute. In other words, events do not replicate themselves. Second, it would be necessary to assume that the observations required to answer clinically relevant questions place approximately equal demands on an investigator's intelligence. Such an assumption would be counter-intuitive, since some observational procedures appear to place greater demands on an investigator's intelligence and ingenuity than others do. Questions that, to be answered, required an observational procedure that was well developed and standarized (such as a standardized test) would not intuitively appear to place as great a demand on an investigator as would those requiring an observational procedure the investigator had to devise and standardize.

The second assumption (probably the more important of the two with reference to the ability of a clinician to function as an investigator) is that the level of intelligence required to answer clinically relevant questions for research purposes exceeds that required to answer such questions for clinical purposes. If a clinician has the ability to answer some clinically relevant questions for clinical purposes, he also should be able to answer some such questions for research purposes. We would suspect that at least some speech pathologists and audiologists who feel they are not sufficiently intelligent to do research would accept this argument if it were presented to them. Probably one reason they do not do research is that they do not understand that the answering of questions is the essence of research. In sum, if they feel sufficiently intelligent to answer *certain* clinically relevant questions for clinical purposes, they could rationally also feel sufficiently intelligent to answer the same questions for research purposes.

Thus far, this section has dealt with attributes and competencies that do *not* appear to be essential for a speech pathologist or audiologist to function successfully as a clinician-investigator. What attributes and competencies *do* appear to be essential for success in this role? How do these abilities differ from those necessary for him to have a reasonable chance for success as a clinician? Since few relevant research data have been reported, the answers given here should be regarded as speculative.

The personal attributes that appear necessary for a speech pathologist or audiologist to have a reasonable chance of functioning successfully as a clinician-investigator also appear, for the most part, necessary for him to have a reasonable chance of functioning successfully as a clinician. Partial support for this conclusion is provided by the findings of a study (Silverman, Halbach, and Palmer, unpublished data) in which a national random sample of speech pathologists ascribed essentially the same attributes to "A speech pathologist who does clinical work" as a second such random sample ascribed to "A speech pathologist who does clinical work and clinical research." While these data generally support the conclusion that the attributes of a successful clinician-investigator are essentially the same as those of a successful clinician, they obviously do not constitute a direct test of this hypothesis. A direct test would require comparing a number of personal attributes of a group of clinician-investigators with those of a group of clinicians who do not function as investigators.

What competencies are essential for speech pathologists or audiologists to function successfully as clinician-investigators? A general answer to this question would be that they must know how to: (1) formulate "answerable" questions and make the observations necessary to answer them with adequate levels of validity and reliability, (2) relate their answers to existing theories and knowledge, and (3) communicate questions, answers, and relations. The information in this book, hopefully, will assist in developing these competencies.

REFERENCES

ADAMS, J., Delayed language development. *Journal of Speech and Hearing Disorders*, 34, 169–171 (1969).

ANDERSON, D., The effect of climate on the incidence of hearing loss. *Journal of Speech and Hearing Disorders*, 30, 66–70 (1965).

BAYNES, R. A., An incidence study of chronic hoarseness among children. *Journal of Speech and Hearing Disorders*, 31, 172–176 (1966).

BURKLAND, M., Use of television to study articulation problems. *Journal of Speech and Hearing Disorders*, 32, 80–81 (1967).

CODY, R. C., Instrumentation: SAL technique with a Grason-Stadler speech audiometer. *Journal of Speech and Hearing Disorders*, 31, 257–258 (1966).

DARLEY, F. L., ARONSON, A. E., and BROWN, J. R., Differential diagnostic patterns of dysarthria. *Journal of Speech and Hearing Research*, 12, 246–269 (1969).

FREEMAN, G. G., An educational-diagnostic approach to language problems. In *Language, Speech, and Hearing Services in Schools 4*, American Speech and Hearing Association, 23–30 (1971).

GOLDSTEIN, R., Presidential address: 1971 national convention. *Asha*, 14, 58–62 (1972).

GOTTMAN, J. M., N-of-one and N-of-two research in psychotherapy. *Psychological Bulletin*, 80, 93–105 (1973).

HAMRE, C. E., Research and clinical practice: A unifying model. *Asha*, 14, 542–545 (1972).

JERGER, J., More on "Who is qualified to do research." *Journal of Speech and Hearing Research*, 7, 4–6 (1964).

JERGER, J., Viewpoint. *Journal of Speech and Hearing Research*, 6, 203–206 (1963).

JERGER, J., Who is qualified to do research? *Journal of Speech and Hearing Research*, 6, 301 (1963).

Johnson, W., *People in Quandaries*. New York: Harper & Row, Publishers (1946).

LaCroix, Z. E., Management of disfluent speech through self-recording procedures. *Journal of Speech and Hearing Research*, 38, 272–274 (1973).

Lauder, E., The laryngectomee and the artificial larynx—A second look. *Journal of Speech and Hearing Disorders*, 35, 62–65 (1970).

Powers, M. H., The dichotomy in our profession. *Journal of Speech and Hearing Disorders*, 20, 4–10 (1955).

Ringel, R. L., The clinician and the researcher: An artificial dichotomy. *Asha*, 14, 351–353 (1972).

Schuell, H., Jenkins, J. J., and Jiménez-Pabón, E., *Aphasia in Adults*. New York: Harper & Row, Publishers (1964).

Schultz, M. C., Roberts, W. H., and Yairi, E., The clinician and the researcher: Comments. *Asha*, 14, 539–541 (1972).

Shore, I., and Kramer, J. C., A comparison of two procedures for hearing-aid evaluation. *Journal of Speech and Hearing Disorders*, 28, 159–170 (1963).

Slipakoff, E., An approach to the correction of the defective /r/. *Journal of Speech and Hearing Disorders*, 32, 71–75 (1967).

Summers, J., The use of the electrolarynx in patients with temporary tracheostomies. *Journal of Speech and Hearing Disorders*, 38, 335–338 (1973).

Tretsven, V. E., Incidence of cleft lip and palate in Montana Indians. *Journal of Speech and Hearing Disorders*, 28, 52–57 (1963).

Wessell, M., A language development program for a blind language-disordered girl: A case report. *Journal of Speech and Hearing Disorders*, 34, 267–274 (1969).

Williams, D. E., Stuttering therapy: An overview. In Hugo H. Gregory (Ed.), *Learning Theory and Stuttering Therapy*. Evanston, Illinois: Northwestern University Press, 52–66 (1968).

Wilson, F. B., The voice-disordered child: A descriptive approach. In *Language, Speech, and Hearing Services in Schools 4*, American Speech and Hearing Association, 14–22 (1971).

THREE

RESEARCH AS A PROCESS OF ASKING AND ANSWERING QUESTIONS

The first two chapters attempted to demonstrate that clinical research in speech pathology and audiology is needed and that speech pathologists and audiologists can help to satisfy this need by functioning as clinician-investigators. This chapter discusses the *scientific method* that underlies research. The primary objective will be to demonstrate that the scientific method, as applied to research, can be viewed as a set of rules for asking and answering questions and for evaluating answers to questions.

It is desirable for speech pathologists and audiologists to have an intuitive understanding of the scientific method. This is true regardless of whether they function as clinicians or clinician-investigators; they are obviously consumers of research in both roles. As such, they have to be able to assess the validity, reliability, and generality of research findings—that is, "answers" to research questions. To do this, they need an intuitive understanding of the method used to generate research findings from the frame of reference both of the philosophy of science (how it is supposed to function) and the history of science (how it has functioned). The methods used by investigators to answer questions (and to arrive, apparently at "correct" answers) are not always those that philosophers of science regard as consistent with the scientific method (Bush, 1974; Kuhn, 1962). What the philosopher of science regards as the method of science is not always what the historian of science has found to be the case. For this reason, the scientific method will be considered in this chapter from both points of view. Several examples relevant to speech pathology and audiology will be presented to illustrate the difference between the two ways of regarding the scientific method, including Gall's discovery of the importance of the anterior portion of the brain for motor speech.

In addition to understanding intuitively the set of rules used to answer questions based on the scientific method, speech pathologists and audiologists should also preferably understand the assumptions (or presuppositions) on which the scientific method, and hence these rules, are based. They should understand what they are required to accept on "faith" when they interpret research findings. This knowledge can enhance their ability to evaluate research reports critically as well as to help them develop an objective attitude toward research.

First, the intuitive understanding. To play a game successfully, you must understand the rules, and the scientific method can easily be viewed as a game. Like any game, it has both objectives and strategies for maximizing the probability of achieving these objectives. In fact, as Agnew and Pyke (1969) pointed out in their provocative and entertaining description of "the science game,"

> The ingredients of any great game can be found in science—massive effort, goals, great plays, mediocre plays, lousy plays; umpires making clear calls, judgment calls, biased calls, and, of course, mistaken calls. There are prizes and penalties. You will find integrity, dignity, and deals, along with good luck and bad luck—but above all you will find commitment (Agnew and Pyke, 1969, pp. vii–viii).

To learn the rules of the "Game," the clinician-investigator should study them from the frame of reference of both the philosophy of science and the history of science. The philosophy of science provides information on strategies that, theoretically, should lead to success at the Game; the history of science provides information on strategies that have lead to success at the Game in the past. Together, they provide a set of guidelines.

Speech pathologists and audiologists need an intuitive understanding of the scientific method just as much in their role as clinician. All else being equal, a speech pathologist or audiologist probably will be a more effective diagnostician and behavior modifier if he has at least some grounding in the scientific method. Diagnosis, particularly differential diagnosis, consists in large part of asking "answerable" questions (or formulating "testable" hypotheses) and making the observations necessary to answer (or test) them. The scientific method offers a set of rules for maximizing the probability of "correct" answers to such questions (or of reliable and valid tests of such hypotheses). As such, it is relevant for the speech pathologist or audiologist who functions as a diagnostician. It is also relevant for the speech pathologist or audiologist who functions as a behavior modifier. Rules associated with the scientific method are applicable both to the administration of therapies (or behavior modification procedures) and to the evaluation of effects produced by them. In fact, most approaches to behavior modification based on learning theory, including Skinnerian Operant Conditioning, are applied and their results evaluated by means of "rules" derived from the scientific method.

WHAT IS THE SCIENTIFIC METHOD?

Now that we have briefly considered the "why" question (Why is a knowledge of the scientific method relevant for speech pathologists and audiologists?), we are ready to deal with the "what" question: What is the scientific method? As a partial answer, some of its objectives, characteristics, and underlying assumptions will be delineated. These objectives, characteristics, and underlying assumptions are not the only ones that have been attributed to the scientific method, nor is there universal agreement that they are a necessary part of the scientific method. However, they are among those that tend to be most frequently mentioned by philosophers and historians of science.

Objectives

We will begin our discussion of the scientific method with its objectives. We will consider the functions it can serve, specifically the question: What can the scientific method do for a speech pathologist or audiologist? How and when might he use it?

The scientific method is a set of rules that can be used for *describing* events, *explaining* events, and *predicting* events. The term "event," as used here, includes anything observable that occurs in time and thus includes phenomena usually classified as objects.

Description. Describing events means partially answering questions beginning with "who," "what," "when," "where," "how," and "which," questions concerning events. The following are examples:

1. *Who* should be examined by an otolaryngologist before being scheduled for voice therapy?
2. *Who* can benefit from a particular type of hearing aid?
3. *What* factors cause a child to begin to stutter?
4. *What* factors influence speechreading ability?

5. *When* is a speech deviation a speech defect?
6. *When* is a hearing loss educationally significant?
7. *Where* do esophageal speakers have most difficulty communicating?
8. *Where* should ear protectors be worn?
9. *How* can a child who "lateralizes" /s/ be taught to produce a "frontal" /s/?
10. *How* can hearing loss be identified most reliably in neonates?
11. *Which* of two aphasia tests yields the most reliable and valid information concerning a stroke patient's ability to communicate?
12. *Which* approach to teaching the deaf is most likely to result in the highest level of ability to communicate with normal-hearing persons, the "oral" method or "total communication?"

The structures of these questions, of course, should be regarded as illustrative rather than exhaustive. Questions that result in answers that describe events can begin with various words. The process of structuring questions is further discussed in Chapter 4.

Speech pathologists and audiologists can use the scientific method whenever they have to describe something. It offers an approach for describing events (e.g., behavior) that both maximizes the reliability and validity of a description and permits its reliability and validity to be estimated. Since the meaningfulness of descriptive data is a direct function of their reliability and validity, the scientific method can perform a useful function for speech pathologists and audiologists in this regard.

Explanation. Explaining events means dealing with the "why" question—i.e., specifying the reason or reasons for events. Once an event has been described, we may be interested in explaining why it occurred. If a therapy approach employed by a speech pathologist or audiologist resulted in a reduction in the severity of a client's communicative disorder, the clinician probably would have some interest in being able to specify the reason or reasons why. If, for example, you could identify the aspect, or aspects, of the therapy that were responsible for the observed change, you might be able to "simplify" the therapy and thereby make it more efficient. Or if you could identify and isolate the active ingredient in the therapy, you might be able to incorporate it into a new therapy approach that would be more effective than the one you originally used. Also, if you could determine why the frequency, duration, and complexity of behaviors that contribute to communicative disorders vary in predictable ways under specified laboratory conditions, you might be able to incorporate the active components of such conditions into programs of therapy for communicative disorders. If, for example, you could explain why the frequency of stuttering decreases under certain laboratory conditions (e.g., reading in chorus), you might be able to incorporate the active components of such conditions into programs of therapy for stuttering. Or if you could explain the reasons for spontaneous recovery following damage to the central nervous system, you might be better able to devise therapy strategies to maximize it.

The scientific method is helpful in establishing the degree of certainty a speech pathologist or audiologist can have in answers to "why" questions—questions of causality. These questions are particularly difficult to answer with a high degree of certainty in the biological and behavioral sciences which, of course, are the areas to which most questions in speech pathology and audiology relate (Perkins and Curlee, 1969). Philosophers of science have pointed out several reasons why questions of causality are difficult to answer with a high degree of certainty, including the following:

First, *more than one explanation for an event may be possible from descriptions of it.* The existing data may support more than one explanation for an event. Even if the existing data support only one of the explanations posited for an event, they could conceivably support as well, or possibly even better, an explanation for the event that has not yet been posited. Also, while existing data may support one explanation of an event more than others, new data may become available that would make one of the other explanations appear more viable. Under these circumstances, no explanation of an event can be accepted as absolutely certain. All we can conclude based on the scientific method is that judging by what we know about an event, the most plausible explanation for it appears to be. . . . As the amount of information we have about an event increases, our judgment on the most plausible explanation for it may change. One of the most important rules, or principles, of the scientific method is that explanations for events *must be* subject to change without notice when new information becomes available.

Second, *because two events are highly correlated does not necessarily mean that one is causally related to the other.* Because auditory memory span is fairly highly related to articulation proficiency, for example, does not necessarily mean that poor auditory memory span is a cause of articulation errors. The two may be correlated because they are both related to a *third variable* such as mental age. If a child were developing mentally at a slower-than-normal rate, both auditory memory span and articulation proficiency would also be developing slowly. The possibility that two variables that appear closely related are actually both causally related to a third variable is another reason why explanations for events must be regarded as tentative and thus subject to change.

Third, *all events in a system are interrelated.* Causation, therefore, is apt to be complex. A system, for example, could be "centered" around a client and could include all events in both his internal and external environments that effect him. Because of the existence of such systems, if a client improves following a period of therapy, we can never be certain that his improvement was due solely to the therapy he received. Even if we isolate one aspect of therapy (event associated with therapy) that always seems to be present when improvement occurs, we can never conclude this is the only event that has to be present for improvement to occur. In fact, we could not be certain that the aspect isolated was related to the observed improvement. There could be other common aspects we have not abstracted, or identified, that were wholly or partially responsible for the observed improvement.

Another possibility that needs to be considered here is that an aspect of therapy might be more likely to result in improvement if it is combined with a particular value of another variable, or variables. Organismic and therapist variables (Edwards and Cronbach, 1966) would be relevant here. A given therapy, for example, might be more effective with clients who have above-average intelligence than with those who have below-average intelligence. Also, this same therapy might be more effective if it were administered by a clinician who expected it to be effective (positive placebo effect) than if it were administered by one who did not expect it to be effective (negative placebo effect).

We can conclude our discussion of the role of the scientific method in explanation with this generalization: answers to "why" questions should be regarded as tentative and subject to change without notice when new information becomes available.

Prediction. Predicting events means making probability statements about the likelihood of their future occurrence—that is, estimating the odds that a specific event will occur during a specific period of time. Once an event has been described and information becomes available concerning the conditions under which it occurs, its future occurrence may be predicted with "greater than chance" accuracy. The degree of accuracy with which such predictions can be made will be at least partially a function of the amount of information available about the conditions under which the event occurs. The greater the available information about these conditions, the more accurately an event can be predicted.

Weather forecasting illustrates the application of the scientific method to predicting events. The weather forecaster estimates the odds a specific event (rain) will occur during a specific time period (next 24 hours). He bases his prediction on available information about: (1) the conditions under which specific weather events occur, and (2) the conditions that are likely to be present during the period for which he is making his prediction. For each event he predicts, he usually makes a probability statement (20 percent chance of rain) about the likelihood of its occurrence.

What kinds of events do speech pathologists and audiologists attempt to predict? One is the probable outcome of therapy. This prediction is incorporated into the statement of prognosis. In this statement a speech pathologist or audiologist attempts to predict the probable impact of a specific program of therapy on a specific client's communicative disorder (possibly within a specific period of time). To make this statement, he consciously or unconsciously uses: (1) information about the conditions that have to be present for improvement to occur in persons who have a given communicative disorder and (2) his judgment on the likelihood that these conditions will be operative for the client. The statement of prognosis could have a statement of either verbal (little chance for further improvement) or numerical (less than a 10 percent chance for further improvement) probability attached to it.

Speech pathologists and audiologists also may have to make predictions relevant to program planning. A speech pathologist, for example, may be called upon to predict which young children who have sound substitutions are likely to correct them on their own and which most likely will require some form of therapy. These predictions usually are based on information about: (1) the conditions under which a child is likely to correct sound substitutions on his own ("error" phonemes are stimulable), and (2) whether these conditions appear to be present for a given group of children. A probability statement probably will be attached to such predictions (kindergarten-age children are quite likely to correct sound substitutions on their own if their "error" sounds are stimulable in both isolation and words).

The scientific method can assist the speech pathologist and audiologist in predicting events in a manner that both maximizes and permits them (at least roughly) to estimate accuracy of prediction. A number of statistical procedures have been developed that can be used for this purpose, including regression analysis and discriminant function analysis (both are discussed in Chapter 8).

Characteristics

We will now delineate some of the characteristics of the scientific method as they relate to speech pathology and audiology. Our primary goal is to help the reader develop an intuitive understanding of the method as an approach to describing, explaining, and predicting events. This discussion can be viewed as an *operational definition* (Bridgman, 1927) of the scientific method, because it describes how one would have to behave to function in a manner consistent with it. The terminology used is that of Feigl (1953).

Intersubjective Testability. This term refers to "... the requirement that the knowledge claims of science be in principle capable of test (confirmation or disconfirmation, at least indirectly and to some degree) on the part of any person properly equipped with intelligence and the technical devices of observation or experimentation" (Feigl, 1953, p. 11). If speech pathologists or audiologists devise therapeutic procedures which purport to reduce the severity of a communicative disorder, or diagnostic procedures which purport to be effective in determining the etiology of a communicative disorder, these claims should be capable of test by another person. Their procedure should be described in sufficient detail so that it can be tested by someone else. Before any claims can be accepted, they must be confirmed by others. They cannot be accepted on the basis of "authority" or appearance in print. Because a person regarded as an authority claims a procedure is effective and his claim appears in print does not make his claim credible. Claims have appeared in speech pathology and audiology literature that could not be confirmed by those who tested them.

That a claim should not be regarded as valid unless it has been adequately tested and reasonably well confirmed has relevance for speech pathologists and audiologists when they are deciding whether to adopt a therapy. Before making such a decision, they should attempt to determine whether the claims made for it have been adequately tested and, if they have, whether the data appear to confirm or disconfirm them. Obviously, it would probably be safer to adopt a therapy that has been tested and its claims confirmed than one that has not been tested. It is probably reasonable to assume that the claims made for some diagnostic and therapy procedures currently used by speech pathologists and audiologists have not been adequately tested. As indicated in Chapter 2, one of the reasons there is a need for speech pathologists and audiologists to function as clinician-investigators is simply to test such claims.

Reliability. The "knowledge-claims" of science are required to have "... a sufficient degree of confirmation. This second criterion of scientific knowledge enables us to distinguish what is generally called 'mere opinion' (or worse still, 'superstition') from knowledge (well-substantiated belief)" (Feigl, 1953, p. 12). Degree of confirmation can vary from none to considerable. Obviously, the weight given to a claim in decision making is partially a function of the degree to which it has been confirmed. The greater the degree to which a claim has been confirmed (and hence the greater its reliability), the more confidence one can place in it and the more weight it can be given in decision making.

The claims, or observations, that speech pathologists and audiologists utilize in clinical decision making have been confirmed to varying degrees. Some have been confirmed beyond reasonable doubt while others are no more than hunches. Examples of claims relevant to speech pathology and audiology that appear to have received enough degree of confirmation to be regarded as well-substantiated belief include:

1. Anticipation of stuttering is somehow involved in precipitating the moment of stuttering.

2. Damage to the anterior portion of the left cerebral cortex in right-handed persons is more likely to result in expressive aphasia than damage to the corresponding portion of the right cerebral cortex.
3. Vocal abuse is a cause of vocal nodules.
4. A characteristic of at least some types of noise-induced hearing loss is a greater degree of loss by air conduction at 4000 Hz than at 2000 Hz and 8000 Hz.

Definiteness and Precision. It is necessary that "... the concepts used in the formulation of scientific knowledge-claims be as definitely delimited as possible. On the level of the qualitative-classificatory sciences this amounts to the attempt to reduce all border-zone vagueness to a minimum. On the level of quantitative science the exactitude of the concepts is enormously enhanced through the application of the techniques of measurement" (Feigl, 1953, p. 12). Speech pathologists and audiologists are concerned with both qualitative-classificatory and quantitative concepts.

Why is it necessary that the concepts dealt with by science be as definitely delimited (and hence as precise) as possible? An event, or phenomenon, referred to by a concept cannot be investigated unless it can be defined with enough precision that it is likely to be identified when it occurs, and unlikely to be identified when it does not occur. Before we can determine the effect of a therapy on the "lateralized" /s/ (concept) we have to be able to detect with precision both when /s/ is and is not being lateralized. The meaning of precision in this context is illustrated by Figure 3.1. If precision is high, /s/ will be identified as lateralized when it is lateralized and will not be identified as lateralized when it is not lateralized. Judgments will fall into one of the two

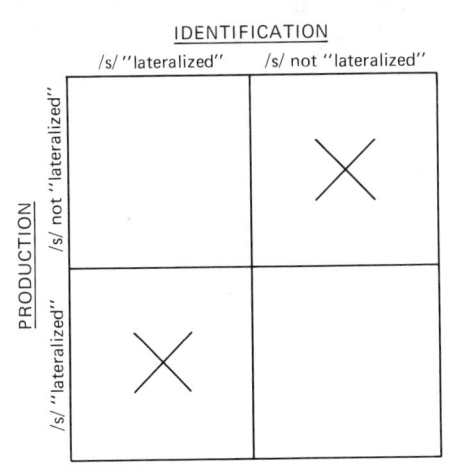

FIGURE 3.1. *A four-cell bivariate table for assessing accuracy of judgments of /s/ lateralization. If accuracy is perfect, all judgments will fall into one of the two cells marked with Xs.*

cells marked with Xs. The more frequently /s/ is judged to be lateralized when it is not lateralized and judged not to be lateralized when it is lateralized, the lower the precision of the judgments (and the lower the percentage of judgments that will fall into one of the two cells marked with Xs). To maximize the precision of such judgments, it would be necessary to define as precisely as possible what is meant by a lateralized /s/ and thereby reduce all border-zone vagueness between what is meant by a lateralized and nonlateralized /s/ to a minimum. Increased definiteness would be expected to lead to increased precision.

The borderline vagueness between categories sometimes can be reduced by supplementing verbal definitions with extensional ones. A category, or term, can be *defined extensionally* ". . . by pointing to or exhibiting somehow the actual objects, phenomena, etc., to which the term refers" (Johnson, 1946, p. 507). Thus, the borderline vagueness between the categories "lateralized" and "nonlateralized" /s/ probably could be reduced by preparing an audiotape recording on which are both labeled examples of Ss that the definer considers lateralized and labeled examples of Ss he does not consider lateralized.

Thus far, we have considered why it is necessary for qualitative-classificatory concepts to be defined as precisely as possible. Speech pathologists and audiologists also deal with quantitative concepts. The events, or phenomena, referred to by such concepts are designated by numerals (rather than words) and hence constitute measurement. (Measurement, which can be defined as the assignment of numerals to events according to rules, is discussed in depth in Chapter 7.) Quantitative concepts of interest to speech pathologists and audiologists include degree of hearing loss (in decibels), language age (in years), and frequency of stuttering (in percentage of words stuttered). Obviously, it is important that quantitative concepts be defined with precision.

How precisely do concepts have to be defined? How definitely delimited do they have to be? How much borderline vagueness can be tolerated? The answers to these questions are dependent upon the purpose for which a conceptual scheme is being used. For some purposes—i.e., to answer some questions—the conceptual scheme must be highly precise (have little borderline vagueness). To answer other questions, a conceptual scheme could have considerable borderline vagueness and still be adequate for the purpose. As Feigl has indicated ". . . there is no point in sharpening precision to a higher degree than the problem in hand requires. (You need no razor to cut butter.)" (Feigl, 1953, p. 12).

Coherence or Systematic Structure. In science we seek "not a mere collection of miscellaneous items of information, but a well-connected account of the facts. . . ." (Feigl, 1953, p. 12). This is true on both descriptive and explanatory levels.

On the *descriptive level*, the need for coherence or systematic structure "...results, for example, in systems of classification or division, in diagrams, statistical charts and the like" (Feigl, 1953, pp. 12–13). An articulation test response form is a way of organizing information concerning the types of articulatory errors (i.e., substitutions, omissions, distortions, additions) a child produces. An audiogram is a diagram for organizing certain information concerning a person's hearing.

Items of information concerning a phenomenon can be viewed as pieces of a puzzle. As such items become available and are fitted together into a coherent whole, our ability to describe the phenomenon increases. When information concerning a person's hearing acuity at various frequencies is plotted on a pure-tone audiogram form and thus is made more coherent, our ability to describe his hearing problem (if one is present) increases. Similarly, when a child's articulation errors are recorded on an articulation test response form, patterns of misarticulations emerge that can be useful in clinical decision making.

To satisfy the need for coherence or systematic structure on the explanatory level, "...sets of laws, or theoretical assumptions, are utilized. Explanation in science consists in the hypothetico-deductive procedure. The laws, theories, or hypotheses form the premises from which we derive logically, or logico-mathematically, the observed, or observable facts" (Feigl, 1953, p.13). Thus, after we had plotted a person's hearing acuity in the left ear at various frequencies by air conduction and bone conduction on an audiogram form, and connected the points for the air conduction curve (see Figure 3.2), we would attempt to explain the mechanisms responsible for the configura-

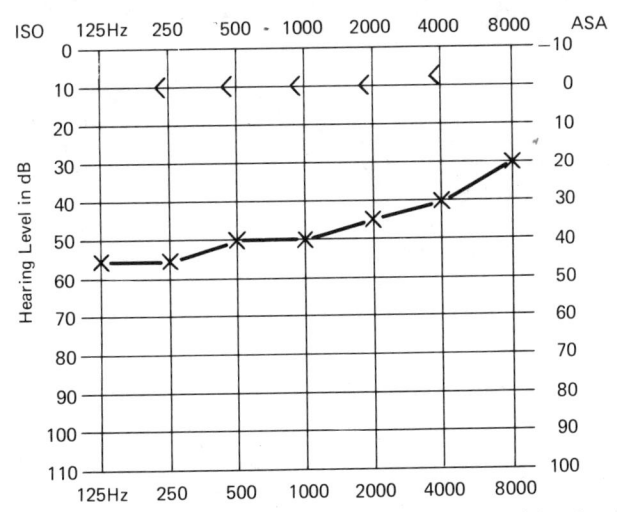

FIGURE 3.2. Pure-tone audiogram indicating degree of hearing in left ear by air conduction (×) and bone conduction (<).

tions of the curves. We could hypothesize one or more mechanisms that could account for the observed configurations and then attempt to determine how well each hypothesized mechanism could explain it. Two hypotheses that might be offered to explain the configurations of the air and bone conduction pure-tone audiogram curves would be: (1) outer or middle ear pathology, and (2) inner ear pathology. We would state by *reasoning deductively* from each hypothesis what we would expect the configuration of the curves to be if it were the mechanism responsible. If this mechanism were pathology in the outer or middle ear, we would expect the air conduction curve to be relatively flat and the bone conduction curve to indicate essentially normal hearing. On the other hand, if the mechanism responsible were pathology in the inner ear, we would expect the configuration of the air conduction curve to indicate greater loss in the high frequencies than in the low frequencies; we would also expect the bone conduction curve to indicate approximately the same amount of loss as the air conduction curve. Since the configurations of the curves in Figure 3.2 more closely approximate what we would expect if the mechanism responsible were outer or middle ear pathology than inner ear pathology, we would conclude that outer or middle ear pathology appears to be the more viable explanation. In other words, we would conclude that the data plotted in Figure 3.2 are *consistent with the hypothesis* that the person has outer or middle ear pathology in his left ear.

Because a hypothesis is consistent with the data concerning a phenomenon does not necessarily mean it explains the phenomenon. There could be other hypotheses as consistent or even more consistent with the data. This dilemma was aptly described by Einstein and Infeld in *The Evolution of Physics:*

> In our endeavor to understand reality we are somewhat like a man trying to understand the mechanism of a closed watch. He sees the face and the moving hands, even hears it ticking, but he has no way of opening the case. If he is ingenious he may form some picture of a mechanism that could be responsible for all the things he observes, but he may never be quite sure his picture is the only one which could explain his observations. He will never be able to compare his picture with the real mechanism and he cannot even imagine the possibility or the meaning of such a comparison. But he certainly believes that, as his knowledge increases, his picture of reality will become simpler and simpler and will explain a wider and wider range of his sensuous impressions. (Einstein and Infeld, 1938)

This statement reinforces the conclusion we reached earlier in this chapter, that explanations for phenomena must be regarded as tentative.

Comprehensiveness or Scope of Knowledge. "Instead of presenting a finished account of the world, the genuine scientist keeps his unifying hypotheses open to revision and is always ready to modify or abandon them if evidence should render them doubtful. This *self-corrective aspect* [italics added] of science has rightly been stressed as its most important characteristic .... It is a sign of one's maturity to be able to live with an unfinished world view" (Feigl, 1953, p. 13).

Speech pathologists and audiologists, whether they function as clinicians or clinician-investigators, have to be able to tolerate living professionally with an "unfinished world view." The "facts" concerning communicative disorders they use are not really facts, but hypotheses subject to revision. Such facts (or beliefs) include those relevant to the symptomatology, incidence, etiology, prognosis, evaluation, prevention, and treatment of communicative disorders. Their beliefs about the etiology of communicative disorders may have to be modified or abandoned if new evidence renders these beliefs doubtful. Many speech pathologists who believed that stuttering resulted from lack of unilateral cerebral dominance, for example, abandoned this view when evidence appeared to render it doubtful (Bloodstein, 1975). Likewise, speech pathologists and audiologists have had to modify or abandon some of their beliefs concerning the symptomatology, incidence, prognosis, evaluation, prevention, and treatment of other communicative disorders.

How do we know when the evidence is sufficiently compelling to require us to modify or abandon a belief? There is no simple answer to this question. Several factors will influence the decision, including: (1) the internal standard of the person on what constitutes compelling evidence, (2) the evidence itself, and (3) the person's ego-involvement with the belief.

People differ in their internal standards of what constitutes compelling evidence. Evidence that one person would regard as compelling another may not. In part, this is a function of how critically you evaluate evidence. A person who did not evaluate the evidence relevant to a hypothesis critically might regard it as more compelling than one who did. (Considerations involved in evaluating evidence critically are discussed in Chapter 9.) One of the reasons, incidentally, why it is important for clinicians to develop an intuitive understanding of research methodology and the scientific method is to maximize their ability to evaluate evidence critically and thereby modify their internal standard of what constitutes compelling evidence.

Another relevant factor is the evidence itself. Some pieces of evidence will be judged stronger and more compelling than others, regardless of individual differences in internal standards among clinicians. Improved performance on a speech discrimination task would probably be considered more compelling evidence that a hearing aid has improved a hard-of-hearing person's ability to understand speech than would the person's own subjective report.

The third, and final, factor influencing the probability that evidence will be judged compelling is the person's ego-involvement with the belief.

The greater his ego-involvement, the stronger the evidence would have to be before he would regard it as sufficiently compelling to modify or abandon his belief. Some persons become quite ego-involved with their beliefs and for this reason have difficulty evaluating them objectively. They tend to filter out evidence that might require them to modify or abandon their beliefs. In extreme cases, the filtering is so complete they communicate (verbally, nonverbally, or both) to anyone they feel might challange their beliefs that *their minds are already made up and they don't wish to be confused by facts.* Whether we function as clinicians, clinician-investigators, or investigators, we have to be constantly on guard against this consequence of ego-involvement. We should regard our beliefs as tentative and thus subject to modification and abandonment.

Underlying Assumptions

Thus far in our discussion of the scientific method we have dealt with its objectives and characteristics. We now will consider its underlying assumptions, or presuppositions. These must be accepted *on faith* by users of the method since they have not been, and presumably cannot be, either proven or disproven. They are being discussed here not only to help you develop an intuitive understanding of the method, but also to help you develop an objective attitude toward it. That is, you must realize that while the method is extremely useful because it provides a "set of rules" for asking and answering questions that maximize the probability of correct answers, it is not completely objective, since it rests upon assumptions that are not empirically verifiable. Three such assumptions will be discussed here: (1) the principle of causality, (2) the principle of uniformity, and (3) the principle of the finitude of relevant factors.

Principle of Causality. One assumption, or presupposition, of the scientific method is that "every event has a cause" (Pap, 1949, p. 403). Without this assumption, two objectives of the scientific method—explanation and prediction—could not be achieved. To explain an event, we must assume it has a cause; otherwise, it would make no sense to try to explain it. Also, predicting an event requires a knowledge of its cause or causes. If events cannot be assumed to have causes, then attempting to predict their future occurrence with greater than chance accuracy makes no sense.

This assumption is implicitly or explicitly made every day by speech pathologists and audiologists, regardless of whether they function as clinicians or clinician-investigators. It underlies, for example, such statements as: "The cause of your speech disorder is. . ." or "The cause of your child's hearing problem is . . ."

Is it reasonable to assume that all events have causes? The success of the scientific method in explaining and predicting events during the past three hundred years offers some support for the reasonableness of this assumption. If events did not have causes, then predicting their occurrence with greater than chance accuracy would be impossible. Whether *every* event has a cause, however, cannot be established until every event has been studied. This is, of course, an impossible condition to satisfy since new events are constantly occurring. The assumption is worth being made, nevertheless, since it has heuristic value. That is, by making it we are more likely to be able to explain and predict events than we are by not making it.

Principle of Uniformity. Another presupposition of the scientific method related to causality is the so-called principle of uniformity—i.e., "... *'same cause, same effect'* [italics added]: it has been remarked that if an experiment, designed to prove a generalization 'if A, B, C, then D' is repeated several times under varied conditions, it is in order to make sure that A, B, C really are the essential conditions on which the effect D depends, and that the appearance of such a dependence was not due to some 'accidental' circumstance" (Pap, 1949, p. 405–406).

This assumption has relevance for speech pathologists and audiologists, since without it they would have difficulty generalizing from their observations about causation. If they observed, for example, that a particular response-contingent reinforcer was likely to have a particular effect on a particular behavior evinced by a particular subgroup of individuals with communicative disorders, they could not conclude without making this assumption that it would probably be as likely to have the same effect on the behavior in other members of the subgroup. Also, therapy outcome research would have limited generality and usefulness if this assumption were not made, since whether the therapy evaluated would have the same effect on other clients who were similar to those studied in all relevant variables would be uncertain.

Principle of the Finitude of Relevant Factors. The third and final presupposition of the scientific method we will discuss—the principle of the finitude of relevant factors—states that "... only a small, and in fact enumerable, set of circumstances is causally related to the observed effect" (Pap, 1953, p. 27). If we did not make this assumption implicitly or explicitly, we would be restricted in our ability to specify the reason or reasons for, or explain, events. We could not conclude with confidence, for example, that a person's communicative disorder probably was due to one or at most a small set of circumstances. We could not deal with causation as if it were relatively simple and employ relatively simple research designs when we wished to establish causation.

Is this assumption viable? Some relatively recent work in several disciplines, including general semantics (Korzybski, 1958) and general systems theory (Buckley, 1968), suggests it might be more reasonable to assume the set of circumstances that are causally related to an observed effect is relatively complex. That is, it might be reasonable to assume that all parts of a system are interrelated—that all events within a system are, to some extent, causally related to all other events in that system. The value of such an assumption has been demonstrated in several fields including ecology and economics. The causes of such events as "environmental pollution" and "inflation" apparently are quite complex.

How crucial is this assumption to the scientific method? If causation could not be assumed to be relatively simple, would this invalidate the method? The assumption does not appear crucial to the validity of the method. However, substituting the opposite assumption would probably necessitate some revision in the methodology used to answer "why" questions. Greater emphasis would be placed, for example, on the use of multivariate statistical techniques—techniques that permit us to assess the combined, or composite, effects of a number of variables. (The rationale for, and application of, such techniques is discussed in Chapter 8.)

Historical Perspective

Thus far, we have discussed the scientific method primarily from the frame of reference of the philosophy of science. There is a second frame of reference through which it may be viewed—that of the history of science. The first is concerned with how the scientific method is *supposed* to function; the second, with how it *has* functioned. The two may not, in fact, be synonymous (Bush, 1974; Kuhn, 1962). Scientists have made the observations necessary to answer questions accurately and to develop and test hypotheses by methods that deviated to some extent from the scientific method as defined by philosophers of science. For example, Gall in 1818 was apparently the first to hypothesize that the "faculty of speech" is located in the anterior portion of the brain. His hypothesis appears to have arisen from the following observations:

> ...he was sent in his ninth year to an uncle who was a *curé* in the Black Forest. Here he was educated with another boy of his own age who excelled him in learning his lessons. The two youths passed on to school at Baden, and Gall discovered that, when it was a question of learning by heart, he was beaten by those who were greatly inferior to him in written composition. Two of his new schoolfellows surpassed even his first companion in the ease with which they learnt by heart, and because they had *large and prominent eyes* [italics added] . . . they received the nickname of "Ox eyes." Three years later at Bruchsal and again at the University of Strasbourg he continued to notice that those who learnt easily by heart had the same sort of eyes. He began to

associate this conformation with a good verbal memory, and so arrived at the conclusion that this faculty was situated in that part of the brain which lay behind the orbits. From such fantastic beginnings sprang the idea that memory for words was situated in the frontal lobes. (Head, 1963, p. 9)

Here we have a classic example of a person arriving at a correct conclusion—i.e., formulating a valid hypothesis—on the basis of observations that were made in a manner inconsistent with the scientific method. Historians of science have reported a number of such cases (Bush, 1974; Kuhn, 1962).

If one can arrive at valid conclusions by using procedures that are not compatible with the scientific method, why is it important to use procedures that are compatible with it? The use of such procedures *maximizes the probability* that answers to questions will be "accurate" and hypotheses formulated, or conclusions drawn, from these answers will be plausible and testable. While these results can also be achieved when the scientific method is not rigorously applied, they are more likely to be achieved when it is. For this reason, researchers usually design and conduct their studies in such a way that their methodology is compatible with the scientific method.

THE SCIENTIFIC METHOD AS A SET OF RULES FOR ASKING AND ANSWERING QUESTIONS

The objective of this final section will be to demonstrate that the scientific method as applied to research can be viewed as a set of rules for asking and answering questions.

The characteristics of the scientific method discussed implicitly or explicitly suggest rules or criteria for formulating questions, making observations to answer them, and relating the answers to the existing body of knowledge. The criterion we referred to as "intersubjective testability," for example, suggests that the observational procedures used to answer questions should be described in sufficient detail that they can be repeated by others. That is, the methodology used to arrive at an answer should be described in sufficient detail that someone else could attempt to replicate the answer—i.e., arrive at the same answer.

The second criterion of the scientific method which we discussed, "reliability," in this context suggests that a sufficient number of observations should be made before we attempt to answer a question so that we can have a reasonable degree of confidence in the accuracy of the answer. It further suggests that we should incorporate into our studies some way of estimating the reliability of the observations we use to answer questions so that we can judge the maximum degree of confidence we can reasonably have in the accuracy of an answer.

The criterion we referred to as "definiteness and precision" also is relevant to the asking and answering of questions. It suggests that concepts referred to in questions formulated for research purposes should be as definitely delimited as possible. If such concepts are not defined precisely (i.e., with minimum borderline vagueness), questions which deal with them may not be answerable. (What makes a question answerable will be discussed in Chapter 4.) It also suggests that the language used to *answer* questions should be as unambiguous as possible. Concepts referred to should be clearly defined. Likewise, it suggests that the language used for *interpreting* answers to questions should be as unambiguous as possible with theoretical constructs clearly defined.

The criterion we referred to as "coherence or systematic structure" also has relevance here. Before we attempt to answer a question, we should organize the pieces of relevant information resulting from the observational process to make them coherent. This increases the probability of a correct answer. (Strategies for organizing qualitative and quantitative information to answer questions are discussed in Chapter 8.)

The final criterion of the scientific method we discussed was "comprehensiveness or scope of knowledge." It indicates that answers to questions should be regarded as tentative and subject to change when new information becomes available.

I have attempted to demonstrate in this chapter why the scientific method can be viewed as a set of rules for asking and answering questions. From this frame of reference, how might research be defined? For our purposes, we will define research as *a process of asking and answering questions that is governed by a set of rules referred to as the scientific method*. My goal in the next seven chapters is to help the reader develop an intuitive understanding of this process as it relates to speech pathology and audiology.

REFERENCES

AGNEW, N. M., and PYKE, S. W., *The Science Game*. Englewood Cliffs, N.J.: Prentice-Hall, Inc. (1975).

BLOODSTEIN, O., *A Handbook on Stuttering*. Chicago: National Easter Seal Society for Crippled Children and Adults (1975).

BRIDGMAN, P. W., *The Logic of Modern Physics*. New York: The Macmillan Company (1927).

BUCKLEY, W. (Ed.), *Modern Systems Research for the Behavioral Scientist*. Chicago: Aldine Publishing Company (1968).

BUSH, S. G., Should the history of science be rated X? *Science*, 183, 1164–1172 (1974).

EDWARDS, A. L., and CRONBACH, L. J., Experimental design for research in psychotherapy. In Arnold P. Goldstein and Stanford J. Dean (Eds.), *The Investiga-*

tion of Psychotherapy: Commentaries and Readings, New York: John Wiley & Sons, Inc., 71–79 (1966).

EINSTEIN, A., and INFELD, L., *The Evolution of Physics*. New York: Simon and Schuster, Inc. (1938).

FEIGL, H., The scientific outlook: Naturalism and humanism. In Herbert Feigl and May Brodbeck (Eds.), *Readings in the Philosophy of Science*, New York: Appleton-Century-Crofts, 8–18 (1953).

HEAD, H., *Aphasia and Kindred Disorders of Speech*, Volume 1. New York: Hafner Publishing Company (1963).

JOHNSON, W., *People in Quandaries*. New York: Harper & Row, Publishers (1946).

KORZYBSKI, A., *Science and Sanity: An Introduction to Non-Aristotelian Systems and General Semantics*. Lakeville, Conn.: Institute of General Semantics (1958).

KUHN, T. S., *The Structure of Scientific Revolutions*. Chicago: The University of Chicago Press (1962).

PAP, A., Does science have metaphysical presuppositions? In Herbert Feigl and May Brodbeck (Eds.), *Readings in the Philosophy of Science*, New York: Appleton-Century-Crofts, 21–33 (1953).

PAP, A., *Elements of Analytic Philosophy*. New York: The Macmillan Company (1949).

PERKINS, W. H., and CURLEE, R. F., Causality in speech pathology. *Journal of Speech and Hearing Disorders*, 34, 231–238 (1969).

part II

Asking and Answering Questions

FOUR

ASKING QUESTIONS THAT ARE BOTH RELEVANT AND ANSWERABLE

The first three chapters attempted to set the stage for our discussion of research design. The primary objective in this chapter and the six that follow is to provide basic information about the process of asking and answering questions that a speech pathologist or audiologist would need to function as a clinician-investigator. This chapter will deal with selecting and formulating questions for research. It also will be concerned with selecting a topic, or area, to research, since the topic selected will obviously determine the questions asked.

A speech pathologist or audiologist who chooses to function as a clinician-investigator must first decide what to investigate—what question or questions to try to answer. This decision is important because it will influence both the impact of this research and the likelihood that the research will be completed. By *impact* here we mean the effect that answering a particular question or group of questions is likely to have on clinical process in speech pathology and audiology. Unfortunately, the amount of impact that answering a particular question is likely to have on clinical process is quite difficult to predict. As Murray Sidman has pointed out,

> It is necessary ... to be wary about using the presumed importance of data as a criterion for evaluating them. Science, like fashion, has its fads and cycles. A discovery that lies outside the current stream of interest may be unrecognized and eventually forgotten, perhaps to be rediscovered at some later date. On the other side of the coin, we often find experiments acclaimed as significant because they resolve a problem of great contemporary concern, but of little lasting interest. It is a characteristic of science that we are seldom able to predict its future course of development. Many of the exciting issues of today will be forgotten tomorrow as the stream of scientific progress shifts into new channels (Sidman, 1960, p. 2).

Sidman's comments obviously have relevance for assessing the probable impact of answers to questions (i.e., experimental results) on clinical process in speech pathology and audiology. While the criterion of "importance" will always be of concern to investigators, it will not be particularly useful either for selecting questions to answer or for evaluating answers to questions.

An investigator's choice of questions to answer influences the likelihood that he will complete the research, for several reasons. The first is the *time required to make the necessary observations*. The longer you take to make these observations, the less likely you are to complete your research. As long as the time necessary does not exceed a year, this probably would not be an important consideration. While I do not wish to imply here that investigators should avoid questions that take a long time to answer—since there are probably many such questions that would be worthwhile answering—you should realize that when you attempt to answer such questions you are less likely to complete your research. This may be one of the reasons, incidently, why so little longitudinal research has been reported.

A second factor likely to influence the probability that research will be completed is the *complexity of the procedures required to make the necessary observations*. The more complex such procedures, the less likely an investigator is to complete the research. If you need electronic instrumentation (particularly, complex electronic instrumentation) to make your observations, you may have difficulty getting the instrumentation to function well enough to make them. The author experienced such difficulty in his own research with a miniature voice-actuated white-noise generator that was designed to be used with stutterers. About 50 percent of the time the device would not function properly, and several electronics technicians who tried to repair it were unsuccessful. While we are not attempting to discourage investigators from answering questions that require instrumentation to answer, you should realize that problems can arise when you attempt to answer such questions.

A third factor is the *availability of subjects*. If subjects are not available in sufficient numbers *within a reasonable time period*, the probability that the research will be completed can be reduced. It should be noted, however, that speech pathologists and audiologists have successfully completed research which has taken a number of years to observe a sufficient number of subjects.

Berry et al.(1974), for example, required fifteen years to observe a sufficient number of persons with Wilson's disease to be able to describe the speech deviations associated with it.

A fourth factor is the *time available for the purpose*. Some questions require more time to answer than others. Before beginning a piece of research, therefore, you should at least roughly estimate both the time required to complete it and the time you are likely to have available for the purpose.

A fifth factor is the *availability of supporting personnel (including consultants) and services*. To make the observations necessary to answer a question may require the cooperation or assistance of persons with expertise in various areas, and such persons may not be available. Special computer programs may be required, for example, to analyze the observations; and the services of a computer programmer may not be available. Or a study of the effect of a therapy program on persons who have vocal nodules may require the services of an otolaryngologist to do indirect laryngoscopy on the subjects before and after participating in the program. The investigator may be unable to locate an otolaryngologist who would be willing to provide this service. An investigator should therefore consider this possibility before beginning a piece of research.

The sixth, and final, factor considered here is *available funding*. To answer some questions, a large research grant may be needed, and to answer others, only minimal funding (less than one hundred dollars) would be required. Many questions of interest to speech pathologists and audiologists, incidentally, would probably require only minimal funding to answer. Such questions may only need funding for supplies, such as recording tapes or test forms. But before you commit yourself to answering a particular question, or questions, you should be reasonably certain that available funding will be adequate.

GENERATING RELEVANT QUESTIONS FOR RESEARCH

Now that we have considered the importance of an investigator's choice of questions to answer, we will deal with how to go about generating relevant questions for research. By a "relevant question" we mean one for which a response to the "so what" or "who cares" question can be provided—in other words, a question for which *a need* for answering can be established.

Need for Selecting Relevant Questions

An investigator ought to select questions to answer that he or she feels are relevant and can convince others are relevant, for several reasons. First, your research is more likely to be publishable if you select such questions. In the introductory section of a research report for a professional journal such as *Journal of Speech and Hearing Research*, *Journal of Speech and Hearing Disorders*, and *Language, Speech, and Hearing Services in Schools*, the author is expected to establish *scientific justification* for the research reported. That is, the author is expected to demonstrate the importance of answering the question or questions proposed. If you understand why it is important and can communicate this to readers of your report, you will increase the probability that your report will be accepted for publication.

A second reason to select questions that both peers and administrators to whom you are responsible will regard as relevant is to increase the possibility that you will receive the support you need for your research. You are more likely to secure funding for research you can justify as relevant than for research for which you can provide no such justification. Also, you are more likely to receive approval from administrators for "released time" for research if they view your research as satisfying an important need. Such approval would be particularly important for speech pathologists and audiologists who are employed in clinical settings and whose primary responsibilities are clinical.

Identifying a Problem Area

What should a speech pathologist or audiologist take into consideration when attempting to identify a problem area from which to generate relevant questions for research? Several factors need to be considered. These factors include: (1) personal interests, (2) competencies, (3) the potential value of the research, (4) the available equipment and facilities for making observations and analyzing data, (5) the "populations" available for study, (6) the financial resources available, (7) the amount of time available, and (8) the possibilities for consultation.

The first factor a speech pathologist or audiologist should consider when attempting to identify a problem area for research is *personal interests* —you should attempt to identify the problem areas within the field of communicative disorders that are of most interest to you. An area could be defined partially by a symptom complex such as aphasia, stuttering, defective articulation, or conductive hearing loss. An area could also be defined partially by a technique such as impedance audiometry, operant conditioning, or articulation testing. You should attempt to identify as many such areas as you can and roughly order them on the basis of your interest in them. It is desirable to identify more than one area initially since factors may be present that would make it quite difficult to pursue certain areas. Several such factors will be discussed in this section.

You should select an area to research in which you have some interest. Your interest in the research will influence both how positively reinforcing you will find the experience and the probability that you will complete it. We all tend to pursue activities we find positively reinforcing and avoid those we find punishing.

A second factor a speech pathologist or audiologist should consider when selecting a problem area for research is *competencies*. Because of your training and experience, the probability that you will be successful in your research endeavors may be greater if you avoid certain problem areas. If you had no training or experience in aphasia testing, for example, you might be wise to avoid questions that required the administration of aphasia tests to answer. While you could probably learn to administer such tests, it might require a considerable investment of time before you would be sufficiently competent to administer them with adequate reliability for your purposes. Of course, you might be able to find someone with whom to collaborate on the research who is competent in aphasia testing. This illustrates one way an investigator can reduce the consequences of a "deficiency" in training or experience. It is not unusual, incidently, for two or more persons to collaborate on a piece of research. In fact, 48 percent of the papers in five randomly selected issues of the *Journal of Speech and Hearing Disorders* were authored by two or more persons. It is desirable, therefore, when attempting to evaluate a potential problem area for research, to specify as completely as you can the competencies necessary to pursue the research and to judge whether you possess each one. If you do not possess some necessary competencies and cannot find a collaborator (or collaborators) who does, you might be wise not to pursue research in the area, particularly if overcoming such deficiencies would require large investments of money or time.

A third consideration when attempting to identify a problem area for research is the *potential value* of the research. As already indicated, it is difficult to predict the impact a piece of research will have on a discipline. Nevertheless, this is almost always a consideration when an investigator chooses an area to research. You will usually choose a problem you regard as worthwhile to investigate. For this reason, you may choose a problem with immediate relevance—e.g., you may attempt to evaluate a therapy program that you are presently using or are contemplating using. Such research could have considerable impact on your own caseload and, if it is communicated to other clinicians, on their caseloads as well.

A fourth factor is the *availability of equipment and facilities for making observations and analyzing data*. An investigator may not be able to pursue a research area of interest because necessary facilities, equipment, or both, are lacking. From one frame of reference this factor could restrict an investigator in exploring certain problem areas. From a second frame of reference additional possible problem areas for research might be suggested. An investigator with equipment and facilities that are not generally available may wish to exploit them—that is, to define a problem area based on questions they would permit to be answered. An audiologist, for example, who possessed some pieces of testing equipment not generally available might choose to ask questions that could be answered through the use of this equipment. Or a speech pathologist employed in a setting with sophisticated biofeedback instrumentation might choose to exploit these instruments in a similar manner. As an investigator, therefore, you might find it worthwhile to prepare an inventory of the equipment and facilities available to you as a preliminary step in defining a problem area for research. Such an inventory could assist you in assessing problem areas you are considering and in identifying additional possible problem areas.

A fifth factor is the *"populations" available for study*. Before you begin to try to identify such an area, you might find it worthwhile to inventory relevant attributes of persons who might be available and willing to serve as research subjects. Relevant attributes might include: (1) sex, (2) whether or not they have particular communicative disorders, (3) chronological age, (4) physical status, (5) intellectual and emotional status, (6) socio-economic status, and (7) therapy history—whether or not they have previously had therapy and if they have what kind or kinds. Such an inventory could provide two types of input into the selection process. First, it could alert you, the investigator, to research areas you would be wise to avoid because subjects who have the necessary attributes would probably not be available to you in sufficient numbers. A speech clinician employed in a school setting, for example, might have a difficult time obtaining adequate numbers of laryngectomized geriatric subjects for a research project. Second, the inventory could suggest problem areas you might want to consider. If you had subjects available in fairly large numbers who were relatively homogeneous in some attribute (e.g., deaf children or mentally retarded children) or if you had small numbers of subjects available who were unusual in some way (e.g., persons with rare diseases or conditions that influence communicative behavior), you might be able to define a problem area in which you could use observations made on such subjects to answer questions. A single subject, incidently, who is unusual in some regard might be used in this manner for an individual case study.

A sixth factor is the *financial resources available*. As previously mentioned, while some research requires only minimal funding, other research can be quite costly. To do research that required more than minimal funding, an investigator would probably have to secure a research grant from a government (state or national) agency, private organization, or private foundation. Many such agencies, organizations, and foundations have funded research on communicative disorders. Nevertheless, a person who is considering applying for such a grant should be aware that they are usually quite competitive. More applications are ordinarily submitted than can be funded. Investigators who have demonstrated research competence by publishing are usually favored for the larger grants; they also are favored for many relatively small grants. A beginning investigator, therefore, would probably be wise to select a project that only requires minimal funding. However, after demonstrating research competence by publishing the results of several such projects, you can consider projects that require outside funding if you so desire.

A seventh factor is the *amount of time available*. Before you decide to do a particular research project, it is a good idea to estimate roughly both the amount of time it would take to complete and the amount of time that is likely to be available. If the amount of time necessary grossly exceeds time available for the purpose, you have several options as an investigator: (1) you can try to locate one or more professional colleagues who would be interested in collaborating with you on the project and sharing the work; (2) you can enlist the aid of persons who are not speech pathologists or audiologists, such as spouses or secretaries, for parts of the project that do not require competence in these areas; (3) you can secure a research grant and hire full- or part-time research assistants to gather data and assist with data analysis; (4) you can attempt to arrange your schedule to have adequate time available for the project; or (5) you can decide not to pursue the project. Many projects, incidentally, require a time investment that would not exceed that available to most clinicians. Among these are projects for which data could be gathered in conjunction with ongoing clinical activities, e.g., therapy evaluation studies.

The eighth, and final, factor is the *possibilities for consultation*. If, to research a problem area, you must consult with persons who have expertise in certain areas such as statistics, electronics, computer programming, and mental measurement, you should be reasonably certain before beginning that such persons will be available for consultation. As previously mentioned, faculty members at local colleges and universities who have the required expertise may be willing to serve as consultants.

Generating Relevant Research Questions

After a problem area has been selected, the next task is to generate one or more questions to answer that are relevant to the area. These questions, implicitly or explicitly, define the research topic. They indicate what the investigator is trying to find out. They also indicate the kinds of information that are apt to result from the research. Since most research questions only can be answered in a finite number of ways, we usually can infer from a question what the possible answers could be. If, for example, the question we sought to answer was, "Do most elementary-school stutterers avoid talking?" our research could lead to three possible answers: (1) it could indicate uneqivocally that the majority of elementary-school stutterers avoid talking; (2) it could indicate unequivocally that the majority of elementary-school stutterers do not avoid talking; or (3) it could be lead to an equivocal result. Finally, the questions asked specify, at least partially, what has to be done to answer them. Suppose, for example, we asked the question, "How likely are persons who are employed as firemen for more than ten years to develop noise-induced hearing losses?" To answer this question, we would have to measure the hearing acuity of persons who have been employed as firemen for more than ten years using methods that were sufficiently reliable and valid to detect noise-induced hearing losses if they were present.

What approaches can be used for selecting a research topic—i.e., generating questions to answer? A number of approaches can be used for this purpose, including the following:

You can do a careful review of the literature in the area selected to identify: (1) questions that have been formulated but only partially answered, (2) questions that have been formulated but not answered, and (3) questions that have not been formulated but should be.

Many questions about communicative disorders have been formulated but only partially answered. A question is rarely answered unequivocally on the basis of a single set of observations, for several reasons. First, in many cases the observations that have been used to answer questions of concern to speech pathologists and audiologists were *not* made on a *random sample* of subjects from the population referred to by the question. To illustrate this point, let us again use the question, "How likely are persons who are employed as firemen for more than ten years to develop noise-induced hearing losses?" The population referred to by this question consists of all firemen who have more than ten years experience. For a sample from this population to be random, all such firemen would have to have an equal chance of being selected. However, it would be unusual for an investigator who sought to answer this kind of question to use a random sample. You would most likely base your observations on a "nonrandom" sample, such as a local group of firemen with more than ten years service who volunteered to have their hearing tested. The likelihood of the subjects in such a sample having noise-induced hearing losses may differ systematically from that for firemen in general. In other words, the answer to the question could be different for this sample than it would have been for a random sample. Hence, the generality of an answer based on a nonrandom sample would be uncertain. In cases where a question has been answered through the use of a nonrandom sample, therefore, the answer should be regarded as equivocal until the observations have been replicated on other samples of subjects from the population. This would be true even if the results were statistically significant. One assumption that underlies almost all tests of statistical significance is that the subjects observed were a random sample from the population of interest. (This concept is further discussed in Chapter 9.)

A second reason why a question may not have been answered unequivocally on the basis of a single set of observations is that they were *not* adequately *reliable*, *valid*, or both. If the observations were not sufficiently reliable, the investigator may not have been able to observe the phenomenon with sufficient clarity to answer the question accurately. Returning to the fireman example again, if the audiometer used had not been properly calibrated, or if the person who administered the test or tests had not been sufficiently proficient, or if the room in which the testing was done had not been adequately sound-treated, the thresholds recorded could have been sufficiently in error that the effect of noise on firemen's hearing might not be detected. On the other hand, if the observations used to answer a question were not sufficiently valid, the answer *might* be incorrect. We use the word "might" here because an investigator could arrive at the right answer for the wrong reason (e.g., Gall's conclusion that the anterior portion of the brain is dominant for speech, discussed in Chapter 3). In our fireman example, an investigator could conclude through the use of an invalid testing procedure (e.g., one that was thought to be able to detect noise-induced hearing losses but was not sensitive to such losses) that the firemen did not have noise induced hearing losses when they did, or that they had noise-induced hearing losses when they did not.

A third reason why a question may not have been answered unequivocally on the basis of a single set of observations is *random*, or chance, *sampling error*. This can influence research results derived from random samples of subjects by methods which were adequately reliable and valid. What happens here is that by chance the behavior of the subjects in the sample is not representative of that in the population from which they were selected, even though appropriate sampling procedures were used. While random sampling is more likely to result in a sample that is representative of the population than are other sampling procedures, it does not always result in such a sample. The sample selected will not be representative of the population from which it was selected a certain percentage of the time. (The reason for this phenomenon is discussed in Chapter 9.) The observations that were made on such a sample of subjects could be sufficiently biased to cause an investigator to answer a question incorrectly. Because of this possibility, research findings should be regarded as suspect until they have been replicated. A question should not be regarded as having been answered unequivocally until the same answer has been obtained with several samples of subjects.

A fourth, and final reason why a question may not have been answered unequivocally on the basis of a single set of observations is *experimenter bias*. A number of studies (e.g., Rosenthal, 1969) have demonstrated that an investigator's expectations and theoretical biases can influence his observations without his being conscious of it. If you expect a question to be answered in a particular way or if your theoretical biases suggest that a question should have a particular answer, you may unconsciously "filter" your observations to obtain the answer you expect. This is particularly apt to be a problem when an investigator has considerable ego-involvement in a theoretical position relevant to the questions he is attempting to answer. This problem is extremely difficult to deal with. With regard to our concern here—selecting questions to answer—the relevance of experimenter bias is that if a question has only been answered by a single investigator (particularly one with an ego-investment in the answer), the answer should probably not be regarded as unequivocal unless it has been replicated by other investigators unlikely to have the same theoretical biases.

In addition to helping identify questions that have been formulated but only partially answered, a search of the literature in the area of interest may reveal questions that have been *formulated but not answered*. There are several places in which such questions might be found. One is the "discussion" sections of research reports in the area. Frequently the author or authors will indicate some implications they feel their findings have for future research in this section. They may even indicate what specific questions they feel should be answered, for a piece of research often raises more questions than it answers.

Another source of questions that have been formulated but not answered is review papers in the area of interest. A review paper is one that summarizes and integrates the research in a particular area. Such papers usually specify what information is needed to improve our understanding of the area, thus suggesting questions that need to be answered. Review papers have been published for many areas of interest to speech pathologists and audiologists. They have appeared in professional journals and monographs as well as in some textbooks. The best way to locate a review paper on a topic of interest (if one has been written) is probably through the use of an abstracts journal, such as: (1) *Psychological Abstracts*, (2) *dsh* (Deafness, Speech, and Hearing) *Abstracts*, (3) *Language and Language Behavior Abstracts*, (4) *Index Medicus*, and (5) *Dissertation Abstracts*. Abstracts of papers relevant to the topic can be scanned to determine if they are review papers. It would be wise to begin a literature search with the most recent volume of an abstracts journal and work backwards. This procedure would maximize the odds of finding the most recent review paper on a topic, if there has been more than one.

A third source of questions that have been formulated but not answered would be publications in which individuals or committees indicate what research they feel is needed in particular areas. One of the most ambitious projects of this type was a monograph entitled *Research Needs in Speech Pathology and Audiology*, which was published as a monograph supplement to the *Journal of Speech and Hearing Disorders* in 1959. Other publications that have indicated research needs in speech pathology and audiology include Darley, 1972; *Human Communication and its Disorders—An Overview*, 1969; Kavanaugh, 1974, Morley, 1962; *Public school speech and hearing services*, 1961; Sheehan, 1970; Sommers, 1967; Templin, 1953. A comprehensive up-to-date list of these publications for a particular area can be compiled through the use of relevant abstracts jounals. Before beginning to answer a question selected from such a publication, of course, you would have to do a search of relevant literature to make certain that it had not been answered unequivocally in the time since its appearance in the publication.

Thus far, we have considered how a review of the literature in the area of interest can help to identify questions that have been formulated but only partially answered and questions that have been formulated but not answered. We now will consider how such a review can suggest *questions that have not been formulated but should be.* The strategy here would be to: (1) do a careful search of the literature in the area to determine what is known (what questions have been answered), and (2) formulate questions which, if answered, would be likely to increase our understanding of the area.

The first task, the literature search, can be facilitated by the use of abstracts journals. *Psychological Abstracts* may be quite useful here, since it goes back to 1927. *Dsh Abstracts* began in 1960, *Language and Language Behavior Abstracts* in 1967, and *Dissertation Abstracts* in 1938. The reference lists of all papers found should be checked for relevant research reports that were not abstracted by the abstract journal or journals used. Such reports would include those published prior to the year in which the literature search began (i.e., prior to the year of the earliest abstract journal used); those that appeared in limited circulation journals such as state speech and hearing journals; those that were presented orally at state, national, and international professional and scientific meetings; those that were reported in unpublished masters' theses and doctoral dissertations; and those that were reported in unpublished papers, including technical reports.

The research reported should be organized in a manner to make it apparent what is known about the area. One approach that can sometimes be used for this purpose is to define a *dependent variable* and indicate what *independent variables* have been shown to influence it. One example of a dependent variable is speechreading ability; examples of independent variables that have been shown to influence it include visual acuity and training in speechreading. Another example of a dependent variable is extent of recovery from aphasia. Independent variables that would be expected to influence it include chronological age, extent and location (e.g., right or left hemisphere) of brain damage, and amount of stimulation received.

After the available data has been organized to make it apparent what is known about the area, the next task is to formulate questions which, if answered, would be likely to increase our understanding of the area. What is required here is first to formulate as many questions as possible that have not been answered, and then to select from these one or more to answer.

Organized in this way, the information available on a topic would facilitate the question formulation process. This would be particularly true if a dependent variable had been defined and independent variables that have been shown to influence it catalogued. One would then attempt to identify independent variables not yet studied that might be relevant. A question, or questions, could be formulated about each such variable. If the dependent variable, for example, were speechreading ability and an independent variable that had not been investigated were telepathic ability, one question that might be asked would be, "Do persons who earn relatively high scores on a Duke University card-guessing telepathy task exhibit greater speechreading ability than those who earn relatively low scores on this task?"

How can we identify uninvestigated independent variables that may influence a particular dependent variable? This question is difficult to answer, since the process of discovery is not fully understood. Perhaps our ability to identify such independent variables involves what Michael Polanyi (1967) has referred to as "tacit knowing." According to Polanyi,

> ... *we can know more than we can tell.* This fact seems obvious enough; but it is not easy to say exactly what it means. Take an example. We know a person's face, and can recognize it among a thousand, indeed among a million. Yet we usually cannot tell how we recognize a face we know (Polanyi, 1967, p. 4).

Polanyi states that tacit knowing guides the scientist to problems worth investigating—i.e., to questions worth answering. Hunches and intuitions resulting from tacit knowing may be the mechanism by which we identify relevant independent variables.

While the process used to identify relevant independent variables is not fully understood, there is a strategy which may facilitate it. This strategy is to identify independent variables that have been shown to influence other dependent behavioral variables that have not been investigated with regard to the dependent behavioral variable of interest. Chronological age is an example of an independent variable that has been shown to influence many dependent behavioral variables of interest to speech pathologists and audiologists. If such an independent variable had not been investigated with regard to the dependent behavioral variable in which you are interested, it might be worthwhile for you to do so. The author worked for several years as a research associate on a project which investigated the variability of stuttering frequency (dependent variable) in school-age children under the same conditions it had previously been investigated in adults. The question we sought to answer was, "Do conditions which have been shown to reduce stuttering frequency in adults also reduce it in school-age children?"

A second general approach for identifying relevant research questions is to examine your clinical experience in the area of interest for questions that seem worth answering and then to search the relevant literature to determine whether they have been answered. You should ask yourself the following question: "To what clinically relevant questions have I sought answers for which I knew of no data to answer?" You also should ask yourself, "To what clinically relevant questions do I feel I have answers where my answers probably are not based on reliable and valid data?" That is, "What questions am I assuming have been answered that haven't?" Things are frequently done clinically not because they have been established effective empirically, but because they have either been recommended by an "authority," make sense theoretically, or are "traditional." What I mean by being traditional can be illustrated by the frequency and duration of therapy sessions assigned to clients. It may be "traditional" in a particular clinical setting for clients with a particular communicative disorder to be scheduled for therapy a particular number of sessions per week, each of which is a particular number of minutes in duration. One might ask whether this number of sessions per week of this length is optimal for reducing the severity of these clients' communicative disorders. Perhaps the sessions either are: (1) longer and more frequent than necessary, or (2) longer but not more frequent than necessary, or (3) less frequent but no longer than necessary, or (4) shorter and less frequent than necessary. One way to answer this question—to determine whether the frequency and duration of therapy sessions are optimal—would be to vary systematically the frequency and duration of sessions for clients who have a given communicative disorder and observe whether better results are obtained when a different frequency or duration is used.

One approach that can be used for identifying questions that have answers based on "authority" or "tradition" rather than empirical data is to subject information on which we operate clinically to the "how do we know?" question. How do we know, for example, that a therapy procedure does what it is supposed to do? If there were no unequivocal empirical evidence a therapy procedure did what it was supposed to do, this circumstance would suggest questions for research.

The available data on clinical procedures of interest can be located through the use of the abstracts journals that I have referred to previously.

A third approach for generating questions that might be worth answering is "brainstorming" with colleagues about their clinical experience in the area and then searching relevant literature to determine whether the questions suggested have been answered unequivocally. The procedure here is much the same as that described for the second approach. The only difference is that questions are abstracted from informal discussions with colleagues about their clinical experience rather than from the clinician's own experience. If you adopt an appropriate set, many potential research questions probably can be abstracted from informal conversations with colleagues.

What specifically might colleagues say that would suggest potential research questions? They might indicate concern over the effectiveness of a particular diagnostic or therapeutic procedure. They might state that they failed to obtain the results reported for this procedure in the literature.

Assuming that they appeared to have applied it as described in the literature, one might ask whether the results reported in the literature can be replicated. Such could be the genesis of a piece of clinical research.

A colleague might raise questions concerning the organization of clinical programs for which no data-based guidelines exist in the literature. Such questions may relate to any of a number of areas, including intake procedures, dismissal procedures, follow-up procedures, and the utilization of sub-professionals.

A colleague might also raise questions concerning the validity of research results reported in the literature. He may state, for example, that the incidence of a particular communicative disorder appears to be considerably higher or lower than reported in the literature. Or he may indicate that most of those clients who have a particular communicative disorder fail to exhibit some aspect or aspects of the symptomatology reported in the literature as characteristic of this disorder.

STRUCTURING RESEARCH QUESTIONS TO MAKE THEM ANSWERABLE

The question considered thus far in this chapter has been, "How can we generate relevant questions for research?" In this section we will consider the question, "How can we structure research questions to make them 'answerable'?" By an answerable question we mean one that can be answered by observations and that implicitly or explicitly (preferably the latter) specifies the observation or observations necessary to answer it.

Not all questions of interest to speech pathologists and audiologists are answerable empirically. There are several reasons why this is so. First, a question may be formulated in such a way to make it uncertain what observations have to be made to answer it. Consider, for example, the following questions:

1. Is hypnosis effective in treating stuttering?
2. Is the post-hypnotic suggestion, "You will not stutter any more," effective in reducing stuttering frequency?

These questions are not equally answerable. The second specifies the observations that would have to be made to answer it more explicitly than the first and hence is more likely to be answerable empirically.

A second reason why a question may not be answerable empirically is that it is not possible to make the observations necessary to answer it. In some cases this would be because the necessary observational procedures have not been developed. When they are, the question would no longer be unanswerable. In other cases, a question may be unanswerable because the instruments required to make the observations are not available to the investigator. While such a question would be unanswerable for him, it might not be for someone else (someone who has the necessary instruments).

How does one structure a question to make it answerable? According to Wendell Johnson,

> One cannot get a clear answer to a vague question. The language of science is particularly distinguished by the fact it centers around well-stated questions. If there is one part of a scientific experiment that is more important than any other part, it is the framing of the question that the experiment is to answer. If it is stated vaguely, no experiment can answer it precisely. If the question is stated precisely, the means of answering it are clearly indicated. The specific observations needed, and the conditions under which they are to be made, are implied in the question itself (Johnson, 1946, pp. 52–53).

For a question to be answerable, therefore, it cannot be vague or ambiguous. The meanings of all words must be made explicit and, if possible, defined operationally. If a question we wished to answer were "Do persons with cleft palates have normal intelligence?" we would have to specify as precisely as possible what segment of the cleft palate population we were referring to (i.e., those with a cleft of the soft palate only, or those with clefts of both hard and soft palates, or both groups) and what we meant by intelligence (i.e., performance on what task or test). The question would be more answerable, for example, if it were structured as follows: Are five-year-old children who have clefts of the palate only more likely to have below normal intelligence as measured by the Stanford-Binet than five-year-old children who do not have this condition?

To develop further your intuitive understanding of what an answerable question consists of, pairs of questions are presented in Table 4.1 in which

TABLE 4.1. Pairs of questions that differ in the degree to which they are answerable.

Less Answerable Version	More Answerable Version
How much can aphasics be expected to improve between one month and one year following trauma?	How many points can receptive aphasics be expected to gain, on the average, on the Minnesota Aphasia Test between one month and one year following trauma?
Does drinking alcholic beverages reduce stuttering?	Does drinking five highballs in a period of two hours reduce the stuttering frequencies of most adult stutterers?
Are home assignments helpful for correcting articulation errors?	Is a particular home assignment at a particular stage of therapy for a particular articulation error helpful for correcting this error?
Is a particular ear-protector effective in preventing noise-induced hearing loss?	Is a particular ear-protector effective in preventing a temporary threshold shift if used in the presence of noise of a particular intensity with a particular spectrum for a particular period of time?

the members of each pair differ in the degree to which they are answerable. The member in column one is less answerable than that in column two. The two versions presented are not necessarily the least and most answerable possible.

REFERENCES

BERRY, W. R., DARLEY, F. L., ARONSON, A. E., and GOLDSTEIN, N. P., Dysarthria in Wilson's disease. *Journal of Speech and Hearing Research*, 17, 160–183 (1974).
DARLEY, F. L., The efficacy of language rehabilitation in aphasia. *Journal of Speech and Hearing Disorders*, 37, 3–21 (1972).
Human Communication and its Disorders—An Overview. National Institute of Neurological Diseases and Stroke (1969).
JOHNSON, W., *People in Quandaries*. New York: Harper & Row, Publishers (1946).
KAVANAUGH, J. F., Issues and needs in research. *Language, Speech, and Hearing Services in Schools*, 5, 258–262 (1974).
MORLEY, D. E., Research needs in communication problems of the aging. *Asha*, 4, 345–347 (1962).
POLANYI, M., *The Tacit Dimension*. Garden City, N. Y.: Doubleday Anchor Books (1967).
Public school speech and hearing services. *Journal of Speech and Hearing Disorders*, Monograph Supplement 8, 114–123 (1961).
Research needs in speech pathology and audiology. *Journal of Speech and Hearing Disorders*, Monograph Supplement 5, 1–78 (1959).
ROSENTHAL, R., Interpersonal expectations: Effects of the experimenter's hypothesis. In Robert Rosenthal and Ralph L. Rosnow (Eds.), *Artifact in Behavioral Research*, New York: Academic Press, Inc., 182–277 (1969).
SHEEHAN, J. G., *Stuttering: Research and Therapy*. New York: Harper & Row, Publishers, 312–350 (1970).
SIDMAN, M., *Tactics of Scientific Research*. New York: Basic Books (1960).
SOMMERS, R. F., Problems in articulatory research: Methodology and error. *Asha*, 9, 406–408 (1967).
TEMPLIN, M. C., Possibilities of research for public school speech therapists. *Journal of Speech and Hearing Disorders*, 18, 355–359 (1953).

FIVE

SELECTING THE APPROPRIATE DESIGN FOR ANSWERING SPECIFIC QUESTIONS

After an investigator has formulated research questions, the next task is to select an appropriate design for making the observations to answer them. There is no one design appropriate for answering all questions. This chapter will describe the two basic types of designs—individual subject and typical subject—and will present criteria for identifying the more appropriate one to answer specific questions.

What are individual subject and typical subject designs? In what ways are they different? What are their advantages and disadvantages? What variations are possible within each type? These questions will be dealt with in turn to help the reader develop an intuitive understanding of the attributes of these two basic types of designs.

An *individual* subject design permits the performance of individual subjects under the experimental condition or conditions to be *reliably* determined. Reliable conclusions can be reached concerning the effects of an experimental condition on the behavior of an individual subject. The question, "Has a client improved following a period of therapy?" would require an individual subject design to answer. The simplest such design would be one that permitted relevant "before and after" measures (e.g., pre-therapy and post-therapy measures) to be made.

A *typical* subject, or group, design *reliably* permits the average (mean, median, or mode) performance of the subjects in a group under the experimental condition or conditions to be determined. Reliable conclusions can be reached concerning the effects of an experimental condition on the behavior of the average, or "typical," member of a group. The question, "Are elementary-school stutterers able to predict their moments of stuttering as accurately as adult stutterers?" would require a typical subject, or group, design. To answer it, the average (i.e., mean or median) performance of a group of elementary-school stutterers on a stuttering prediction task could be compared to that of a group of adult stutterers on the same task.

Thus far, these two types of designs have been discussed as if they were mutually exclusive. This is not the case. Some designs perform both functions. They permit the average performance of a group as well as the performance of the individual subjects in that group under the experimental condition or conditions to be *reliably* determined. Such designs are useful when it appears likely that subjects will respond differently to an experimental condition. In fact, they permit the investigator to determine whether subjects do, in fact, respond differently to such a condition. It might be suspected, for example, that a particular approach to teaching speechreading would be more effective with some hard-of-hearing persons than with others. It probably would be worthwhile, therefore, to gather sufficient data on each person with whom the approach is used so that the amount each learned could be *reliably* estimated. From these data could be determined: (1) the amount the "average" person in the group learned, and (2) the degree of variability in the amount learned. Also, if considerable variability occurred, an attempt could be made to identify the factor or factors responsible through the use of correlational procedures. (These are described in Chapter 8.)

Considerable emphasis has been placed here on the word "reliability," particularly with regard to the individual subject design. The types of data usually gathered when group designs are used—i.e., each subject run only once under each experimental condition—usually are not sufficiently reliable for determining the responses of individual subjects to experimental conditions. A subject may not always respond to an experimental condition in the same manner, because of the effects of extraneous variables that have not been controlled and in many cases would be quite difficult to control even if we wished to. A subject's emotional state and degree of motivation would be examples of such variables.

Another reason for the lack of reliability of such data is that descriptions of behavior (both numerical and verbal) are subject to error of various kinds. The human observer is not an error-free describer of events. The more observations on which a description is based, the more reliable it is apt to be. Suppose that we wished to determine the effect of speaking in the presence of masking noise on stuttering. Our description would probably be more reliable if each stutterer spoke five times without masking noise and five times with masking noise and stuttering frequencies during the five speeches under each condition were averaged than it would be if each spoke only once under each condition.

DIFFERENCES BETWEEN INDIVIDUAL SUBJECT AND TYPICAL SUBJECT DESIGNS

To clarify the distinction between individual subject and typical subject designs, we have indicated in Table 5.1 eight of the more important differences between them. The order in which they appear in the table is not necessarily related to their importance.

TABLE 5.1. Differences between individual subject and typical subject designs.

Individual Subject Designs	Typical Subject Designs
Provide data concerning the "typical" behavior of an individual subject under an experimental condition	Provide data concerning the behavior of the "typical" member of a group under an experimental condition
Not necessary to assume that subjects respond similarly to an experimental condition	Necessary to assume that subjects in a group respond similarly to an experimental condition
Necessary for subjects to be run more than once under each experimental condition	Not necessary for subjects to be run more than once under each experimental condition
Generalize to "typical" behavior of individual studied under experimental condition	Generalize to "typical" behavior of mean or median group member under experimental condition
May not be relatively easy to control for order and sequence effects	Usually relatively easy to control for order and sequence effects
Statistical procedures for assessing the reliability of research findings are not as well developed as for typical subject designs	Statistical procedures for assessing the reliability of research findings are well developed
Minimum number of subjects necessary is 1	Minimum number of subjects necessary is approximately 10
Generalize to population from which subjects are selected on logical basis	Generalize to population from which subjects are selected on statistical basis

One of the more important differences between these two designs is the nature of the data provided. Individual subject designs provide data on the *typical* response of *one person* to an experimental condition. The typical response referred to here would be the mean, median, or most frequently occurring (modal) response. Typical subject designs, on the other hand, provide data on the mean, median, or most frequently occurring (modal) response of the *members of a group*.

With both designs, it is possible for the typical response to an experimental condition not to be typical. This is particularly likely to occur when the mean is used. With an individual subject design, a subject's mean response to an experimental condition may represent behavior that did not occur even once. This has been demonstrated, for example, with the mean response of individual aphasics to aphasia test subtests (Silverman, 1974).

The typical response to an experimental condition also may not be typical when a group design is used. The mean response of the typical group member may not correspond to that of any group member. The mean number of stutterings produced by 25 stutterers during their reading of a 100-word passage, for example, might be 10.5. Since no stutterer could stutter a fraction of a stuttering, this stuttering frequency would not correspond to that produced by any of the 25 stutterers. The lack of "representativeness" of mean data would be of considerable importance for answering some questions since it would lead to incorrect answers.

A second difference between individual and typical subject designs is the necessity of assuming that subjects respond differently to an experimental condition—that is, the necessity of assuming that observed differences in the responses of subjects to an experimental condition result from the effects of extraneous variables or from "chance" (random) fluctuation rather than from real differences in their responses to that condition. While individual subject designs do not require such an assumption, typical subject designs implicitly or explicitly do. Without such an assumption, it would not be particularly meaningful to talk about the typical response of a group to an experimental condition. This would be particularly true when an experimental condition had opposite effects on different persons. An example of such a condition would be consecutive readings of a passage. This condition has been shown to result in some stutterers becoming progressively more disfluent (adaptation effect) and others becoming progressively more fluent (Bloom and Silverman, 1973). The only circumstance under which it would probably be meaningful to talk about a typical response to an experimental condition when people differ in their responses to that condition is when the differences are of degree rather than kind—that is, when an experimental condition changes the behavior of all subjects in the same direction but to different degrees. A particular obturator may reduce the hypernasality of all persons with cleft palates who are fitted with it, but not to the same degree. It would be meaningful, therefore, to talk about the effect of this obturator on the speech of the typical person who was fitted with it.

A third difference between individual subject and typical subject designs is the minimum number of times it is necessary to run a subject under each experimental condition. With a typical subject design, reliable results are frequently obtainable when a subject is run only once under each such condition. With an individual subject design, on the other hand, reliable results would rarely be obtainable if a subject were run only once under each condition. The reason for this difference is that with a typical subject design, factors that reduce reliability (e.g., measurement error, effects of extraneous variables, and random fluctuation) can be kept from biasing the results by using as a measure of performance (criterion measure) the average of the measures from a number of subjects under each condition. Such factors usually would not bias the performance of the majority of subjects in a group under an experimental condition in the same manner.

With an individual subject design, the previously mentioned factors that can reduce reliability can be prevented from biasing the results by using as a measure of individual performance (criterion measure) under each condition the average of the measures made under each condition. These factors usually will not bias measures of a subject's performance under a given experimental condition in exactly the same manner. Hence, answers to questions will tend to be more reliable with an individual subject design if they are based on a subject's average performance under a condition rather than on any single performance under it.

A fourth difference between individual subject and typical subject designs is what answers to questions, strictly speaking, can be generalized to. For research findings to be useful, they must be applicable outside of the experimental situation in which they were generated. With an individual subject design, the behavior of a subject under an experimental condition can be used to predict his most probable behavior under that condition.

With a typical subject design, the behavior of the mean or median group member under an experimental condition can be used to predict the most probable behavior of the mean or median member of such a group under such a condition. It also can be used to predict the response to an experimental condition of the mean or median member of a population from which a group was selected, if it was randomly selected from that population. A population consists of all individuals who are classified in a particular manner. Thus, the population referred to by the question, "Are adults who have anomia helped by a particular therapy?" consists of all adults who have anomia. If a group were not randomly selected from a population, this type of generalization would be questionable. (The rationale and methodology for random sampling are described in Chapter 8.)

A fifth difference between individual subject and typical subject designs is related to the control of order and sequence effects. An *order effect* is one that systematically improves or impairs a subject's performance on a series of tasks. An example of an order effect that could impair performance would be fatigue. If an aphasic were to perform a series of ten tasks one after the other, his performance might systematically worsen as a function of fatigue.

This could occur regardless of the ordering of the tasks. An example of an order effect that could enhance a subject's performance on a series of tasks would be learning. A client may score higher on a test following a period of therapy than he did on the same test prior to therapy not because he improved, but because of what he learned during his first exposure to the test.

A *sequence effect* occurs when a subject's performance on a task is enhanced or impaired by his or her doing another task before it. An investigator who sought to determine the effect of a drug on stuttering, would have to obtain samples of stutterers' speech both while they were and while they were not under the influence of the drug. If both speech samples were elicited during the same day, it might make a difference whether the "drug" or "no-drug" speech sample was elicited first. If the "drug" speech sample was made first and if the effects of the drug had not worn off completely before the "no-drug" sample was made, this could result in a different stuttering frequency during the "no-drug" condition than probably would have occurred if it had come first. For a sequence effect, then, the ordering of tasks, or experimental conditions, is critical. One ordering may result in sequence effect contamination, while a second ordering may not.

Both order and sequence effects are easier to eliminate in a typical subject design than in an individual subject design. In a typical subject design, they can be controlled by administering only one experimental condition to each subject. An investigator who wished to determine the effect of a drug on stuttering could take a group of stutterers and randomly assign them to one of two conditions—i.e., speaking without being under the influence of the drug and speaking while under the influence of the drug. Since each subject would only speak under one condition, there would be no possibility of order or sequence effect contamination.

Order and sequence effect contamination is always a possibility with an individual subject design, since subjects are run under more than one condition and often more than once under each condition. These effects can sometimes be prevented by having fairly long intervals between treatments. An investigator who wished to determine the effect of a drug on stuttering with an individual subject design could separate drug and no-drug speech samples by 24 hours. This would prevent a sequence effect if the effects of the drug wore off in less than 24 hours. Some order effects, such as fatigue, could probably be eliminated with this same strategy.

A sixth way that individual subject and typical subject designs differ is related to statistical procedures for assessing the reliability of research findings. These are less well developed for individual subject than for typical subject designs.

A seventh way that individual subject and typical subject designs differ is in the minimum number of subjects necessary. With an individual subject design, research can be done with a single subject (N of 1). Therapy outcome research, for example, can be done with an N of 1 (though a larger N usually would be desirable). "Pure" research also is sometimes possible with an N as small as 1. In some of the research on teaching "language" to chimpanzees, only a single chimpanzee was used.

The minimum number of subjects necessary when a typical subject design is used almost always exceeds that necessary for an individual subject design. Studies that use a typical subject design usually require an N of greater than 10. The minimum N necessary for a particular study is a function of several factors, including how reliable answers to questions have to be. The more reliable they have to be, the larger the N required. An investigator who wished to determine whether a particular therapy resulted in a particular behavioral change would need a larger N if he wished to be 99 percent certain of the accuracy of the conclusion than if it were adequate to be 95 percent certain. (Factors that should be considered when estimating the N necessary for a particular study are discussed in Chapter 8.)

The eighth, and final, difference between individual subject and typical subject designs to be considered here is the basis on which generalizations are made to the population from which subjects are selected. A typical subject design usually employs a statistical basis, and an individual subject design usually employs a "logical" basis.

In a typical subject design, if the sample of subjects selected approximates a random sample from the population to which one wishes to generalize, then one could generalize to the population through the use of *inferential statistical procedures*. (These are discussed in Chapter 8.) These procedures permit us to infer characteristics of a population from characteristics of a sample (or samples) from that population. If the population of interest were speech pathologists who hold the Certificate of Clinical Competence in Speech Pathology from the American Speech and Hearing Association, and the sample consisted of a group of speech pathologists randomly selected from this population (from the American Speech and Hearing Association Membership Directory), the attitudes of speech pathologists in the population could probably be inferred reliably from those in the sample through the use of inferential statistics.

In an individual subject design, generalizations to the population from which subjects are selected usually are made on a "logical" rather than statistical basis. While a single subject from a population cannot be assumed to respond similarly to the majority of persons in the population to an experimental condition, it is unlikely that he or she would be the only person in the population who would respond in this way to the condition. Thus, the behavior of this single subject would represent that of a segment of the population. The size of this segment, however, could not be specified. All that could be concluded is that, based on laws of probability, the subject is more likely to represent a relatively large segment of the population than a relatively small one.

ADVANTAGES AND DISADVANTAGES OF EACH DESIGN

Advantages and disadvantages of individual subject and typical subject designs will be summarized in this section. Much of this discussion is based upon material in Table 5.1.

Individual Subject Design

Advantages. The individual subject design has several advantages. First, this design makes it possible to detect individual differences. It does not require an investigator implicitly or explicitly to assume that all persons in a population respond similarly to particular experimental conditions. In fact, it offers a means of testing this assumption. If subjects respond differently to an experimental condition and their responses are adequately reliable, this is evidence that the assumption that all persons in a population respond similarly to an experimental condition is not viable. This characteristic of individual subject designs is of particular importance in therapy outcome research, since most clinicians are usually not willing to assume *a priori* that particular therapies affect all clients with similar communicative disorders in the same manner.

A second advantage of the individual subject design is that it permits generalization to real persons in a population rather than an abstraction—i.e., the "typical" member of a population—who might not exist. A speech pathologist may never encounter an aphasic who responds to a particular stimulus as does the "typical" aphasic. This is because of the problem with mean data discussed previously.

A third advantage of the individual subject design is that it does not require a large N. The N needed, in fact, can be as few as 1.

Disadvantages. Several characteristics of the individual subject design may be disadvantageous under certain circumstances. The first, and perhaps most important, is that the design may be difficult to control for order and sequence effects. The possibility of such effects should be considered when you are planning a study in which an individual subject design may be used. If they seem possible and it seems unlikely they can be controlled (e.g., by spacing experimental conditions), you should probably not use an individual subject design.

A second possible disadvantage is that statistical procedures may not be available for assessing the reliability of answers. These are available for a wider variety of typical subject designs than individual subject designs. Before deciding to use an individual subject design, you would probably be wise to determine whether an appropriate statistical procedure is available for assessing the reliability of answers, assuming you feel it necessary to assess the reliability of answers. In some types of research (e.g., operant conditioning research), this is rarely done.

A third possible disadvantage is that generalizing to a population may not be "neat" if appropriate statistical procedures are unavailable.

Typical Subject Design

Advantages. The main advantages of typical subject designs are that statistical procedures usually are available both for assessing the reliability of answers and for generalizing to the population from which subjects are selected. Also, such designs usually make it possible to control for order and sequence effects and, through randomization, for the effects of extraneous variables. In addition, it is often possible to infer from these data characteristics of the "typical" member of a population or characteristics of the majority of members of a population (statistical procedures for doing both are described in Chapter 8).

Disadvantages. A typical subject design *may* be disadvantageous for several reasons. First, it usually requires an investigator implicitly or explicitly to assume that all members of a population respond similarly to an experimental condition. Observed differences in response would be regarded as a function of extraneous variables, random fluctuation, measurement error, and so on, rather than differences in response to the condition. Without this assumption, it usually would not make sense to average together the responses of individual subjects. The qualifier *usually* was used here because a few typical subject designs, such as analysis of variance, may not require this assumption.

A second possible disadvantage of a typical subject design is that it may require more subjects from a particular population to answer a particular question than are available. A speech pathologist who wished to determine the impact of a particular therapy on elementary-school stutterers and had only six such children in his or her caseload would probably have too small an N to use a typical subject design. This N would probably be adequate, however, for an individual subject design.

A third possible disadvantage of typical subject designs is that the characteristics of a "typical" subject may not be typical. Mean measures of the characteristics of the subjects in a sample may not be similar to those of most, if not all, subjects in that sample. Suppose we wished to evaluate the effects of an articulation therapy on the speech of ten children who had multiple articulation errors. As a criterion measure, we might use the number of errors each child made on an articulation test before and after receiving the therapy. Suppose the numbers of articulation errors produced by these children before and after therapy were as follows:

Subject Number	Number of Errors before Therapy	Number of Errors after Therapy
1	3	3
2	11	4
3	4	4
4	1	1
5	3	3
6	9	6
7	2	2
8	2	2
9	4	4
10	1	1
Mean	4	3

It would be reasonable to conclude from these means that the typical child in this group had fewer articulation errors following therapy than before therapy. Actually, the therapy only appeared to influence the articulation of two of the ten children and the magnitude of the effect for these children was considerably more than one error. Thus, the mean performance of the children in this group is not representative of the "typical" performance of these children.

A fourth possible disadvantage of the typical subject design pertains to generalizing to the population from which subjects are selected on statistical grounds. If a sample of subjects who were observed did not at least closely approximate a random sample from the population of interest, generalizations to this population on the basis of statistical inference would be of uncertain validity and possibly misleading. If, for example, the children in a kindergarten classroom did not approximate a random sample of kindergarten children in general, attempts to generalize the results of a speech improvement program conducted in this classroom to the population of kindergarten children through the use of statistical inference would be of uncertain validity and possibly misleading. The children in a particular classroom may not approximate a random sample because the suburbs or the inner city are underrepresented. A speech improvement program which is effective in the suburbs may not be in the inner city, and vice versa.

VARIATIONS POSSIBLE WITHIN EACH CATEGORY OF DESIGN

Thus far two basic types of designs have been described, differences between them pointed out, and advantages and disadvantages of each summarized. Some of the variations possible within each category of design will be described in this section.

Individual Subject Design

Individual subject designs can vary considerably in complexity. The simplest such design would require a single measure to be made twice—once preceding a treatment and once following it. This design could be diagrammed as follows:

$$X \ O \ X$$

where O indicates a treatment and X indicates a measure. The application of this design that would probably be encountered most frequently by speech pathologists and audiologists is assessment of the effects of therapies. An attribute of a client's communicative behavior would be measured both before and after his receiving a therapy, and the two measures would be compared. If a change occurred, and if it was in the direction of improvement, we might conclude that the improvement resulted from the therapy. Unfortunately, research that utilizes this design is difficult to interpret, since it contains no way of assessing reliability or controlling for the effects of extraneous variables. (For an in-depth discussion of the limitations of "before and after" designs, see Campbell and Stanley, 1966.)

The level of reliability of the "before and after" design can be increased by using the means of several measures as criterion measures. The design diagrammed here could be used to generate such criterion measures:

$$X \ X \ X \ X \ X \ O \ X \ X \ X \ X \ X$$

Each subject's behavior would be measured ten times—five times preceding the treatment and five times following it. The "before" criterion measure would be the mean (or median) of the five measures that were made prior to the treatment being administered, and the "after" criterion measure would be the mean of the five measures made following the treatment. The mean of several measures almost always would be more reliable than a single measure. Suppose the behavior you wished to measure was frequency of stuttering. Since stuttering frequency tends to vary considerably on a situational basis, you probably could obtain a more reliable estimate of a stutterer's pre- and post-therapy stuttering frequencies by using as a criterion measure the mean (or median) of several measures rather than a single measure.

Another approach to increasing the level of reliability of "before and after" individual subject designs (and other types of individual subject designs as well) involves measuring, or describing, a behavior of interest in more than one way. Rather than making a single measure of a behavior at specified points in time, you would make more than one measure at each point in time. A representative design of this type would be:

$$X_1 \quad X_1 \quad X_1 \quad X_1 \quad X_1 \quad X_1$$
$$O$$
$$X_2 \quad X_2 \quad X_2 \quad X_2 \quad X_2 \quad X_2$$

Each of the two measures (X_1 and X_2) would be made three times before a treatment is administered and three times following its administration. Again, suppose that the behavior you wish to measure is stuttering. X_1 might be the percent of words stuttered and X_2 might be a physiological measure of anxiety level (e.g., GSR). Both measures would be made three times before a treatment is administered and three times following its administration. Here the assumption is made that X_1 and X_2 are both valid measures of the behavior of interest. The mean pre-therapy measures and mean post-therapy measures would then be compared to determine whether the treatment had any effect on stuttering. If both measures indicated change in the same direction (e.g., reduced stuttering frequency and reduced anxiety level), this would be more convincing evidence of the effectiveness of a treatment than change in a single measure if only a single measure were made. On the other hand, if one measure indicated change in a certain direction and the other indicated either no change or change in the opposite direction, the reliability of the data would be uncertain and any conclusions based on the data concerning the effect of the treatment on stuttering would be equivocal.

Another approach that sometimes can be used to increase the reliability of data from individual subject designs is to replicate the treatment, or experimental condition. The experimental condition, or treatment, could be administered more than once to determine whether it had a consistent effect on a behavior of interest. A representative design of this type would be:

$$X \quad X \quad X \quad O \quad X \quad X \quad X \quad O \quad X \quad X \quad X \quad O \quad X \quad X \quad X$$

The criterion measure would be made twelve times at specified intervals. Between the third and fourth, sixth and seventh, and ninth and tenth measures an experimental condition, or treatment, would be administered. If the treatment changed the behavior being measured, the fourth, seventh, and tenth measures would be related in a consistent manner to the third, sixth, and ninth measures. They would either be higher than those preceding or lower. This type of design could be used to demonstrate the effect of speaking in the presence of masking noise on a stutterer's anxiety level. His skin resistance (GSR) could be measured twelve times at five-minute intervals. He could read a different randomly selected passage between each measure. The readings between the third and fourth, sixth and seventh, and ninth and tenth measures would be in the presence of masking noise. It would then be determined whether the fourth, seventh, and tenth measures differed systematically from the preceding ones (i.e., were either higher or lower).

A variation of this "replication" design involves administering the treatment at *randomly selected* rather than fixed intervals. Following a decision regarding the number of times a treatment would be administered to a subject, the temporal points at which the treatment would be administered would be selected by a table of random numbers. This design could be substituted for the one used in the previous example. That is, the three intervals between measures during which the subject would read in the presence of masking noise could be randomly selected. This could be done by numbering the eleven possible intervals (i.e., 1-2, 2-3, 3-4, 4-5, 5-6, 6-7, 7-8, 8-9, 9-10, 10-11, and 11-12) from one to eleven consecutively and selecting three intervals by means of a table of random numbers (see Appendix B). Some persons would regard a demonstration of a phenomenon as more convincing if the "random" approach were used—i.e., if following a treatment, regardless of when it was administered, a predictable change in a measure occurred.

One other strategy that has been used in communicative disorders research to increase the reliability of the individual subject design is to measure two behaviors at given points in time—one that the treatment should modify and one that the treatment would not be expected to modify. If the treatment modified the one and not the other, this would be interpreted as evidence of its effectiveness. This strategy has been used to evaluate the effectiveness of articulation therapies (Elbert, Shelton, and Arndt, 1967). The behavior measured here that the treatment might be expected to modify would be the articulation error being treated. The behavior measured that would not be expected to be modified by the treatment would be a dissimilar "control" error for which the subject has received no therapy. Thus, if a clinician were administering a therapy to a child to achieve correct production of /s/ and the child were receiving no therapy for his defective /r/ production, the clinician could estimate periodically the percent of time /r/ and /s/ were produced correctly. If /s/ were produced correctly a higher percentage of the time following therapy than before, and /r/ were produced correctly approximately the same percentage of the time following therapy as before, this would be interpreted as evidence of the effectiveness of the therapy. Note that this design differs from multiple measure designs discussed previously in that the measures made are of behaviors that are *assumed* to be different rather than of the same behavior.

The individual subject designs described here have been illustrated with quantitative rather than qualitative data. These designs can also be used with observational procedures that result in qualitative data. The "before and after" design,

$$X \ O \ X$$

could be used to assess qualitatively how a person had been influenced by a treatment (such as a therapy). Relevant aspects of behavior could be described (written down) both before and after the treatment was administered. To assess the impact of the treatment, these descriptions could be compared. Estimates of behavioral change based on qualitative data tend to be no more or no less reliable and valid than those based on quantitative data. Some behavioral phenomena can be more reliably and validly described in words than in numbers, or in a combination of words and numbers than in words or numbers alone. A person's language behavior at a given point in time usually can be described more reliably and validly in a combination of words and numbers than in either alone. Speech pathologists and audiologists tend to use both types of data when describing a client's communicative behavior.

The variations of the individual subject design discussed in this section should be regarded as representative rather than exhaustive. Several sources that describe other variations and further discuss the variations presented here are included in the reference list (Campbell, 1963; Campbell and Stanley, 1966; Dukes, 1965; Gottman, 1973; Holtzman, 1963; Jerger, 1964; Sidman, 1960).

Typical Subject Designs

Hundreds of designs have been devised that can be classified as typical subject, or group, designs. Many of those that are useful in behavioral research are included in books by Guilford (1954), Hays (1963), Keppel (1973), Lindquist (1953), and Winer (1962).

Two general categories of typical subject designs can be identified: (1) those intended to determine whether a *difference* exists, and (2) those intended to determine whether a *relationship* exists. The designs in these categories permit different kinds of questions to be answered. Those in the first category permit the answering of such questions as:

1. Is vocal rest effective in reducing the size of vocal nodules?
2. Does hearing aid A tend to result in better speech discrimination ability for persons with conductive losses than hearing aid B?

Designs in the second category, on the other hand, permit the answering of such questions as:

3. Is auditory discrimination ability positively related to articulation proficiency?
4. Are scores on audiometric test A negatively related to scores on audiometric test B?

The first of these questions can be answered by determining whether there is a *difference* in the average (mean or median) size of the vocal nodules of a group of persons following vocal rest. The second can be answered by determining whether there is a *difference* in the average (mean or median) speech discrimination scores of a group of persons who have conductive hearing losses when hearing aid A and hearing aid B are used. The third can be answered by determining whether there is a *positive relationship* between scores on auditory discrimination tests and scores on tests of articulation proficiency—that is, it would be necessary to determine whether persons who earn high scores on one tend to earn high scores on the other, and whether those who earn low scores on one tend to earn low scores on the other. Finally, the fourth question can be answered by determining whether persons who earn *high* scores on audiometric test A tend to earn *low* scores on audiometric test B, and vice versa.

Designs for Detecting Differences. To answer some questions, it is necessary to determine whether one or more differences exist. These differences can be of several kinds. They can, for example, be differences between percentages (or proportions), as in these questions:

1. Are stutterers more likely to have articulation errors than nonstutterers?
2. Do more children who have hearing losses fail audiometric screening test A than audiometric screening test B?

The first question can be answered by determining whether a higher percentage (or proportion) of stutterers than nonstutterers have articulation errors; the second, by determining whether the same percentage (or proportion) of children who have hearing losses fail audiometric test A as audiometric test B.

Other kinds of differences that can be detected by a typical subject design are those between means, or medians, as in these questions:

1. Do kindergarten children tend to have fewer articulation errors after participating in a particular speech improvement program than before?
2. Does the level of academic achievement of elementary-school stutterers tend to differ from that of their nonstuttering peers?

The first question can be answered by comparing the mean (or median) number of articulation errors of a group of kindergarten children after participating in the program to that before participating in the program; the second, by comparing the mean (or median) academic achievement scores of a group of elementary-school stutterers with that of a matched group of nonstutterers. Note that the first requires a comparison between two measures on the *same* subjects and the second requires a comparison between single measures made on *different* subjects.

The questions that illustrated typical subject designs for detecting differences involved comparisons between two measures. Such designs also can be used to compare more than two measures. Suppose we wished to determine whether there was any difference in the percentage of children in kindergarten through sixth grade who had chronic hoarseness. A typical subject design could be used for comparing these seven percentages. Similarly, such a design could be used to compare mean auditory discrimination scores earned by a group of persons who have conductive hearing losses while using five different hearing aid models.

Typical subject designs for detecting differences differ in several dimensions, including: (1) the type of measure for which they are appropriate, (2) the number of measures that can be compared, and (3) their appropriateness for dependent measures, independent measures, or a combination of the two. The type of measure for which a design is appropriate refers to the nature of the criterion measure—whether it is a percentage, a proportion, a frequency count, a mean, a median, a mode, or some other derived measure. A design appropriate for detecting differences between percentages may not be appropriate for detecting differences between means. (Typical subject designs appropriate for detecting differences between various types of criterion measures are described in Chapter 8.)

A second dimension in which typical subject designs for detecting differences differ is the number of measures that can be compared. Some such designs only are appropriate for comparing two measures and others, more than two measures. (Typical subject designs appropriate for various numbers of measures are described in Chapter 8.)

A third dimension in which these designs differ is their appropriateness for dependent measures, independent measures, and combinations of the two. Dependent measures are measures made on the same subjects or on matched groups of subjects. Independent measures are measures made on unmatched groups of subjects. "Before and after" therapy measures would be examples of dependent measures, since they are made on the same persons. Measures made on unmatched groups such as stutterers and nonstutterers would be examples of independent measures.

Some designs only are appropriate for dependent measures or independent measures, and others are appropriate for combinations of the two. A design appropriate for dependent measures would be necessary to answer this question: "Do dysarthrics who have been fitted with palatal lift prostheses tend to be more intelligible with the device than without?" Such a design would be needed because two measures on the same subjects would have to be compared—one with the prostheses and one without it.

Answering other questions requires a design appropriate for independent measures. Consider the question, "Do dysarthrics who have been fitted with palatal lift prostheses tend to be more intelligible than those who have had pharyngeal flap surgery?" A design appropriate for comparing independent measures would be needed here because two groups are being compared, one consisting of dysarthrics who have been treated surgically and the other consisting of dysarthrics who have been fitted with a prosthesis.

To answer some questions, a design appropriate for both dependent and independent measures is necessary. For example, consider the question, "Do palatal lift prostheses tend to increase the intelligibility of the speech of dysarthrics who have inadequate velo-pharyngeal closure more than pharyngeal flaps?" One design appropriate for answering this question, known as the Type I analysis of variance design (Lindquist, 1953), can be diagrammed as follows:

| | DEPENDENT MEASURES ||
	Before Management	After Management
Palatal Lift Group		
Pharyngeal Flap Group		

INDEPENDENT MEASURES

If this design were used, measures of the intelligibility of the speech of two groups of dysarthrics would be made before and after physical management. Between-group comparisons would involve independent measures, and "before and after" treatment comparisons would involve dependent measures.

Designs for Detecting Relationships. Answering some questions requires a design for detecting relationships rather than differences. There are several kinds of questions about relationships that such designs can help to answer if relationships are found to exist, including those related to: (1) the *direction* of the relationships, (positive or negative), (2) the *strength* of the relationships, and (3) the *nature* of the relationships, (linear or nonlinear). Suppose you wished to describe the relationship between children's speech disfluency levels in two situations—that is, you wished to determine whether those who tended to be the most disfluent in one situation also tended to be the most disfluent in the other, and vice versa. You might sample the speech of ten children in the two situations and determine the frequency of speech disfluency per 100 words spoken by each child in each situation. Suppose the disfluency frequencies you obtained were as follows:

Child	Situation I	Situation II
1	6.3	10.1
2	5.6	9.4
3	4.5	10.1
4	9.0	22.5
5	4.5	8.7
6	3.9	6.1
7	6.8	17.5
8	5.5	10.4
9	12.5	35.4
10	3.4	5.6

To permit the relationship between the disfluency frequencies in the two situations to be visualized, they were plotted on a two-dimensional graphical display known as a *scattergram* (see Figure 5.1). The configuration of this scattergram provides data for answering the following four questions (assuming the answer to the first is "yes"):

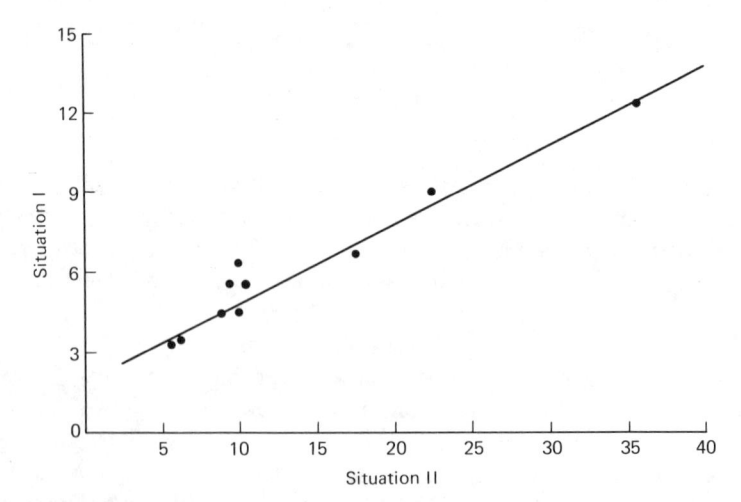

FIGURE 5.1. Scattergram depicting a relatively strong positive relationship between two variables.

Selecting the Appropriate Design for Answering Specific Questions 83

1. Does a relationship exist between these children's disfluency frequencies in the two situations?
2. What is the *direction* of the relationship between the disfluency frequencies in the two situations?
3. Does the relationship appear to be *linear* or *nonlinear*? If nonlinear, what does the *nature* of the relationship appear to be?
4. How *strong* does the relationship between the disfluency frequencies in the two situations appear to be?

What would be the answer to each question based on the configuration of the scattergram in Figure 5.1? The answer to the first question would be "yes", since the points are not randomly distributed on the scattergram but are confined to a relatively small segment of it. The configuration of Figure 5.2, incidently, illustrates what a scattergram might look like if little or no

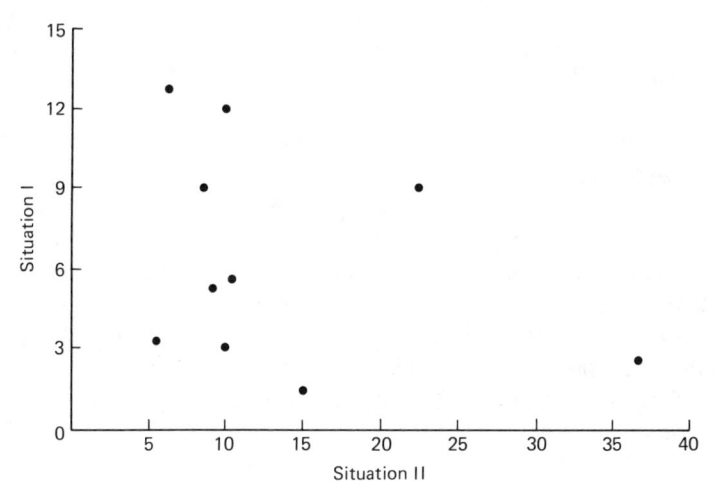

FIGURE 5.2. Scattergram depicting little or no relationship between two variables.

relationship existed between the variables. The points are not confined to a segment of the graph, they are scattered throughout the graph. A child who had a relatively high disfluency frequency in one situation would be about as likely to have a relatively high as a relatively low frequency in the other.

From the configuration of the points in Figure 5.1, it would appear that the *direction* of the relationship between the children's disfluency frequencies in the two situations is "positive." The ordering of the children with regard to disfluency frequencies is quite similar in the two situations. Children who had relatively high disfluency frequencies in one tended to have relatively high disfluency frequencies in the other, and vice versa. If the direction of the

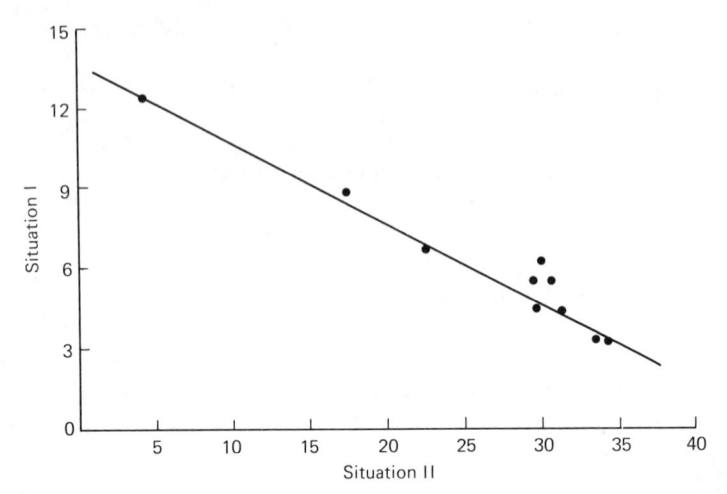

FIGURE 5.3. *Scattergram depicting a relatively strong negative relationship between two variables.*

relationship had been "negative," the configuration of the points might have been similar to that in Figure 5.3.

To answer the third question, it would seem reasonable to assume from the configuration of the points in Figure 5.1 that the relationship between the disfluency frequencies in the two situations for these children is *linear*. The line that could be drawn on the scattergram from which the points would deviate least and which could be the least complex would be a straight line. When two variables are linearly related, an increase (or decrease) in the magnitude of one is associated with a *proportional* increase (or decrease) in the magnitude of the other. This proportional increase (or decrease) will occur throughout the range of possible values. If two variables are *not linearly related*, on the other hand, an increase (or decrease) in the magnitude of one will not be associated with a proportional increase (or decrease) in the magnitude of the other throughout the range of possible values. Two common nonlinear relationships between variables are depicted in Figures 5.4 and 5.5. The relationship depicted in Figure 5.4, which is *curvilinear*, is the least complex of the possible nonlinear relationships between variables. That depicted in Figure 5.5, which is *cubic*, is one step up in complexity from curvilinear.

To answer the fourth question, it would appear from the configuration of points in Figure 5.1 that the relationship between the relative disfluency frequencies in the two situations for these children is *fairly strong*. The points are not scattered very much; they deviate little from the straight line which best describes the relationship between them. The greater the deviation of the points in a scattergram from the line which best describes the nature of the relationship between two variables, the weaker the relationship between

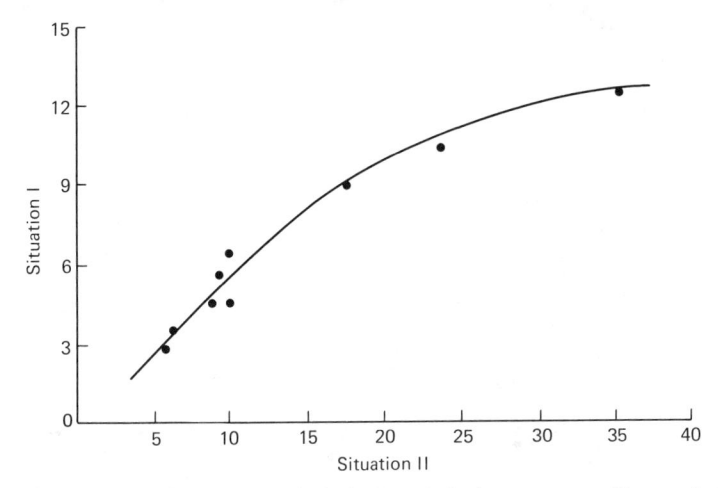

FIGURE 5.4. Scattergram depicting a relatively strong curvilinear relationship between two variables.

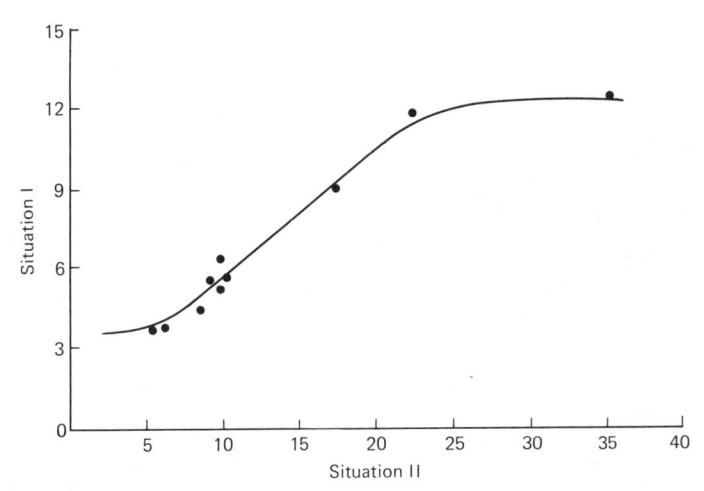

FIGURE 5.5. Scattergram depicting a relatively strong cubic relationship between two variables.

them. The scattergrams in Figure 5.6 illustrate two degrees of linear relationship. The relationship depicted in the scattergram on the top is stronger than that depicted in the scattergram on the bottom.

The discussion thus far has been limited to detecting and describing relationships between two variables. There are typical subject designs for detecting and describing more complex relationships—that is, those involving more than two variables. Such designs could be used for answering such questions as:

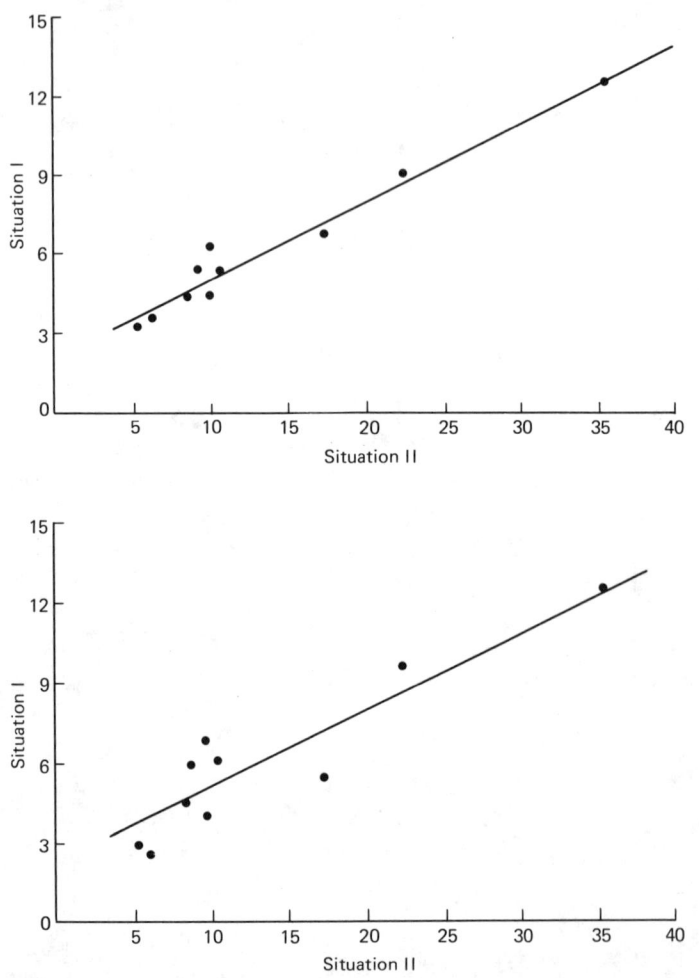

FIGURE 5.6. *Scattergrams depicting two degrees of linear relationship. The relationship depicted in the scattergram on the top is stronger than that depicted in the one on the bottom.*

1. How well do clinicians agree on how severe stutterers are?
2. What factors influence how severe a stutterer is perceived as being?
3. What factors best differentiate the speech of a child beginning to stutter from that of his peers?

The first question could be answered by determining the extent to which a sample of clinicians would order a group of stutterers in the same manner in the severity of their stuttering. The second could be answered by identifying factors that are related to judgments of stuttering severity. And the third could be answered by identifying factors that are more likely to be related to the speaking behavior of children known to be beginning to stutter than to the speaking behavior of peers who have no history of a stuttering problem. Statistical procedures that could be used to answer these questions (the Kendall coefficient of concordance, multiple regression and correlation, and discriminant function analysis for questions one through three respectively) are discussed in Chapter 8.

WHICH TYPE OF DESIGN SHOULD YOU USE?

It should be fairly apparent from the discussion in this chapter that usually a number of factors must be considered when you decide whether to use an individual subject or typical subject design to answer a question. For some questions, however, only one of these two types would be appropriate because of a single consideration. Such questions include those

1. that state unequivocally whether they refer to individuals or to typical members of groups,
2. for which all treatments could not be administered to individual subjects, and
3. for which an insufficient N would be available for a typical subject design.

For questions where the choice is not clear-cut, you must weigh the advantages and disadvantages of each design and select the one that seems most likely to yield data of adequate validity, reliability, and generality to answer the question. If neither design seems likely to yield data of adequate validity, reliability, and generality to answer a question (or questions), it might be wise to search for some other question (or questions) for which the prospects of collecting such data seem better.

REFERENCES

BLOOM, C. M., and SILVERMAN, F. H., Do all stutterers adapt? *Journal of Speech and Hearing Research*, 16, 518–521 (1973).

CAMPBELL, D. T., From description to experimentation: Interpreting trends as quasi-experiments. In C. W. HARRIS (Ed.), *Problems in Measuring Change*, Madison: University of Wisconsin Press, 212–242 (1963).

CAMPBELL, D. T., and STANLEY, J. C., *Experimental and Quasi-Experimental Designs for Research*. Chicago: Rand McNally (1966).

DUKES, W. F., $N = 1$. *Psychological Bulletin*, 64, 74–79 (1965).

ELBERT, M., SHELTON, R. L., and ARNDT, W. B., A task for evaluation of articulation change: I. Development of methodology. *Journal of Speech and Hearing Research*, 10, 281–288 (1967).

GOTTMAN, J. M., N-of-one and N-of-two research in psychotherapy. *Psychological Bulletin*, 80, 93–105 (1973).

GUILFORD, J. P., *Psychometric Methods*. New York: McGraw-Hill Book Company (1954).

HAYS, W. L., *Statistics for Psychologists*. New York: Holt, Rinehart and Winston (1963).

HOLTZMAN, W. H., Statistical models for the study of change in the single case. In C. W. HARRIS (Ed.), *Problems in Measuring Change*, Madison: University of Wisconsin Press, 199–211 (1963).

JERGER, J., Subject-orientated research. *Journal of Speech and Hearing Research*, 7, 207–208 (1964).

KEPPEL, G., *Design and Analysis: A Researcher's Handbook*. Englewood Cliffs, N.J.: Prentice-Hall, Inc. (1973).

LINDQUIST, E. F., *Design and Analysis of Experiments in Psychology and Education*. Boston: Houghton Mifflin Company (1953).

SIDMAN, M., *Tactics of Scientific Research*. New York: Basic Books (1960).

SILVERMAN, F. H., The Porch Index of Communicative Ability (PICA): A psychometric problem and its solution. *Journal of Speech and Hearing Disorders*, 39, 225–226 (1974).

WINER, B. J., *Statistical Principles in Experimental Design*. New York: McGraw-Hill Book Company (1962).

SIX

TYPES OF DATA

This chapter will deal with the observations, or data, that serve as the raw material for answering questions. Such observations can be viewed as raw material because they have to be organized in some manner before they can be used for answering questions. (This topic is discussed in Chapter 8.)

WHAT ARE DATA?

Data can be viewed as an abstraction from the observational process. When you observe an event, you do not attend to, or abstract, all aspects of it. You simply attend to a small number (in some cases only one) that are relevant for answering a particular question. If, for example, you wished to determine whether a child had articulation errors, you could administer an articulation test. Most such tests require the child to say a number of words in which the phonemes of the language occur in various positions. The child's production of each word constitutes an event. This event would have a number of attributes, including accuracy of production of each phoneme, voice quality, pitch level, intensity, etc. During the child's production of each word, you would probably only attend to the phoneme (or possibly two phonemes) the word was included in the test to sample. This illustrates what is meant, therefore, by abstracting only those aspects of an event that are relevant for answering a question, which in this case would be: Is the phoneme (or are the phonemes) which the word was intended to sample produced correctly in the position in which it occurs in the word? The information abstracted about the accuracy of production of the phoneme that could be communicated would constitute *data*.

There may be more than one aspect of an event which, if abstracted, could serve as data for answering a particular question. The accuracy of production of a phoneme in a word, for example, could be described in several ways. First, it could be described on the basis of how it sounds to an observer (or observers). Second, it could be described on the basis of how accurate the postures of the articulators look during production of the phoneme through the use of cinefluorography (i.e., X-ray motion pictures). Third, it could be described on the basis of action potentials recorded from the speech musculature during production of the phoneme by means of electromyography. Finally, it might be described on the basis of oral and nasal pressure and flow measurements made during production of the phoneme through the use of appropriate transducers and electronic amplifiers and recording devices. (The use of instrumentation for observing aspects of events is discussed in Chapter 7.)

Strictly speaking, data are symbolic representations of attributes of events. They are not what is abstracted from events, but abstractions of what is abstracted from events. As the general semanticists have pointed out (e.g., Johnson, 1946), you cannot express in words or numbers everything you observe. If, for example, the event you were observing was a child telling a story about a picture and the attribute you were attending to was phonological development, the data resulting would be your description of what you observed—in words, or numbers, or both. It would not be what you observed per se.

What relationship should exist, then, between the symbolic representation of what is observed (data) and what is observed? The answer is that the two should be similar in structure. By this we mean that the relationship between data and what is observed should be analogous to that between a *map* and the *territory* it represents. If a map that included Illinois and Wisconsin were similar in structure to the territory represented, Chicago, Illinois would be north of Champaign, Illinois and Milwaukee, Wisconsin would be north of both Champaign and Chicago. If the map indicated that Milwaukee was south of Chicago, the structure of the map would not be similar to that of the territory. (For further discussion of the map-territory analogy see Johnson, 1946, pp. 131–133.)

The relationship between map and territory, or between what is observed and its symbolic representation, can be further illustrated by means of the relationship between a pure-tone audiogram and what it depicts. A pure-tone audiogram can be regarded as a *partial* symbolic representation of one aspect of hearing, i.e., threshold for pure tones. It is a partial representation because thresholds are not plotted for all frequencies in the audio range. If the configuration of the audiogram is similar in structure to the territory it is supposed to depict—i.e., a person's thresholds for pure tones at selected frequencies—it will accurately indicate the person's thresholds at the frequencies tested. The ordering of these frequencies for threshold would correspond to the person's relative ability to detect the presence of pure tones at the frequencies tested. Not only would the ordering of frequencies for threshold correspond to that in the territory, but the relative degrees of hearing loss at the frequencies tested would also. If a pure tone of one frequency, to be detected, had to be made 10 dB louder than a pure tone of a second frequency, this would be indicated by the configuration of the audiogram.

A second illustration of the map-territory relationship that is relevant to communicative disorders is the relationship between articulation test results and articulation errors. For articulation test results to be similar in structure to the territory they are supposed to depict—i.e., the articulation errors of the person tested—they have to indicate the speech sounds that are produced incorrectly and how they are produced incorrectly (i.e., omitted, distorted, or substituted for).

The extent to which a data map is similar in structure to the territory it represents determines its validity. The greater the structural similarity, the more valid the data. A description of something is valid if it accurately describes that which it is intended to describe. Aphasia test results are valid to the extent that they accurately describe an aphasic's language deficits. A description of a therapy session would be valid to the extent that it accurately portrayed what occurred during the session. Assessing the validity of data, therefore, involves estimating the degree of structural correspondence between map and territory—between the description of an event and the event itself.

Speech pathologists and audiologists use many types of data for answering questions. The following data, for example, were reported in a single issue of the *Journal of Speech and Hearing Disorders:*

1. transcriptions of samples of stuttered speech,
2. linguistic analyses of normal speech disfluencies,
3. children's scores on the Environmental Language Inventory,
4. anecdotal reports of parents functioning as language trainers,
5. numbers of syllables spoken per minute,
6. judgments of "normalcy" of speech,
7. stutterers' self-ratings of reactions to speech situations,

8. personality test scores,
9. frequency of use of specific syntactic structures,
10. scores on the Elicited Language Inventory,
11. verbal descriptions of expressive language,
12. chronological ages,
13. scores on Porch Index of Communicative Ability,
14. pure-tone audiometric test results,
15. verbal descriptions of apraxics' use of American Indian Sign,
16. mean values of temporal integration in dB,
17. verbal descriptions of "cocktail party speech" accompanying myelomeningocele and shunted hydrocephalus,
18. auditory localization test scores,
19. verbal description of person with a contact granuloma of the vocal cords,
20. measures of respiratory function (e.g., tidal volume),
21. measures of speaking pitch level,
22. verbal descriptions of X-rays,
23. verbal descriptions of the communicative behavior of a young deaf child,
24. nasality scores, and
25. articulation error frequencies.

Actually, thousands of different kinds of verbal and numerical descriptions have been used by speech pathologists and audiologists to map territories of interest to them.

TYPES OF DATA

There are two basic types, or classes, of data—qualitative and quantitative. *Qualitative* data are *verbal* descriptions of attributes of events, and *quantitative* data are *numerical* descriptions of attributes of events. Both are used by speech pathologists and audiologists to answer questions.

Qualitative Data

Some attributes of events can be more adequately described through words than through numbers. Verbal descriptions of such attributes could be less abstract—that is, could include more information—than numerical ones. Suppose, for example, you wished to describe the response of an aphasic to an aphasia test item. A highly abstract description of such a response would be to assign it a 1 if it were appropriate and a 0 if it were inappropriate. A less abstract description would be to assign it a number that would indicate how close it was to being appropriate, e.g., a number from 0 to 16 as is done with the PICA scoring system (Porch, 1971). The level of abstraction could be reduced even more by describing the aphasic's behavior when the item was presented in as much detail as possible. (Excellent examples of such descriptions of aphasics' response to aphasia test items can be found in Head's classic work, *Aphasia and Kindred Disorders of Speech*, published in 1926.)

Verbal descriptions of attributes of events vary in the degree to which they are similar in structure to the territory they are intended to map. This topic has been dealt with in considerable depth by the general semanticists (e.g., Johnson, 1946). They have indicated how the use of language can cause some verbal maps to be more similar in structure to the territory being mapped than others. The following sets of statements illustrate several of the ways in which verbal descriptions of attributes of events can vary in the extent to which they are similar in structure to the territory they are intended to depict. The second statement in each set would probably be judged to be more similar in structure than the first.

1a. John said his first word when he was 10 months old.
1b. John's parents first remembered hearing him produce sounds which they interpreted as a meaningful word when he was 10 months old.
2a. John is a moderately severe stutterer.
2b. John's stuttering was judged moderately severe in the situation in which he was observed.
3a. John's study was rejected by the *Journal of Speech and Hearing Research* because it was poorly designed.
3b. An associate editor for the *Journal of Speech and Hearing Research* felt that John's study was poorly designed and rejected it.
4a. John is a good clinician.
4b. John behaves in a manner that is consistent with my internal standard regarding what constitutes a good clinician.
5a. Stutterers do not stutter when they are alone.
5b. Some stutterers report they do not stutter when they are alone.
6a. The articulation test results indicated that John had a relatively severe articulation problem.
6b. Based on the articulation test results, I felt that John had a relatively severe articulation problem.

Qualitative data (i.e., verbal descriptions of attributes of events) vary with regard to level of validity, reliability, and generality. The greater the structural similarity between the description of an attribute of an event and what occurred, the more valid the description. The "b" descriptions in the preceding paragraph, therefore, would probably be regarded as more valid than the "a" descriptions.

The level of reliability of qualitative data is a function of the interaction between the observer and the observed. Some persons tend to be more reliable observers than others. They are more likely to abstract relevant aspects of an event. They have fewer "filters" (i.e., biases) that would tend to distort their observations. They usually exert very little influence on what they observe. The latter trait is particularly important in determining reliability. It has been demonstrated that the act of observing an event can change it (e.g., Webb, Campbell, Schwartz, and Schrest, 1966). Placing a microphone in front of a client in an interview situation, for example, can influence his verbal behavior. Taking notes while he is speaking also can have this effect. Some persons are better able than others to avoid or minimize this type of influence.

The level of generality of qualitative data is a function of the representativeness of the sample of events observed. Samples selected by a random procedure (i.e., table of random numbers) that are relatively large usually are the most representative. They permit relatively accurate inferences to be made regarding the class of events of which they are representative. If you wished to determine the distribution of attitudes of A.S.H.A. certified speech pathologists and audiologists toward a piece of legislation before the Congress, you could select a random sample of such individuals from the most recent American Speech and Hearing Association *Directory* and ask each to complete a questionnaire. Assuming your sample was adequately large, the distribution of attitudes in the sample would probably correspond closely to that in the population (i.e., the total group of A.S.H.A. certified speech pathologists and audiologists). The distribution of attitudes in the sample would serve, therefore, as a fairly accurate "map" of the distribution of attitudes in the population. The data in the sample thus would have some generality.

Is qualitative data inferior, or less scientific, than quantitative data? While there is no reason for regarding one form of data as intrinsically inferior or superior to the other, the answer to this question would depend on the territory being described. Verbal descriptions would be more similar in structure to some territories than numerical descriptions would be. For such territories, verbal descriptions would be superior to numerical ones. On the other hand, some territories can probably be described more precisely through numbers than through words. For such territories, qualitative data would be inferior to quantitative data. An investigator's choice would be expected to depend on which he feels provides the most accurate map for the territory.

Quantitative Data

Some attributes of events can be described and communicated more adequately through numbers than through words. This is particularly likely to be true for those attributes which involve quantities, or magnitudes. The following statements concern the frequency of occurrence of an articulation error:

1. During the session John produced /s/ correctly most of the time.
2. During the session John produced /s/ correctly 80 percent of the time.

The second would probably be regarded as more adequately describing John's production of /s/ during the session than the first, since the meaning of "80 percent" is less ambiguous than that of "most." Hence, the second would be a more adequate map of the territory than the first.

The defining characteristic of quantitative data is that they consist of number symbols, or numerals. Numerals function semantically in the same manner as words—i.e., they have *assigned* meanings. Meanings are assigned to both classes of symbols; they do not exist in nature. To identify the meanings that have been assigned to a given word, you can look it up in a dictionary. If it has more than one meaning, its meaning in a particular situation has to be inferred from context. Numerals function similarly in that each can be assigned several meanings; to determine their meaning in a given situation you have to know the context in which they are being used. The numerals 3, 6, and 9, for example, would have different meanings in the following five contexts:

1. They could be used to designate classes of communicative disorders with 3 being stuttering, 6 being hypernasality, and 9 being aphasia.
2. They could be used to designate positions in a rank ordering for hypernasality. The numeral 1, for example, could be used to designate the individual who was most hypernasal and 9 the one who was least hypernasal.
3. They could be used to designate points on an equal-appearing interval scale of articulation defectiveness.
4. They could be used to designate frequencies of occurrence of stuttering.
5. They could be used to designate degrees of hearing loss in *DB*.

The first context illustrates the *nominal* meaning of numerals, or number symbols. In this context they are used merely to designate, or label, categories. Letters of the alphabet, words, or other symbols could be substituted for them. The numerals on the backs of football players' jerseys would have this meaning.

The second context illustrates the *ordinal* meaning of numerals. In this context they are used to designate locations in a rank order. They indicate the amounts of an attribute given individuals possess relative to the amount possessed by the other individuals ranked.

The third context illustrates the *interval* meaning of numerals. In this context they designate points on a continuum which have equal amounts of the attribute being measured between them. If the numerals 3, 6, and 9 had interval meaning, the amount of increase in articulation defectiveness between a speech sample assigned the numeral 3 and one assigned the numeral 6, for example, would be equal in magnitude to the amount of increase in articulation defectiveness between a sample assigned the numeral 6 and one assigned the numeral 9. If these numerals had ordinal rather than interval meaning, the amount of increase in articulation defectiveness between them would not be assumed equal.

The fourth context illustrates the *ratio* meaning of numerals. In this context they designate points on a continuum which both have equal amounts of an attribute between them and are related to an *absolute* 0. Because of the presence of an absolute 0, the magnitudes between points, as well as those represented by the points themselves, have meaning. A speech sample assigned the numeral 6, for example, would contain articulation that is twice as defective as one assigned the numeral 3. And one assigned the numeral 3 only would be one-third as defective in articulation as one assigned the numeral 9. These relationships would not hold for numerals with ordinal or interval meanings, since such numerals are not related to an absolute 0.

The fifth context illustrates the logarithmic meaning of numerals. In this context numerals designate points on a continuum which have *unequal*, but known, mathematically defined amounts of an attribute between them. Such numerals differ from ordinals in that the amounts of an attribute between ordinal numerals are unknown and not mathematically defined. They are similar to interval numerals in the respect that interval widths are known and mathematically defined. However, rather than being equal in magnitude, they decline in magnitude—i.e., the larger the numerals, the smaller the interval widths between them. One advantage of logarithmic numerals is that they permit a wide range of magnitudes to be compactly displayed graphically. The numerals on the decibel scale have logarithmic meanings.

These five meanings of numerals (nominal, ordinal, interval, ratio, and logarithmic) are the ones most often encountered by speech pathologists and audiologists. They will be further discussed in the final section of this chapter, which is concerned with measurement.

Quantitative data, like qualitative data, vary in validity, reliability, and generality. The factors that influence these are the same for quantitative data as for qualitative data.

The validity of quantitative data is a function of the degree of structural similarity, or isomorphism, between the meanings of the numerals used to describe, or quantify, an attribute of an event and the attribute being described. The more valid the data, the greater the degree of similarity, or isomorphism. If ordinal numerals are used to describe the ordering of a group of individuals on the basis of a particular attribute, and the individuals are orderable on the basis of that attribute in the manner designated by the numerals, then the numerals are isomorphic to the attribute being described and hence validly describe that attribute. Suppose you had five stutterers who varied considerably in severity, and you assigned each an ordinal numeral between 1 and 5 to describe his severity in relation to the others, with 1 designating mildest stuttering and 5 most severe stuttering. The numerals would be isomorphic to the territory and hence valid if, for example: (1) the stutterer assigned the numeral 2 was more severe than the stutterer assigned the numeral 1 and less severe than the stutterers assigned the numerals 3, 4, and 5; (2) the stutterer assigned the numeral 5 was more severe than any of the others; and (3) the stutterer assigned the numeral 1 was less severe than any of the others. For the numerals to be a valid map of the territory, therefore, they would have to rank order the stutterers in a manner that would be consistent with the relative severities of their stuttering.

The reliability level of quantitative data, like that of qualitative data, is a function of the interaction between the observer and the observed. The factors mentioned as influencing this interaction in the discussion of qualitative data also apply here. The main difference between the two is that the level of reliability of quantitative data can usually be estimated more precisely than that of qualitative data.

The factors mentioned as influencing the generality of qualitative data also influence the generality of quantitative data. Random sampling and a sufficiently large N maximize the probability of adequate generality for both types of data. The main difference between the two for generality is similar to that for reliability—i.e., the generality of quantitative data usually can be estimated more precisely than that of qualitative data. Statistical inference, which is the approach used to estimate the generality of quantitative data, is discussed in Chapter 8.

MEASUREMENT-RELATED PROPERTIES OF QUANTITATIVE DATA

The measurement-related properties of the five most frequently encountered types of quantitative data in speech pathology and audiology research —nominal, ordinal, interval, ratio, and logarithmic—were summarized briefly in the preceding section. These properties will be discussed here in greater depth. It is essential for speech pathologists and audiologists to develop as good an intuitive understanding of them as they can. Without such an understanding, quantitative data cannot be validly interpreted or applied.

The Nature of Measurement

Measurement can be defined as *the assignment of numerals to attributes of (objects and) events according to rules.* This definition is a slightly modified version of one formulated by the late S. S. Stevens (1951, p. 1), who was a pioneer in psychological and psychophysical measurement. There are several terms in this definition to which particular attention should be paid. The first is the term "numeral." Numerals are number symbols. Their meanings are determined by the rules used to assign them. Numerals on nominal, ordinal, interval, ratio, and logarithmic scales have different meanings because they are assigned by different rules. Therefore, it is necessary to know the rules by which a particular set of numerals are assigned in order to understand their meaning.

The second important aspect of this definition is that numerals are assigned to *attributes* of objects and events rather than to objects and events per se. When you describe an object or event, you only describe certain attributes, not all possible ones. Since measurement is description, when you measure an attribute or event you describe only one (or at the most a limited number) of its attributes. There are always attributes that are not being measured, or described.

The third, important point of this definition is that the term "objects" is in parentheses, to indicate that it could be deleted from the definition. Objects can be classified as events. What you abstract as an object on the macroscopic, observable level would be classified as an event on the submicroscopic, molecular level since its configuration would be constantly changing (Johnson, 1946). The eventness, or process nature, of objects is apparent even if they are observed on the macroscopic level over a relatively long period of time (Johnson, 1946). The author's 1963 Dodge did not have the same attributes in 1974 when he junked it that it had when it was new. The attributes (or characteristics) of a hearing aid after two years of use are probably not identical to what they were when it left the factory. Since the attributes of phenomena classified as objects vary as a function of time on both macroscopic and submicroscopic levels, they are not sharply differentiable from phenomena classified as events. It would appear justifiable, therefore, to classify them as events rather than to place them in a separate category.

The rules used to assign numerals to attributes of events on nominal, ordinal, interval, ratio, and logarithmic scales are presented and discussed in the following sections.

Nominal Scales

Numerals on a nominal scale are assigned to categories, or subclasses, of attributes of events by means of the rule "...do not assign the same numeral to different classes or different numerals to the same class" (Stevens, 1960, p.26). They merely label, or identify, such categories or subclasses. The particular numeral assigned to a particular category or subclass is *arbitrary*. It is desirable, however, that the categories or subclasses be *mutually exclusive* and *exhaustive* with regard to the attribute being scaled. That is, all events that possess the attribute being scaled should be (1) assignable to only one category or subclass, and (2) assignable to a category or subclass. Suppose the attribute you wished to scale was articulation errors. The following three categories, or subclasses, could be used for this purpose, and a numeral could be assigned arbitrarily to identify each:

1. sound substitutions,
2. sound omissions, additions, and inversions, and
3. sound distortions.

These categories would probably be regarded as both mutually exclusive and exhaustive, since individual articulation errors would be assignable to only one category and all such errors could be assigned to a category. The specific ordering of the numerals that is used to label the three categories is completely arbitrary. Any of the six—i.e., $(N)(N-1)$—possible permutations of these three numerals (see Figure 6.1) would serve equally well.

$$\begin{array}{c}1\ 2\ 3\\ 3\ 2\ 1\\ 1\ 3\ 2\\ 2\ 3\ 1\\ 2\ 1\ 3\\ 3\ 1\ 2\end{array}$$

FIGURE 6.1. Permutations of numerals on a nominal scale.

The events assigned to any one category must be equivalent with regard to the attribute being scaled, or fall within the defined domain of that category. They do not have to be equivalent, however, with regard to any other attributes. The relation between such events for the attribute scaled is referred to as *equivalence* and is symbolized by the familiar sign: $=$. The equivalence relation is defined logically as being *reflexive, symmetrical,* and *transitive* ($x = x$ for all values of x; if $x = y$, then $y = x$; and if $x = y$ and $y = z$, then $x = z$). (These qualities are further defined in the section on ordinal scales.)

Nominal scales have been constructed for a variety of attributes of interest to speech pathologists and audiologists. Some such scales are an end in themselves and others are a means to an end. Several examples of the first type would be Angle's (1907) three classes of malocclusion—i.e., Class I (Neutrocclusion), Class II (Distocclusion), and Class III (Mesiocclusion); Jerger's four types of Békésy audiogram tracings (Jerger, 1960); and Schuell's five major diagnostic categories of aphasia (Schuell, Jenkins, and Jiménez-Pabón, 1964). The second type would include instances where qualitatively defined categories, or subclasses, are arbitrarily assigned numerals to facilitate statistical, computer, and punch-card analyses. The category "male," for example, might be assigned the numeral 1, and "female" the numeral 2, to facilitate the coding of sex data on computer cards or punch cards. Or the numeral 1 might be assigned to conductive hearing loss, 2 to sensori-neural hearing loss, and 3 to mixed hearing loss to facilitate the coding of type of peripheral hearing loss data on such cards. The assignment of numerals to such categories not only facilitates the summarizing and storing of data, but their statistical analysis as well. Various statistical analyses can be performed on observations that have been categorized and coded on computer cards or punch cards, including the determination of the number of observations and the percentage of total observations that fall into each category.

Ordinal Scales

Numerals on an ordinal scale are assigned to N categories, or subclasses, of events to designate a *rank order*. The categories, or subclasses, ordered may contain only a single event (e.g., a person). While the ordering of the N numerals designates the ordering of the N categories with regard to the amount of the target attribute they possess, it is arbitrary whether 1 or N is used to designate the greatest amount of the attribute.

With an ordinal scale, the differences in the amount of the target attribute between the categories ranked are not necessarily the same. There are not necessarily equal intervals between scale points. This is illustrated in Figure 6.2. The difference in the amount of the target attribute between the

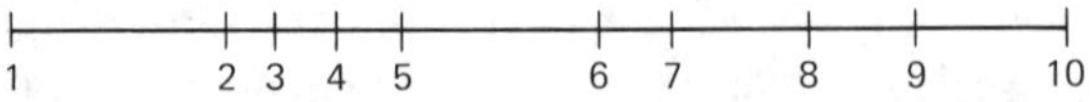

FIGURE 6.2. An ordinal scale.

category assigned the numeral 1 and that assigned the numeral 2 in this figure is greater than the difference between the category assigned the numeral 2 and that assigned the numeral 3. If the ten numerals on this scale had been assigned to ten samples of speech to designate an ordering on the basis of articulation defectiveness, the difference in degree of articulation defectiveness between the sample assigned the numeral 1 and that assigned the numeral 2 would be greater than the difference in degree of articulation defectiveness between the sample assigned the numeral 2 and that assigned the numeral 3.

Categories on an ordinal scale can be labeled by words and certain other symbols rather than (or in addition to) numerals. The labels "mild," "moderate," and "severe" can be attached to categories on an ordinal scale, as can the labels "poor," "fair," "good," "very good," and "excellent;" and A, B, C, D, E. The labels "correct" and "incorrect"; "+" and "−"; and "+", "±", and "−" also can be attached to categories to define ordinal scales.

For a scale to have ordinal properties, the numerals have to be assigned by rules that result in a specific relationship between the categories ranked. This relationship, according to Hempel (1952, pp. 58–62), is based on the relations of *coincidence* (sharing the same place or being equal to another) and *precedence* (being less than or greater than another). For the relationship between categories on a scale to be ordinal, Hempel states that the two relations have to meet the following conditions.

1. Coincidence must be *transitive*, i.e., whenever x stands in coincidence to (or in the same category as) y and y stands in coincidence to (or in the same category as) z, then x stands in coincidence to (or in the same category as) z. In other words, if John lives in the same state as Jim and Jim lives in the same state as Joe, then John lives in the same state as Joe.

2. Coincidence must be *symmetric*, i.e., whenever x stands in coincidence to (or is included in the same category as) y, then y stands in coincidence to (or is included in the same category as) x. In other words, if John lives in the same state as Jim, then Jim lives in the same state as John.

3. Coincidence must be *reflexive*, i.e., any event x stands in coincidence to (is includable in the same category as) itself with regard to the attribute being measured. Another way of stating the same thing is that $x = x$ for all values of x. In other words, all events included in a category are equivalent with regard to the attribute on the basis of which they were assigned to the category.

4. Precedence must be *transitive*, i.e., whenever x stands in precedence to y and y stands in precedence to z, then x stands in precedence to z. In other words, if Bloodstein's (1975) Phase II stuttering is more severe than his Phase I stuttering, and his Phase III stuttering is more severe than his Phase II stuttering, then his Phase III stuttering should be more severe than his Phase I stuttering.

5. Precedence must be *coincidence-irreflexive*, i.e., if x stands in coincidence to (or is equal to) y, then x does not stand in precedence to y. In other words, if John has the same threshold for a 1000 Hz tone as Jim, then John does not have a higher threshold or lower threshold for this tone than Jim.

6. Precedence must be *coincidence-connected*, i.e., if x does not stand in coincidence to (or is not equal to) y, then x stands in precedence to y or y stands in precedence to x. In other words, if John does not have the same threshold for a 1000 Hz tone as Jim, then John either has a higher threshold or a lower threshold for this tone than Jim.

There are six conditions, then, that Hempel indicates need to be satisfied for numerals to have ordinal properties. The first three, incidently, also need to be satisfied for numerals to have nominal properties (see section on nominal scales).

Ordinal scales are the type that has probably been used most frequently to measure, or quantify, attributes of events of interest to speech pathologists and audiologists. There are at least three reasons for the frequent use of this type of scale. First, ordinal scales are simpler to construct than other types which indicate magnitudes, or quantities (i.e., interval, ratio, and logarithmic scales). The reason for this is that the other types require the six conditions for ordinal measurement to be satisfied in addition to some others. (These additional conditions are indicated in the sections in which the three types are discussed.)

A second reason for the frequent use of ordinal scales is that ordinal level measurement is all that is required for answering many questions. Such questions often are similar in form to one of the following:

1. Does Person A (or Group A) *have more of (or less of)* an attribute than Person B (or Group B)? Other phrases that could occur instead of the italicized one include: (a) have a higher (or lower) score on a task, (b) have a longer (or shorter) response time, and (c) exhibit a higher frequency (or lower frequency) of a behavior.

2. Do persons who exhibit a relatively high level (or relatively low level) of an attribute under one condition (or on one task) also tend to exhibit a similar level under one or more other conditions (or on one or more other tasks)? Another way of phrasing this question would be: Does Condition A (or Task A) tend to rank order persons in the same manner as Condition B, etc. (or Task B, etc.)?

A third probable reason for the frequent use of ordinal scales is that some attributes, or dimensions, do not lend themselves to higher than ordinal level measurement—i.e., they do not lend themselves to interval or ratio level measurement. An example would be a scale in which the categories, or points, include several dimensions, such as Bloodstein's (1975) four-phase scale for describing the development of stuttering. It would be extremely difficult, if not impossible, to construct such a scale so there would be equal intervals between points for all dimensions included.

Interval Scales

Numerals on interval scales are assigned by the same rules as those on ordinal scales, *plus* one additional rule: they must be assigned in such a manner that the interval widths between successive numerals are equal in magnitude with respect to the attribute being scaled. This requirement is graphically portrayed in Figure 6.3 for the attribute "distance." The distance between the numerals 1 and 2 in this figure is equal to that between the numerals 2 and 3, 3 and 4, 4 and 5, 5 and 6, 6 and 7, 7 and 8, 8 and 9, and 9 and 10. The equality of these interval widths can be checked with a ruler.

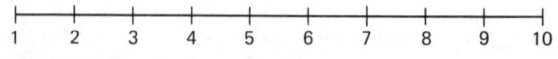

FIGURE 6.3. *An interval scale.*

Interval scales can be constructed for psychological attributes as well as physical ones. In addition to equal physical distances between points, there can be *equal-appearing* perceptual distances between points—distances that appear approximately equal based on observer judgments. The Lewis-Sherman Scale of Stuttering Severity (Lewis and Sherman, 1951) represents an attempt to develop a scale on which the perceptual distances between points are equal-appearing. This scale consists of nine sets of speech segments, each of which has been assigned a numeral between 1 and 9. The segments assigned the numeral 1 contain the mildest stuttering and those assigned the numeral 9 the most severe. The segments were selected from a larger group that were rated by the method of equal-appearing intervals for "degree of stuttering severity." This method, which is described in Chapter 7, is thought to result in measurement that approximates interval level. Theoretically, differences in stuttering severity between speech segments assigned the numeral 1 and those assigned the numeral 2 would be approximately equal to those between speech segments assigned the numerals 2 and 3, 3 and 4, 4 and 5, 5 and 6, 6 and 7, 7 and 8, and 8 and 9. The interval widths on this scale, incidently, were estimated by means of a rating procedure and with a few exceptions were found to be fairly equal (Berry and Silverman, 1972).

Because of the equality of interval widths, the *differences* between numerals on interval scales can be manipulated arithmetically. That is, they can be added, subtracted, multiplied, and divided. The difference in the amount of an attribute between events designated by the numerals 1 and 3 would be twice that between events designated by the numerals 1 and 2 and half that between events designated by the numerals 1 and 5. If these numerals were points on an interval scale of stuttering severity, the difference in severity of stuttering between a speech segment designated by the numeral 1 and one designated by the numeral 3 would be twice that between speech segments designated by the numerals 1 and 2 and half that between speech segments designated by the numerals 1 and 5.

While the differences between numerals on an interval scale can be manipulated arithmetically, the numerals themselves can not be manipulated arithmetically. The reason for this restriction is that the numerals on such a scale are not related to an absolute, or "true," zero. Thus, a speech segment that was assigned the numeral 2 would not necessarily contain stuttering that was twice as severe as that in a segment assigned the numeral 1 nor half as severe as that in a segment assigned the numeral 4.

Scales that have been regarded either implicitly or explicitly as having interval properties have been developed for a number of attributes of interest to speech pathologists and audiologists. Such scales would include those which were constructed by the method of equal-appearing intervals, e.g., the Lewis-Sherman Scale of Stuttering Severity. They also might include scales based on age ratios such as I.Q. (i.e., $MA/CA \times 100$). Numerals on I.Q. scales could be regarded as having either ordinal or interval properties. The interpretation would depend on whether you were willing to assume, for example, that the increase in "intelligence" from an I.Q. of 60 to an I.Q. of 70 is equivalent to the increase from an I.Q. of 95 to one of 105. If you were willing to assume that the intervals between points on the I.Q. scale are approximately equal throughout the *entire* range of possible I.Q.s, then you would be justified in regarding numerals on this scale as having interval properties. On the other hand, if you would not be willing to make this assumption, it would be safest to regard such numerals as having ordinal properties. The viability of the equal interval assumption probably would depend, in part, on the specific test used to estimate mental age (MA). Individual intelligence tests such as the Stanford-Binet would probably be more likely than group intelligence tests to result in I.Q.'s with interval properties.

Scales that are claimed to have interval properties should probably be regarded as having ordinal properties unless it has been demonstrated reasonably unequivocally that the equal interval assumption is viable. Regarding them as such in most instances would probably not cause any problems. Most questions asked by speech pathologists and audiologists appear to require only ordinal data to answer.

Ratio Scales

Numerals are assigned by the same rules on ratio scales as on interval scales with the exception that they are required to be related to an absolute, or true, zero. This requirement is portrayed graphically for the attribute "distance" in Figure 6.4. Because ratio scales have as their origin a true zero

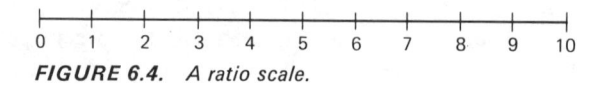

FIGURE 6.4. A ratio scale.

point, the numerals on such scales, as well as the intervals between them, are isomorphic to the structure of arithmetic and can be manipulated arithmetically. A speech segment assigned the numeral 4 on a ratio scale of stuttering severity would contain stuttering that is twice as severe as that in a speech segment assigned the numeral 2 on this scale. A ratio scale theoretically could be constructed for the attribute stuttering because it would be possible to have a speech segment which contained zero stuttering. It might not be possible, on the other hand, to construct a ratio scale for the attribute "intelligence" because it would be difficult to define zero intelligence.

The decision on whether a scale has ratio properties may not be unequivocal. Frequency of articulation errors would probably be regarded as a scale with ratio properties if it were viewed as a *frequency* scale, since the numeral 4, for example, would indicate twice as many articulation errors as the numeral 2. On the other hand, it would probably not be regarded as a ratio scale of *articulation defectiveness*, since 4 errors would not necessarily be judged to represent twice the degree of articulation defectiveness as 2 errors. It would probably not be regarded even as an interval scale of articulation defectiveness since interval widths between successive numerals are unlikely to be judged equal. The change from 1 to 2 articulation errors, for example, would probably be judged to represent a greater increase in articulation defectiveness than would the change from 15 to 16 such errors. Hence, a scale of articulation defectiveness based on frequency of articulation errors would probably be regarded as having ordinal properties.

While one measure of a particular attribute might not result in a scale that has ratio properties, another such measure might result in scale with these properties. It might be possible, for example, to construct a ratio scale of articulation defectiveness by using a psychological scaling procedure such as *direct magnitude-estimation* (see Chapter 7) rather than frequency counts of articulation errors. With this approach, each of a group of speech segments that contained a wide variety of frequencies and types of articulation errors would be assigned a number by a panel of listeners that would be instructed to indicate how defective the articulation was in it as compared to the articulation in a "standard" speech segment. The standard speech segment would be arbitrarily assigned a point value, e.g., 100. Each listener would be instructed to assign a point value to each speech segment that would indicate how defective he considers the articulation in it to be as compared to that in the standard speech segment. A listener who felt, for example, that the articulation in a particular speech segment was twice as defective as that in the standard segment would assign that segment 200 points. On the other hand, a listener who felt the articulation in a particular speech segment was half as defective as that in the standard segment would assign it 50 points. The listener could assign any number of points desired to a speech segment as long as it reflected a judgment on how defective the articulation was in it as compared to that in the standard segment. The mean of the point values assigned to each segment could be computed and used as its *scale value*—i.e., the point, or value, on the scale to which it is assigned. Assuming the listeners rated the speech segments as instructed, the resulting scale would at least come close to having ratio properties. A segment with a mean point value of 100, for example, would be approximately twice as defective in articulation as one with a mean point value of 50, and approximately half as defective in articulation as one with a mean point value of 200.

The unit of measurement on a ratio scale is arbitrary. For the attribute "length," for example, you can convert from inches to feet (or from feet to inches) by multiplying (or dividing) all numerals by the *positive constant* 12. The conversion, or transformation, from one unit of measurement to another by *multiplying* or *dividing* all numerals by a positive constant does not influence the ratio properties of a scale.

Ratio scales for attributes of interest to speech pathologists and audiologists have been developed from several types of measures, including the following:

1. Frequency counts. One attribute that has been scaled by this measure is frequency of moments of stuttering.
2. Temporal (time) measures. One attribute that has been scaled by this type of measure is duration of moments of stuttering.
3. Length (distance) measures. The amount of opening between the posterior surface of the velum and the anterior surface of the posterior pharyngeal wall during the production of /s/ has been measured in millimeters from lateral headplates (X-rays) to assess velopharyngeal closure.
4. Voltage measurements. Output voltages from some types of electroacoustical instrumentation used in audiology (e.g., Békésey audiometers) are recorded and measured.
5. Observer judgments. Scales for attributes of communicative behavior which at least approximate ratio measurement have been constructed through the use of psychological scaling methods such as direct magnitude-estimation. (Several such scales are described in Chapter 7.)

Logarithmic Scales

Logarithmic scales, like ratio scales, are constructed from numerals that meet the conditions for ratio level measurement. To construct a logarithmic scale from such numerals you multiply each by a particular *base* number. (Only numerals with ratio properties can be used to construct logarithmic scales because numerals with nominal, ordinal, and interval properties can not be manipulated arithmetically.) The base numbers used most often for scaling attributes of communicative behavior are 2 and 10. Relationships between ratio scale values and logarithmic scale values for the base numbers 2 and 10 are illustrated below:

Ratio Scale Value	Logarithmic Scale Value (Base 2)	Logarithmic Scale Value (Base 10)
0	(2^0) 1	(10^0) 1
1	(2^1) 2	(10^1) 10
2	(2^2) 4	(10^2) 100
3	(2^3) 8	(10^3) 1000
4	(2^4) 16	(10^4) 10000
5	(2^5) 32	(10^5) 100000
6	(2^6) 64	(10^6) 1000000
7	(2^7) 128	(10^7) 10000000
8	(2^8) 256	(10^8) 100000000
9	(2^9) 512	(10^9) 1000000000

These relationships demonstrate one of the main advantages of logarithmic over ratio scales. A logarithmic scale can present data more compactly than a ratio scale. Scale values up to 10,000 are included in the logarithmic scale depicted in Figure 6.5 in the same space as for scale values up to 10 in the ratio scale depicted in Figure 6.4. The compactness of logarithmic scales in comparison to ratio scales is illustrated further in Figure 6.6.

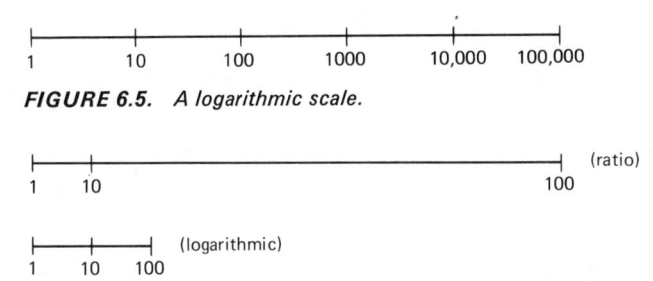

```
├────────┼────────┼────────┼────────┼────────┤
1       10      100     1000    10,000  100,000
```
FIGURE 6.5. *A logarithmic scale.*

```
├────┼──────────────────────────────────────┤  (ratio)
1   10                                     100

├────┼────┤  (logarithmic)
1   10  100
```
FIGURE 6.6. *Comparison between ratio and logarithmic scales.*

Because logarithmic scales are derived from numerals with ratio scale properties, the numerals on such scales can be manipulated arithmetically. Logarithmic scales can be transformed into ratio scales for the same reason.

Logarithmic scales have been used to quantify a number of attributes of interest to speech pathologists and audiologists, including the intensities and fundamental frequencies of voices. They also have been used to record the effects of speech therapies on articulation errors over time (Mower, 1969).

REFERENCES

ANGLE, E., *Malocclusion of the Teeth* (7th Edition). Philadelphia: S. S. White Dental Manufacturing Company (1907).

BERRY, R. C., and SILVERMAN, F. H., Equality of intervals on the Lewis-Sherman scale of stuttering severity. *Journal of Speech and Hearing Research*, 15, 185–188 (1972).

BLOODSTEIN, O., *A Handbook on Stuttering*. Chicago: National Easter Seal Society for Crippled Children and Adults (1975).

HEAD, H., *Aphasia and Kindred Disorders of Speech*. New York: Cambridge University Press (1926).

HEMPEL, C. G., *Fundamentals of Concept Formation in Empirical Science*. Chicago: The University of Chicago Press (1952).

JERGER, J., Békésy audiometry in analysis of auditory disorders. *Journal of Speech and Hearing Research*, 3, 275–287 (1960).

JOHNSON, W., *People in Quandaries*. New York: Harper & Row, Publishers (1946).

LEWIS, D., and SHERMAN, D., Measuring the severity of stuttering. *Journal of Speech and Hearing Disorders*, 16, 320–326 (1951).

Mower, D., Evaluating speech therapy through precision recording. *Journal of Speech and Hearing Disorders*, 34, 329–244 (1969).

Porch, B., Multidimensional scoring in aphasia testing. *Journal of Speech and Hearing Research*, 14, 776–792 (1971).

Schuell, H., Jenkins, J., and Jiménez-Pabón, E., *Aphasia in Adults*. New York: Harper & Row, Publishers (1964).

Stevens, S. S., Mathematics, measurement, and psychophysics. In S. S. Stevens (Ed.), *Handbook of Experimental Psychology*, New York: John Wiley & Sons, Inc., 1–49 (1951).

Webb, E. J., Campbell, D. T., Schwartz, R. D., and Schrest, L., *Unobtrusive Measures: Nonreactive Research in the Social Sciences*. Chicago: Rand McNally & Company (1966).

SEVEN

APPROACHES TO GENERATING QUANTITATIVE DATA

This chapter describes some approaches (or strategies) for generating the types of quantitative data necessary to answer questions of relevance to speech pathology and audiology—specifically, approaches that have proved useful for measuring, or quantifying, attributes of communicative behavior, with particular attention to psychological scaling techniques. It will attempt to develop in the reader an intuitive understanding of these approaches and of the types of questions they can answer, and to indicate factors to be considered in designing (and interpreting the results of) studies utilizing these approaches.

ROLE OF THE OBSERVER IN THE MEASUREMENT PROCESS

Before beginning our discussion of approaches for quantifying, or measuring, attributes of events of interest to speech pathologists and audiologists, we will consider the measurement process itself, particularly the role of the observer in this process. The observer is a component of all schemes for generating quantitative data, since all measurement relies on observer judgment to some extent. In psychological scaling, or rating, procedures (such as equal-appearing intervals and direct magnitude-estimation), the importance of the observer in the measurement process is obvious. It may not be as obvious, however, for physical measurement, i.e., measurement of physical attributes of events that utilizes electronic or other types of instrumentation. Examples of such instruments would be rulers and voltmeters. Both may appear to result in "objective" measurement, i.e., measurement not influenced by observer judgment; distances may appear to be indicated by the marks on rulers and voltages by the position of the pointer on voltmeter dials. Rulers and voltmeters do not read themselves, however. Someone has to decide which mark on a ruler corresponds to the distance being measured and which number of the voltmeter dial the indicator is pointing at. Also, the accuracy of the calibration of such devices obviously influences the accuracy of the measurement it is possible to obtain from them. And the accuracy of their calibration is partially a function of observer judgment, since they are calibrated by some human agent. For these reasons, observer judgment is an unavoidable component of any measurement process or scheme.

The presence of an observer (or observers) in the measurement process introduces error into this process. A group of observers who measure the same thing may not record the same measurement. This can be demonstrated by means of a relatively simple task such as measuring the length of a line with a ruler. How long is this line?

To answer this question, ten students at Marquette University were handed a card on which a line of this length had been drawn and a foot ruler graduated in sixteenths of an inch. All measured the line with the same ruler. They were told to measure the line and record their measurement on a blank card which they had been given. Their length estimates ranged from 2.00 inches to 2.25 inches, with a mean of 2.07 inches. While the differences between estimates are relatively small, they could be large enough in some instances to make a difference that would result in a difference in an answer to a question.

The presence of an observer in the measurement process can introduce two types of error: random and systematic. Both were described in Chapter 5. *Random error*, as indicated previously, is present to some degree in all measurement processes. It can arise from several sources, including insufficient accuracy in making measurements and in recording (writing down) measurements. If, for example, you were measuring distances with a ruler, random error could result occasionally from not placing the ruler at the exact point from which you wished to begin to measure, or from reading distances from the ruler incorrectly, or from writing down distances inaccurately after you had read them. The nature of random error is such that if you were to remeasure an aspect of an event (or object) after you had made an error (or errors), you would be unlikely to make the same error (or errors) again.

Because random error does not replicate itself—i.e., does not occur whenever a measurement process is repeated—it does not bias the data resulting from a measurement process. It does not cause the numerals to be consistently larger or smaller than they should be. While random error can be reduced by such means as making all measurements twice, it is doubtful whether it ever can be completely eliminated.

The second type of error, *systematic error*, is usually of more concern to investigators than the first because it *biases* measurement processes. It causes the numerals generated by such a process to be consistently larger or smaller than they should be. In the case of measuring distances with a ruler, systematic error could result from consistently placing the end of the ruler at a point that was not the one from which you wished to begin to measure, or consistently misreading the ruler in the same manner (e.g., interpreting the gradations as occurring every $\frac{1}{16}$ inch rather than every $\frac{1}{8}$ inch), or consistently recording distances incorrectly after reading them (e.g., indicating inches rather than millimeters after numerals).

Observer-related systematic error can be introduced into the measurement process from several sources, including:

1. A measuring "instrument" or process being improperly administered or conducted. An investigator, for example, may not administer an educational or psychological test in the manner in which it was supposed to be administered. An investigator who deviated from the instructions in the test manual for administering the test might obtain scores that are biased—i.e., consistently higher or lower than they should be.

2. Subjects not performing a task as instructed. They may, for example, not make the judgment they were instructed to make. Suppose a group of subjects were told to rate a series of speech segments from cleft palate speakers for degree of nasality, thus requiring them to ignore articulation errors and other deviations of speech, voice, and language usage. They may not be able to keep the other deviations present in the speech segments from influencing their nasality ratings, which would cause these ratings to be biased.

3. Experimenter bias. An experimenter's outcome expectations or hypotheses can bias the measurements he makes (Rosenthal, 1969). For example, a speech pathologist who expected a particular treatment to be effective in reducing stuttering severity might rate stutterers as less severe after the administration of the treatment than before more often than the effects of the treatment would justify. Such errors would not represent deliberate, or conscious, attempts to deceive, but "wishful thinking." (This topic is further discussed in Chapter 9.)

4. Subject bias. This phenomenon is closely related to, and is sometimes the result of, experimenter bias. Subjects may respond to experimental conditions in the manner which they feel the experimenter either would like them

to respond or expects them to respond. That is, they have thoughts about an experiment that can influence their performance on an experimental task. As Orne (1969, p. 146) has pointed out:

> Insofar as the subject cares about the outcome, his perception of his role and of the hypothesis being tested will become a significant determinant of his behavior. The cues which govern his perceptions—which communicate what is expected of him and what the experimenter hopes to find—can therefore be crucial variables.... They include the scuttlebutt about the experiment, its setting, implicit and explicit instructions, the person of the experimenter, subtle cues provided by him, and of particular importance, the experimental procedure itself. All of these cues are interpreted in the light of the subject's past learning and experience. (Orne, 1969, p. 146)

If clients were asked, for example, to rate the effects a particular therapy had on them on a number of dimensions as part of a study of the effectiveness of that therapy, and if they surmised that the person who was conducting the study either expected (or hoped) to find it effective on certain of these dimensions, they might be more likely to indicate that it had at least "a little" of this effect than they would if they had had no information concerning the expected (or hoped for) effects of the treatment. Hence at least some of their ratings could be biased.

While the observer is a component of all measurement schemes, his or her role, or function, is not the same in all such schemes. Measurement schemes used by speech pathologists and audiologists can be divided into two groups on the basis of the function performed by the observer. The *first group* would consist of those that use an "instrument" to supplement observer judgment. The instrument helps the observer to "abstract" the attribute he wishes to measure. A speech pathologist who wished to measure the extent of increase in sympathetic nervous system activity in response to a feared stimulus as part of a desensitization procedure could use a psychogalvanometer to assist in observing and measuring this activity. Or an audiologist who wished to measure thresholds for pure tones could use a pure-tone audiometer to help abstract this phenomenon.

An instrument used to supplement observer judgment need not be electronic. Most, if not all, educational and psychological tests, for example, could probably be used for this purpose. Included here would be articulation tests, aphasia tests, language development scales, auditory discrimination tests, speechreading ability tests, etc.

The *second group* of measurement schemes includes those that rely primarily upon observer judgment. The observer is the most important component in such schemes, since he makes the judgments on the basis of which numerals are assigned. Psychological scaling techniques, which have been used a great deal by speech pathologists and audiologists for quantifying attributes of interest, are representative of the measurement schemes included in this group. These techniques require the observer to make various kinds of judgments, including:

1. deciding to which of a group of categories an event should be assigned,
2. deciding which member of each of a series of pairs of events possesses the greater amount of an attribute,
3. rank ordering a group, or series, of events on the basis of the amount of an attribute they possess,
4. assigning numerals between 1 and a specified upper limit (usually 7 or 9) to events on the basis of the amount of some attribute they possess, so that the intervals between successive numerals will be equal-appearing with respect to that attribute,
5. assigning numerals between 1 and a specified upper limit (usually 7 or 9) to events on the basis of the amount of some attribute they possess, so that each event is assigned the numeral of the category on the scale that comes closest to indicating the amount of the attribute it possesses (the amount of the attribute possessed by each category on the scale would be specified either verbally or nonverbally),
6. assigning points to each of two events which sum, or add up, to a particular constant (e.g., 100) so that the points assigned to each of the two correspond to the relative amount of the attribute being measured that it possesses in relation to that possessed by the other (e.g., if one member of a pair were judged to possess twice the amount of an attribute as the other, it would be assigned 66.67 points and the other would be assigned 33.33 points), and
7. assigning points to events on the basis of the amount of an attribute they possess as compared to that possessed by a "standard" event, or stimulus (this is the type of direct magnitude-estimation judgment described in Chapter 6).

Each of these tasks is associated with a psychological scaling technique that is described in the final section of this chapter.

Measurement-related considerations in designing and evaluating research that utilizes each group of measurement schemes will be discussed in the remaining two sections of this chapter.

MEASUREMENT SCHEMES THAT UTILIZE AN INSTRUMENT TO SUPPLEMENT OBSERVER JUDGMENT

A number of measurement-related considerations exist for schemes that utilize an instrument to supplement observer judgment. Such schemes can be divided for purposes of discussion into two groups. The first consists of those that utilize electronic or other instruments for physical measurement; the second, those that utilize a psychological or educational measuring instrument or instruments.

Schemes That Utilize Electronic or Other Physical Measurement Instrumentation

Various types of instruments are used by speech pathologists and audiologists to measure physical attributes of communicative behavior. A general discussion of such instruments can be found in the chapter by Hanley and Peters in *The Handbook of Speech Pathology and Audiology* (1971). Other discussions dealing with the use of physical measurement instrumentation in speech and hearing research (which though "dated" in several instances may nevertheless be helpful) include those of Abbs and Gilbert (1973) on strain gage transduction systems; of Carroll (1952), Fletcher, *et al.* (1960), and Moll (1960) on cinefluorographic and other X-ray techniques; of Dempsey, *et al.* (1950) on the Purdue Pitch Meter; of Gay and Harris (1971) on electromyography; of Hoshiko and Holloway (1968) on radio telemetry; of Kelsey, *et al.* (1969) on ultrasound; of Ladefoged (1957) on palatography; of Moore, *et al.* (1962) and Soron (1967) on high-speed photography; of Sanders (1968) on lingual strength measurement; and of Stewart (1954) on the galvanic skin response.

Most instrumentation schemes for measuring attributes of events that are electrical signals or can be transduced (i.e., converted) into electrical signals contain certain components. These components, which are diagrammed in Figure 7.1, can be regarded as defining a series of stages for the process of measuring such signals.

The first stage in the process is *detection*. Its purpose is to detect the presence (and absence) and possibly the magnitude of the signal of interest.

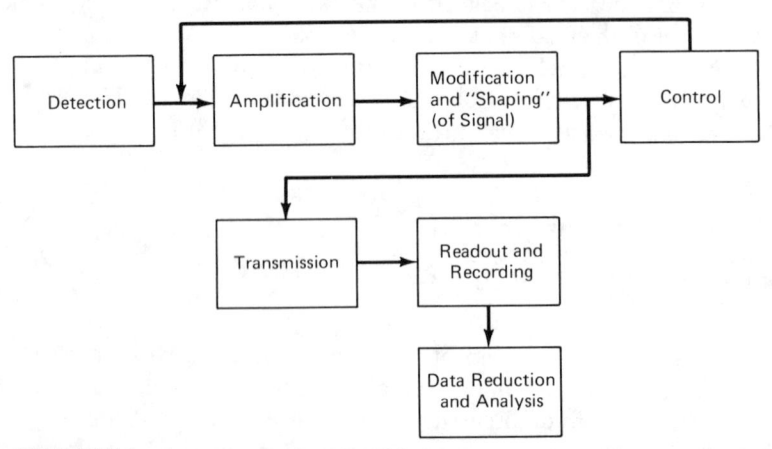

FIGURE 7.1. Instrumentation scheme for measurement.

If the phenomenon is not an electrical signal, it is transduced into an electrical signal.

The detection stage for measuring speech and other acoustical signals consists of a microphone and possibly a preamplifier. The microphone transduces acoustical signals into electrical signals. The function of the preamplifier is to amplify the electrical signals (i.e., voltages) generated by the microphone, with very little distortion, to the point where their magnitude is within the sensitivity range of the "amplifier" stage.

The detection stage for measuring biological electrical signals such as those resulting from muscle action potentials, brain waves, and changes in skin resistance consists of electrodes which either would be attached to the surface of the skin (i.e., surface electrodes) or inserted into muscle fibers or other tissue (i.e., needle electrodes) and an appropriate preamplifier. The function of the preamplifier here would be to increase the magnitudes of the electrical signals detected by the electrodes, with very little distortion, to the point where their magnitude is within the sensitivity range of the "amplifier" stage.

While these two types of detection stages are probably the ones most frequently used in speech and hearing research, several other types have also been used. These would include: (1) strain gages that transduce mechanical pressures, or stresses, into electrical signals, (2) pneumotactographs that transduce rates of air flow into electrical signals, and (3) photoelectric cells that transduce light intensities into electrical signals. An appropriate preamplifier would be fitted to each such transducer.

The second stage in instrumentation schemes for measuring electrical signals is *amplification*. The function of this stage is to increase the magnitude of the electrical signal from the detection stage to the point where it is within the sensitivity range of the readout and recording device being used. The electrical signal from the detection stage may have to be passed through a series of amplifiers, rather than a single amplifier, to increase its magnitude to the point where it is within the sensitivity range of this device. It may also modify the output of the detection stage in such a way that the "noise" (i.e., extraneous signals) in the system will be reduced.

A third stage that may be included in instrumentation schemes for measuring electrical signals is the *modification and shaping* of the signals outputed by the amplifier stage. One of the primary functions of such a stage would be to remove "noise" (extraneous information to what is being measured) from these signals—i.e., to make the figure, or what the investigator wishes to observe, stand out better from the background (other information in the signal).

A modification and shaping stage may consist of a filter network. There are three basic types of filter networks—high pass, low pass, and band pass. Their function is to emphasize or deemphasize specific frequency components of a signal. A *low pass* filter network is used to reduce or eliminate from a signal frequency components *above* a specified frequency. A low pass filter network thus would emphasize the low frequency components of a signal. A high pass filter network is used to reduce or eliminate from a signal frequency components *below* a specified frequency. A high pass filter network thus would emphasize the high frequency components of a signal. A *band pass* filter network is used to reduce or eliminate from a signal *both* frequency components above a specified frequency and below a specified frequency; it consists of a high pass and a low pass filter network. A band pass filter network thus would emphasize a particular "band" of the frequency components of a signal—those between specified upper and lower frequency limits.

The next stage usually included in instrumentation schemes for measuring electrical signals is *control*. Its function is to keep the amplitude or some other attribute of the electrical signal outputed by the amplification stage (or modification and shaping stage, if one is used) *within certain limits*. This is a feedback component that functions in much the same manner as a thermostat on a furnace and an automatic record level control on a tape recorder. It measures the average amplitude (or other attribute) of the output signal from the amplification stage (or possibly that of the shaping stage if one is used). If the amplitude (or value of some other attribute of the signal) is too great, it adjusts the amplification stage to attenuate, or weaken, it. If, on the other hand, the magnitude is insufficient, it adjusts the amplification stage to increase it. This process keeps the amplitude (or other attribute) of the signal within the sensitivity range of the device used to record the signal.

The next stage consists of a device for *transmitting* the signals outputed by the amplification stage (or shaping stage if one is used) to a readout and recording device. The simplest such device would be an electrical cable (i.e., jumpcord) that would connect the output of the amplification stage (or a modification and shaping stage if one were used) to the input of a readout and recording device. Radio telemetry instrumentation also could be used for this purpose. The output signals from the amplification stage (or modification and shaping stage if one were used) would be fed into a radio transmitter and beamed to a radio receiver that could be anywhere from a few feet to hundreds of thousands of miles (e.g., astronauts in space) away. The radio receiver would be connected to a readout and recording device.

The next, and possibly last, stage in such instrumentation schemes consists of a device for *recording and reading out*, or displaying, the output signals from the transmission stage. Without such a device, these signals could not be measured.

Several types of readout and recording devices can be used in instrumentation schemes for measuring electrical signals. The simplest type consists of a *meter*, which indicates the value of the attribute of the signal being measured at given moments in time. This value may be indicated by a pointer (Figure 7.2) or a digital display (Figure 7.3).

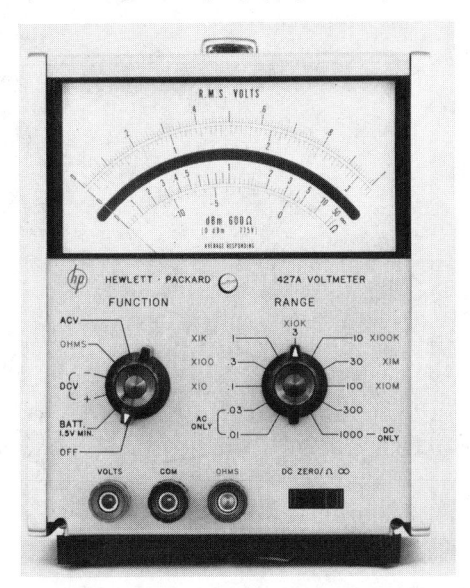

FIGURE 7.2. *A typical meter that indicates values of the attribute being measured by a pointer (Hewlett-Packard Multi-Function Meter, Model 427A).*

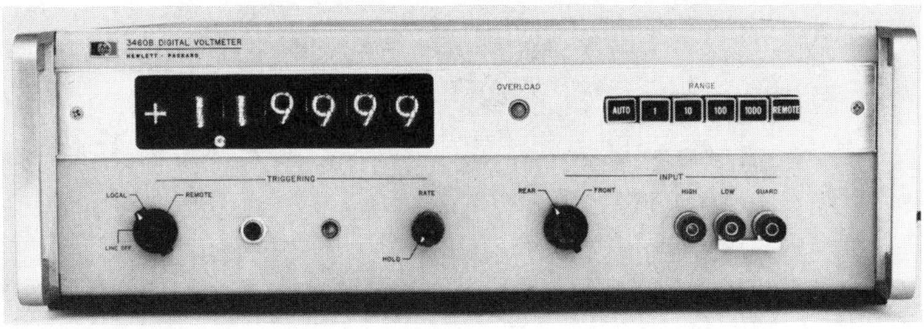

FIGURE 7.3. *A typical meter that indicates values of the attribute being measured by a digital display (Hewlett-Packard Digital Voltmeter, Model 3460B).*

Another class of readout and recording devices that can be used in such schemes include *oscillographic recorders* (see Figure 7.4) and *strip chart recorders* (Figure 7.5). Both will indicate changes in the configuration of a signal during a specified period of time by means of a continuous line drawn on a strip of paper. The primary difference between them is that an oscillographic recorder can handle a wider range of rates of change in the configura-

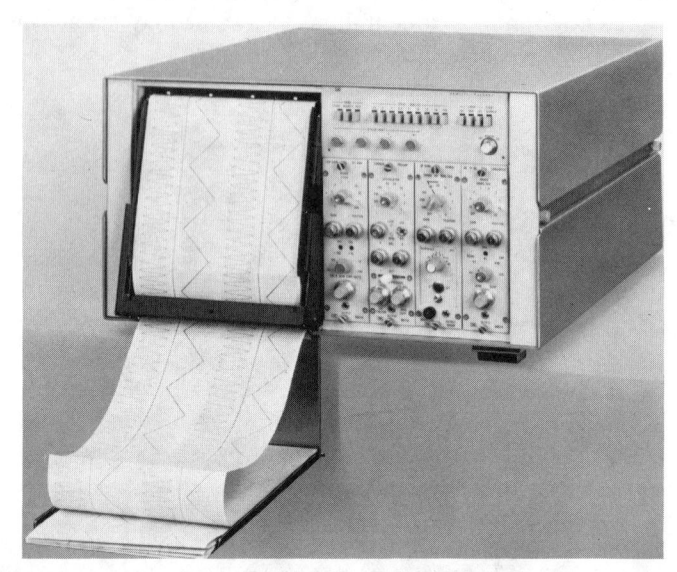

FIGURE 7.4. A typical multi-channel oscillographic recorder (Hewlett-Packard 4-Channel Thermal Tip Oscillographic Recorder, Model 7414A).

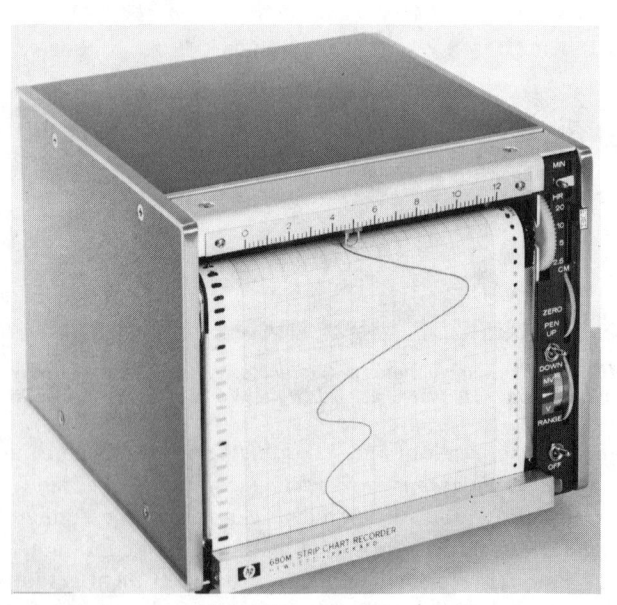

FIGURE 7.5. A typical single-channel strip chart recorder (Hewlett-Packard 5-Inch Compact Recorder, Model 680).

tion of a signal than a strip chart recorder can. Strip chart recorders are most useful when the rate of change in the configuration of a signal is relatively slow. The line may be drawn in ink by a pen, by a light on photosensitive paper, or by a heated stylus on heat-sensitive paper. The strip of paper may be in a roll or in a Z-fold pack (i.e., folded in a fan-like manner similar to computer readout paper). Some such recorders have more than one channel—that is, they can indicate changes in the configurations of several signals simultaneously on the same strip of paper.

A third class of devices for displaying changes in the configurations of electrical signals are *oscilloscopes* (Figure 7.6). The oscilloscope display is

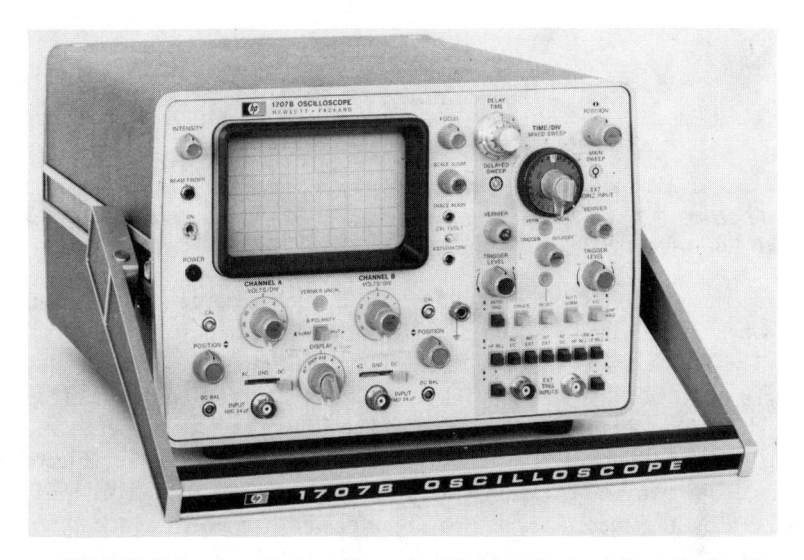

FIGURE 7.6. A typical oscilloscope (Hewlett-Packard Portable Oscilloscope, Model 1707B).

similar to an oscillographic recorder display. The only real difference is that the signal is "painted" with light on a glass television-like screen, not inscribed on a strip of paper. A signal displayed on an oscilloscope screen can be photographed if a permanent record of it is desired.

A fourth class of devices are *magnetic tape recorders*. Two general types can be used for this purpose. The first is the familiar type of audiotape recorder that is used to record speech, music, and other signals (including "noises") within the audio range. The second is an *instrumentation magnetic tape recorder* (Figure 7.7). These can be used to record biological electrical signals and electrical signals from certain types of transducers (e.g., strain gages). They usually have more than one channel (i.e., they can record signals from

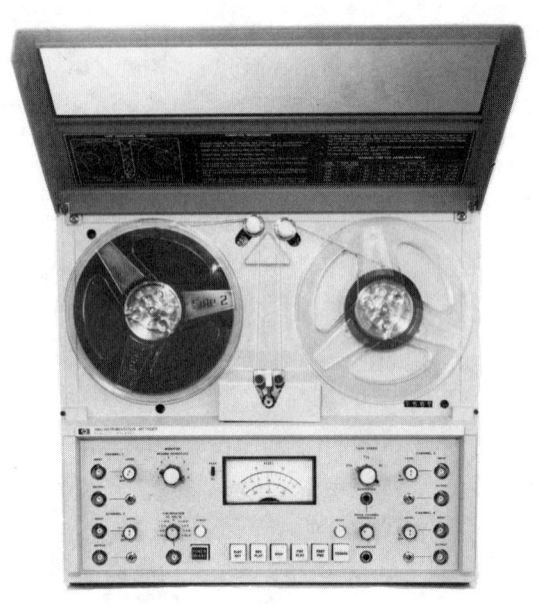

FIGURE 7.7. *A typical instrumentation magnetic tape recorder (Hewlett-Packard 4-Channel Portable Tape Recorder, Model 3960A).*

several transmission stages simultaneously). Such recorders are frequently used when signals are to be fed into a computer for analysis.

The final class of devices that will be mentioned here for displaying changes in the configurations of electrical signals are *X-Y recorders* (Figure 7.8). These recorders automatically plot the value of an independent variable versus a dependent variable directly on sheets of graph paper. Electrical signals from two transmission stages are inputed into the recorder. Plots produced by *X-Y* recorders can provide information concerning the *nature* of the relationship (e.g., linear or nonlinear), the *direction* of the relationship (i.e., positive or negative), and the *strength* of the relationship (i.e., degree of correlation) between the two signals, or variables, being measured. A plot from such a recorder could, for example, provide information on how thresholds for pure tones (X) vary as a function of their frequency (Y). The readout device used on Békésy audiometers is a relatively unsophisticated *X-Y* recorder.

The readout and recording devices mentioned here are not the only such devices that have been used in instrumentation schemes for measuring attributes of events relevant to speech pathology and audiology. However, they are probably the ones that have been used most often for this purpose.

The readout and recording stage is the final stage of some instrumentation schemes for measuring electrical signals. The signals plotted by an oscilloscope, *X-Y* recorder, strip chart recorder, oscillographic recorder, or

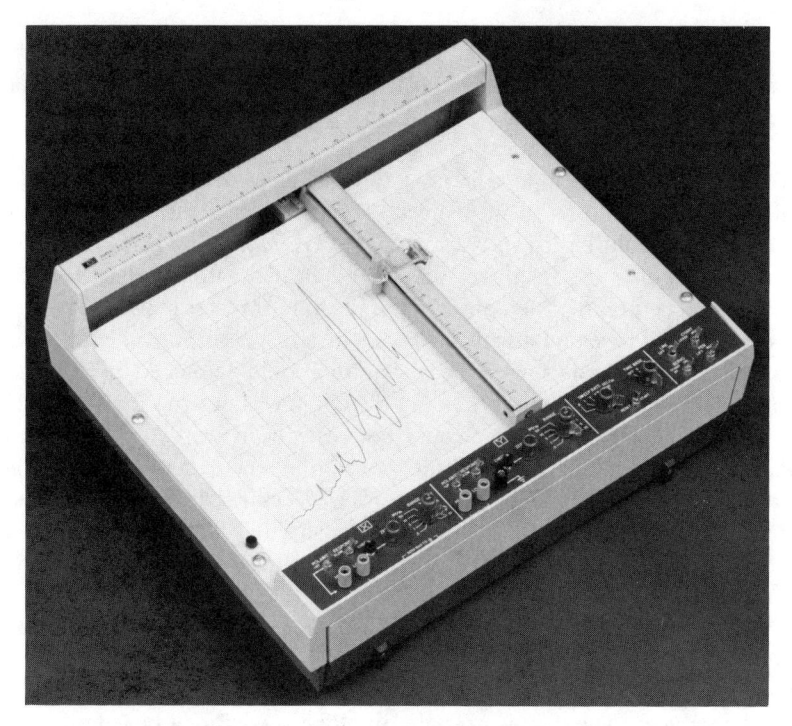

Approaches to Generating Quantitative Data 121

FIGURE 7.8. *A typical X-Y recorder (Hewlett-Packard General Purpose X-Y Recorder, Model 7045A).*

recorded on an audiotape recorder are measured by an observer (or observers). Other such schemes possess an additional stage that is concerned with *data reduction and analysis*. The output of the "readout and recording" stage, for example, could be fed into a computer for organization, measurement, and statistical analysis. Computer data reduction and analysis is particularly likely to be incorporated into an instrumentation measurement scheme when it produces too many signals to be measured by an observer in a relatively short period of time, or when the statistical analyses to be made of the data are relatively complex.

Signals that have been recorded on an instrumentation magnetic tape recorder usually are the simplest to input into a computer. However, they first have to be passed through an *analogue to digital converter*. The function of this device is to assign numerals, or digits, to attributes of electrical signals. These numerals may indicate, for example, the relative magnitudes of such signals at given points in time. This analogue to digital conversion is necessary because computers used for data reduction and analysis require a digital (i.e., numerical) input.

Now that the functions of individual components of instrumentation schemes for measuring electrical signals have been described, we can indicate how such a scheme might be used to measure an attribute of communicative behavior. Suppose we wished to measure a stutterer's anxiety level in certain situations outside the clinic. One measure of anxiety that could be used would be the galvanic skin response (GSR). To *detect* changes in skin resistance (associated with changes in anxiety level) electrodes could be attached to the stutterer's skin in an inconspicuous place. The electrical signals from the electrodes could be fed into a miniature *preamplifier* and possibly into a miniature *amplifier*. From there, they could be fed into a miniature *radio transmitter*. The preamplifier, amplifier, and radio transmitter could be fitted into a very small case and attached to the stutterer's clothing so that it would not be visible. The signals from the transmitter could be picked up by a *radio receiver* located at the clinic (providing the clinic was not too far away). The signals detected by the receiver could be fed into an *amplifier* (or series of amplifiers) to increase their magnitude to the point where they would be within the sensitivity range of a strip chart recorder. A *control* device could be used to keep the level of the signals within the sensitivity range of the strip chart recorder. If the baseline magnitude of the signals transmitted became weaker because the stutterer moved further away from the location of the radio receiver, the degree of amplification would be increased. On the other hand, if the baseline magnitude of these signals became stronger because the stutterer moved closer to the location of the radio receiver, the degree of amplification would be reduced. The signals from the amplifier stage might be fed through a *filter* before being transmitted by means of an electrical cable to a *strip chart recorder*. The function of the filter would be to remove extraneous signals, or "noise," from the output of the amplifier stage so that it would not influence the strip chart recorder plot. Changes in skin resistance could be measured from the strip chart recorder plot.

This instrumentation scheme is obviously not the only one that could be used for measuring changes in skin resistance that occur outside a clinic setting. It is merely intended to illustrate how such a scheme might function.

Measuring Readouts from Instrumentation Schemes. This section will describe how quantitative data are abstracted from meter dials, oscilloscope screens, and the displays from such devices as strip chart recorders, oscillographic recorders, and *X-Y* recorders.

The quantification of electrical signals involves the assignment of numerals to one or more of their attributes (i.e., their amplitudes, frequencies, phase relationships, etc.). The numerals assigned usually have *ratio* properties and for this reason can be manipulated arithmetically. The process by which numerals are assigned may be relatively simple. This is usually the case when the readout device is some sort of meter, e.g., a VU meter. VU meters are used by both speech pathologists and audiologists to measure the loudness levels of auditory signals, including speech. They usually have a dial with numerals around its perimeter ranging from −20 to +3 and a pointer. The position of the pointer indicates the numeral that corresponds to the loudness level of the signal. This numeral is used to designate its loudness level at that moment in time. Since the loudness level of a signal may vary considerably during a relatively short period of time, the pointer may be moving almost continuously. The fact that the loudness level of a signal may not remain constant can create problems when it is necessary to assign a single number to designate it for a particular period of time. One approach that could be used to generate such a value would be to average the numerals indicated by the pointer at specified intervals during this period of time. If this time interval were 60 seconds, for example, the dial might be read every five seconds and the mean of these values computed.

The measurement of displays from strip chart recorders, oscillographic recorders, *X-Y* recorders, and oscilloscopes usually involves a *distance measuring*, or *frequency counting*, or *both* a distance measuring and frequency counting operation.

A *distance measuring operation* involves determining how far (in inches or millimeters) a particular point in a display deviates from a baseline. The numeral assigned to that point is this value. The *baseline* could be the magnitude, or level, of the phenomenon being measured prior to the administration of an experimental treatment. The baseline for measuring the degree of reaction to a feared stimulus through changes in skin resistance, for example, could be the level of skin resistance immediately prior to the presentation of this stimulus. (Such a baseline is used, incidently, in galvanic skin response audiometry.) The deviation from a baseline can be estimated in several ways. It can be measured with a ruler, or by counting the number of squares in the grid printed on the readout paper between the baseline and the point on the display you wish to measure. The amount of deviation from a baseline following administration of a treatment is apt to vary to some extent. If it is necessary to assign a single number to designate the amount of deviation from a baseline during a specific period of time, the mean of a series of deviation measures made during this period of time could be used. The amount of change in skin resistance during a one-minute period following the presentation of a feared stimulus could be designated by the mean amount of deviation from the baseline measured at five second intervals. It would be necessary to attach + and − signs to the deviation measures if they occurred in both directions from the baseline (i.e., + if the signal were above the baseline and − if it were below the baseline). For the point on the section of strip chart in Figure 7.9 marked with an arrow, the deviation from the baseline would be approximately 13 millimeters. The direction of the deviation would be "negative" since the signal falls below the baseline. (Note that the readout has a one-millimeter grid printed on it.)

The measurement of displays could involve a *frequency counting opera-*

124   *Asking and Answering Questions*

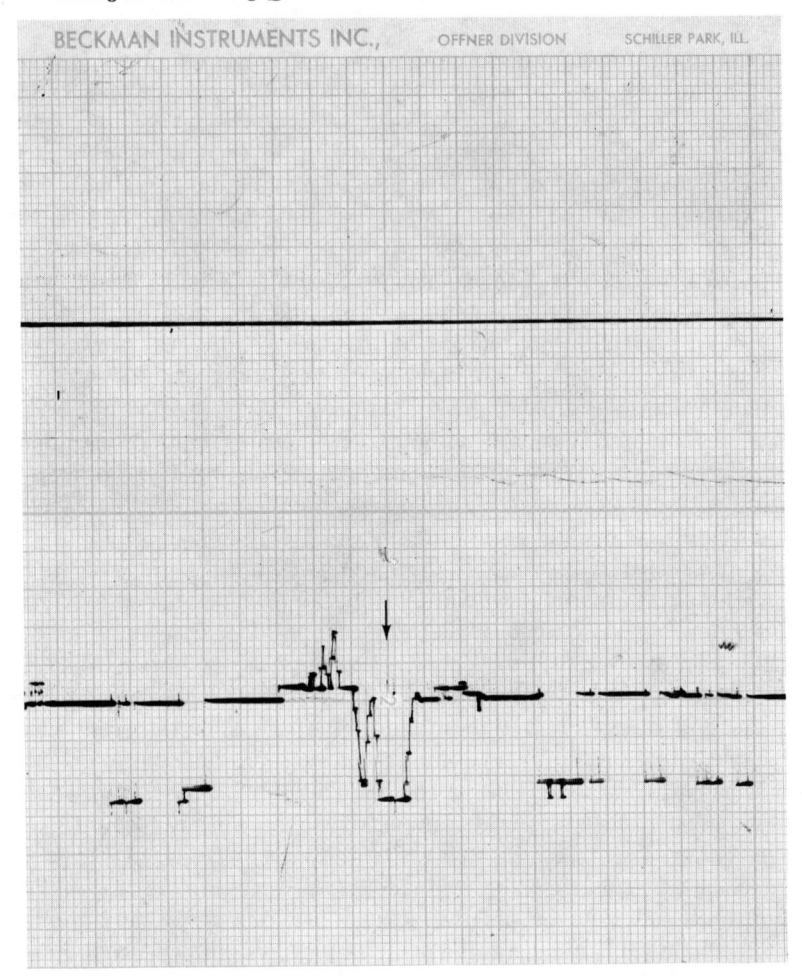

FIGURE 7.9. *Section of a "readout" from a two-channel strip chart recorder.*

tion. This involves determining the number of times a particular attribute, or configuration, of a signal occurs. Frequency of occurrence usually is specified with relation to a particular time interval. Thus, a frequency counting operation may also require a distance measuring operation. The frequency of occurrence of an attribute may be related to a particular time interval that would correspond to a particular distance on the readout paper strip—i.e., the number of inches (or millimeters) of the readout marked by the pen or stylus during the time interval to which the frequency count is related. The frequency of a tone could be determined from an oscillographic recorder readout by counting the number of cycles that were inscribed by the stylus during a one-second time interval. The number of inches of paper that passes under the stylus during a given time interval is estimated from information supplied by the manufacturer of the readout device concerning the speed at which the paper is moving. If six inches of paper passed under the stylus each second, the frequency of a tone would correspond to the number of cycles that were inscribed on a six-inch strip of the paper.

The measurement procedures for oscilloscope screen tracings are essentially the same as those for oscillographic recorder readouts. The attributes of signals that can be measured from oscilloscope screen tracings include frequency and amplitude. Frequency can be estimated by counting the number of cycles displayed on the screen with the oscilloscope set to display a particular time interval. If the interval were 50 milliseconds (i.e., $\frac{5}{100}$ second) and 10 cycles were displayed on the screen, the frequency of the signal (e.g., tone) would be 200 cycles per second. Amplitude can be estimated by a grid inscribed on the oscilloscope screen. It can be measured in millimeter deviation from a baseline, as with an oscillographic recorder, or in volts (a measure of the electrical magnitude of a signal). Measurements can be made directly from the screen display or from photographs of the screen display.

Measurements of attributes of speech and other auditory signals from magnetic tape recordings are made in a variety of ways. In some cases, such signals are fed into an instrumentation measurement scheme before being measured. They are passed through an amplifier stage and a modification and shaping stage and then are transmitted to a readout and recording device such as a strip chart recorder, X-Y recorder, oscillographic recorder, oscilloscope, or meter. The instrumentation scheme helps to abstract the target attribute from the taped signal and thus facilitates the measurement process. A taped speech signal might be fed into a sound spectrograph (e.g., Sonograph) to analyze and display its spectral characteristics—i.e., the amount of energy present at specific frequencies during given moments in time. Several characteristics of the speech spectra could be measured from the resulting spectrogram, or Sonogram (e.g., vowel formant frequencies).

Measurements of attributes of communicative behavior from magnetic tape recordings also are made by means of rating procedures. A number of such procedures, classified as *psychological scaling methods*, are described in the final section of this chapter.

Sources of Error in Measurements from "Readout" Devices. There are several sources of random and systematic error that can influence the accuracy of quantitative data derived from meter dials and from strip chart recorders, X-Y recorders, oscillographic recorders, oscilloscopes, and similar types of displays. These can be grouped under three main headings: (1) gross errors, (2) systematic errors, and (3) random errors (Stout, 1962, pp. 21–26).

Gross errors consist of mistakes in reading meters and other readout displays and in recording numbers resulting from measurement processes.

Misreading a meter would be an example of such an error. The pointer on a VU meter indicates −2, but it is read as indicating −3. Perhaps the person misread the meter because the signals measured previously were −3 and he or she expected further −3 readings. It is well known that your expectations can influence your perceptions (Johnson, 1946). Gross errors also include mistakes in recording (e.g., writing down or typing) the numbers that result from a measurement process. One of the commonest errors of this type is transposition. The person making and recording the measurements from a meter may read 35.2 and write down 32.5. Gross errors can be reduced by making each measurement several times, preferably with one measurement not immediately following the next.

Systematic errors can be grouped under three main headings: (1) instrumental errors, (2) environmental errors, and (3) observational errors. *Instrumental errors* include those that result from shortcomings of the instrument or misuse, or loading effects, of the equipment. The performances of all components of instrumentation measurement schemes probably deviate to some degree from their nominal values (i.e., those specified by their manufacturers) even when they are new. If the instruments included in such schemes are not recalibrated periodically, this deviation is likely to increase because of use and age. If the deviation is fairly small, it may not bias the measurement process in any meaningful way. (It may not make a difference that is a difference.)

The problem of instrumental errors resulting from shortcomings of equipment can be illustrated by means of the pure-tone audiometer. All such audiometers, even when they are new, would not measure exactly the same thresholds at given frequencies, because of factory calibration error. Differences in threshold measurements arising from factory calibration error are likely to be quite small. However, if pure-tone audiometers are not recalibrated periodically, error due to use and age may increase to the point where thresholds will be sufficiently inaccurate to make a difference that *is* a difference.

Instrument calibration errors can be handled in two ways. The best, but usually the most expensive, is to have the instrument recalibrated. The second is to determine the extent of the calibration error and apply a *correction factor*. If you knew, for example, that the amount of hearing loss indicated by a pure-tone audiometer at 1000 Hz was 5 dB too great, you could subtract 5 dB from the degree of hearing loss indicated by this audiometer at this frequency.

Instrumental error also can result from *misuse* or from *loading effects* of components of instrumentation measurement schemes. Failure to use or maintain an instrument according to manufacturers' instructions can cause instrumental error. Failure to use the recommended type of earphones on an audiometer, for example, could result in an impedance mismatch that would probably cause the loudness levels of the pure tones generated by that audiometer to deviate from their nominal values. Such errors can be reduced or eliminated by following manufacturers' recommendations regarding the use of their instruments.

The *loading effects* of components of instrumentation measurement schemes is another source of instrumental error. What sometimes happens is that the measurement process influences what is being measured. The circuitry of a measuring instrument (e.g., a volt meter) can interact with that of the instrument producing the signal being measured (e.g., a pure-tone audiometer), altering this signal and hence producing inaccurate measurements. To avoid this source of error, it is essential to "isolate" the circuitry of measurement instruments from the circuitry of the instruments producing the signals being measured.

The second subclass of systematic errors is *environmental errors*. These result from factors external to a measuring device (i.e., in the environment in which it is being used) which can influence the functioning of one or more of the components within it and thus influence the accuracy of measurements made with it. Environmental factors that can influence the functioning of the components of such schemes include temperature, humidity, barometric pressure, and stray electrical and magnetic fields. The accuracy of the calibration of many electronic instruments is dependent on their being used in an environment in which the temperature is maintained within a specified range. If such an instrument is used in a room in which the temperature either is above or below this range, measurements may be biased. It may be possible to use this instrument in such an environment if the effect of the temperature in the room where the measurements are being made on the resulting measurements is known. A correction factor can be applied to measurements made in this environment. If they are too high, a constant can be subtracted from them; and if they are too low, a constant can be added to them. The most direct way to control for the effects of environmental factors is to use instrumentation measurement schemes in environments that conform to manufacturers' recommendations.

The third subclass of systematic errors are *observational errors*. Different persons measuring the same phenomenon with the same instrumentation under identical environmental conditions will not necessarily produce duplicate results. An observer may consistently record values from a VU meter that are higher or lower than they should be because of the angle at which he or she views the meter. For these values to be accurate, the meter must be read from directly in front. If it is viewed at an angle, the indicator may appear to be pointing to a different number on the scale than that which it would appear to be pointing to if it were viewed from in front. (You can prove this to yourself by viewing the minute hand on a wrist watch from various angles and noting the numbers [or gradations] to which it appears to be pointing.) This source of error can be reduced or eliminated by having measurements made by more than one observer and by using the average of the measurements made of a particular phenomenon as the measure of that phenomenon.

The third, and final, classification of measurement error based on Stout's scheme is *random error*. The sources of this type of error were described at the beginning of this chapter and in Chapter 5.

Schemes That Utilize Psychological or Educational Measuring Instruments

Speech pathologists and audiologists have used a great many psychological and educational measuring instruments, or tasks, to facilitate the observation and quantification of attributes of communicative behavior. The performance of such a task permits the target attribute either to stand out sufficiently from other behavioral attributes or to occur at an appropriate time for it to be observed and measured. If, for example, the target attribute were "accuracy of articulation of certain consonant phonemes in initial, medial, and final positions in words," having a child respond to the stimulus items on a picture articulation test would make it possible for the production of these phonemes in the desired contexts to be observed at an "appropriate" time and their accuracy assessed. On the other hand, if the target attribute were "level of ability to comprehend spoken words," performance on the *Peabody Picture Vocabulary Test* (Dunn, 1959) might provide useful information. Finally, if the target attribute were "approach to coping with a 'new' situation," observing a person's approach to the Rorschach "inkblot" test (Rorschach, 1942) could provide useful clues to that person's habitual manner of responding to such situations. Does the person, for example, study each blot carefully and then give a few "good" associations, or does the person begin to give associations (some "good" and some "bad") machine-gun fashion almost immediately after being presented with each stimulus blot?

The numerals (i.e., scores) assigned to target behavioral attributes by psychological and educational test instruments may be on any level of measurement. However, while such scores could have nominal, ordinal, interval, ratio, or logarithmic properties, they rarely exceed those for ordinal measurement. The intervals between them (with regard to the attribute being measured) are usually not equal *throughout the range of possible scores*, and they are usually not related to an absolute zero. Interpretations of the magnitudes of the differences between test scores, therefore, have to be made with considerable caution. Because one child's performance on an articulation test improved by four points while a second child's performance on the same test improved by two points does not necessarily mean that the first child's articulation improved twice as much as the second child's. In fact, it may not even be true that the first child's articulation improved more than the second child's. The first child's four-point increase may have resulted from learning to produce /s/ blends in the initial positions in words, while the second child's two point increase may have resulted from learning to produce /s/ and /r/ correctly in the initial positions of words. Regardless of the score differences, many speech pathologists would probably regard the second child as having improved more than the first.

Test scores, like all numerals assigned to attributes of events, are subject both to random and to systematic measurement error. The sources of random and systematic error which influence test scores are the same as those indicated for instrumentation measurement schemes, i.e., gross errors, systematic errors, and random errors.

Gross errors include mistakes in reading test and subtest scores and in recording such scores. Recording subtest scores incorrectly on a test profile summary sheet or a data sheet would be an example of such an error. Scores could be recorded incorrectly either because they are misread or because they are written down incorrectly (e.g., numbers are transposed).

Systematic errors, as previously indicated, are of three types: instrumental errors, environmental errors, and observational errors. *Instrumental errors* include those that result from shortcomings of the test instrument. Age norms developed for interpreting test scores, for example, may not be accurate. If the normative group used to standardize a language development scale was not representative of the population of which it was supposed to have been representative, scores from this scale may be consistently interpreted as indicating higher (or lower) language ages than would be the case. Hence language age estimates based on this scale would be biased.

Instrumental errors also include those resulting from *misuse* of test instruments. If an educational or psychological test is not administered according to the instructions in the test manual, the scores obtained may be systematically higher (or lower) than they should be.

Environmental errors include those due to factors external to the device which influence the accuracy of measurements made with it. If a test were administered in an environment that caused the testee to become "anxious," this could cause his score to be lower than it would have been in a relatively "relaxed" environment.

Observational errors include those which result from differences in internal standards among test administrators. All testers would not necessarily evaluate a given test performance in the same manner. A response that one tester would consider to be "within normal limits" another may regard as "not within normal limits." One tester may classify a slightly lateralized /s/ production on an articulation test as "within normal limits" and another may classify it as "not within normal limits." Thus, one tester may consistently identify higher percentages of children as having a lateral lisp than would another.

The third, and final, source of error that can influence test scores is *random error*. While this type of error, as previously indicated, will not bias measurements (i.e., cause them to be consistently higher or lower than they should be), it will reduce their reliability. One source of random error in a test situation may be inconsistency of response by the testee to the test stimuli. It *sometimes* is possible to reduce this source of error by administering test items more than once.

MEASUREMENT SCHEMES THAT RELY PRIMARILY UPON OBSERVER JUDGMENT: PSYCHOLOGICAL SCALING METHODS

This section will describe in considerable detail the use of psychological scaling methods for quantifying observable aspects of communicative behavior. It considers psychological scaling methods as measurement schemes, describes six representative psychological scaling methods, and, finally, deals with the design of scaling experiments, including:

1. preparation of auditory and visual stimuli for scaling,
2. considerations in writing instructions to judges,
3. considerations in the selection of a judging panel,
4. modes of stimulus presentation, and
5. analysis of judges' ratings.

This section attempts to provide information needed both to interpret the results of experiments in which scaling methods are used and to design such experiments.

Need for Psychological Scaling Techniques in Speech and Hearing Research

We will attempt to indicate the need for psychological scaling techniques in speech and hearing research through answers to the following questions:

1. What are the *purposes* of scaling techniques?
2. What can scaling techniques *do* for a researcher interested in speech and hearing?
3. In what ways have scaling techniques been used in speech and hearing research?

Psychological scaling techniques provide a methodology for quantifying a variety of attributes of events of interest to speech pathologists and audiologists with levels of validity and reliability that are sufficiently high for most purposes. An *event* is a phenomenon that occurs in a certain place during a particular interval of time. All events have attributes, or measurable properties. Speech can be classified as an event, since it is a "phenomenon that occurs in a certain place during a particular interval of time." Since all events have attributes, or measurable properties, what are the attributes of the event "speech" and how are they defined? Literally hundreds of attributes of speech have been delineated. (To prove this to yourself, examine the indices of representative speech pathology and speech science texts.) Most have been defined on the basis of observer judgment. In fact, they *are* observer judgments. The observer is the "instrument" by which such attributes are abstracted from the speech signal. After an attribute of this type has been identified, investigators may attempt to identify the physical attributes of the speech signal that results in observers detecting it. They may even attempt to synthesize the configuration of physical attributes they identify (through the use of a computer) and have observers listen to the synthesized signal to determine whether they detect the target attribute. An example of an attribute that has been studied in this manner is hypernasality. This attribute was initially detected in the speech signal by observers and hence was an observer judgment. Later, investigators attempted to identify the physical aspects of the speech signal that cause observers to hear hypernasality and to generate a synthesized signal base on the aspects identified. The taped synthesized signal was then played for groups of observers to determine whether it sounded hypernasal to them. Since hypernasality is an observer judgment, it follows that the most valid indicator of its presence would be observer judgment.

If you are willing to accept the assumption that at least some attributes of speech events are observer judgments—i.e., are the result of the interaction between the observer and the speech event—then for an instrumentation scheme for measuring, or quantifying, such attributes to have *at least* face validity (or appear intuitively to be valid), it would have to involve observer judgment. It would have to require one or more observers to indicate in some manner the amount of the target attribute present in each speech stimulus. Thus, the observer (or panel of observers) would function as a "measuring instrument" with his or her (their) judgments being the "readout." This readout can be of any type that reflects the relative amount of the target attribute present in the stimuli, including words, numbers, and marks on a line.

Psychological scaling techniques are methodologies that can be used for "measuring" the relative amounts of target attributes present in speech events through the use of observer judgments. With these methodologies, an observer (or panel of observers) is instructed to indicate in some manner the relative amount of a target attribute present in each of a group of stimuli (e.g., speech segments). Since they provide instrumentation measurement schemes in which the readout is an observer judgment, these methodologies have *at least face validity* for measuring attributes of speech events which are observer judgments.

Thus in response to the first two questions presented at the beginning of this section, the *purpose* of psychological scaling techniques is to provide methodologies for measuring, or quantifying, attributes of events which are observer judgments. Such techniques can *do* a great deal for investigators in speech and hearing, since many attributes of events of interest to speech pathologists and audiologists are observer judgments.

How have psychological scaling techniques been used in speech and hearing research? What attributes have they been used to measure, or quantify? Due in large part to the pioneering methodological research of Professor Dorothy Sherman of the University of Iowa, psychological scaling methods have been used for quantifying numerous attributes of speech events. A partial list of such attributes is presented in Table 7.1. This list was compiled from a search of the first thirteen volumes of the *Journal of Speech and Hearing Research* for papers in which psychological scaling methods had been used. It includes most of the attributes that were scaled in the studies reported in these papers. The studies cited in Table 7.1, in addition to indicating applications that have been made of psychological scaling methods in speech and hearing research, provide information that could be useful to investigators who wish to rate a set of stimuli for one or more of the attributes listed. Aspects of the scaling methodologies used by the investigators in the studies cited may be utilized by other investigators who wish to quantify these same attributes.

Psychological Scaling Methods as Measuring Instruments

Psychological scaling methods are measuring instruments in the same sense that rulers and thermometers are, because they result in numerals being assigned to attributes of events which have certain "logical" characteristics (see Chapter 6). They have these characteristics because of the rules that are used to assign them. As indicated in Chapter 6, the rules used to assign numerals to attributes of events determine the meaning of the numerals—i.e., the "level of measurement" of the scale which they define. A *scale* consists of a succession or progression of steps or degrees, or a graduated series of categories. The "rules" incorporated into the six psychological scaling methods to be discussed *theoretically* result in one of three types of scales: ordinal, interval, or ratio. (The characteristics of each of these three scale types is described in Chapter 6.) We emphasize "theoretically" to highlight

TABLE 7.1. Representative attributes of events of interest to speech pathologists and audiologists that have been quantified by means of psychological scaling methods.

Attribute	References
Abstraction of words, level of	II, 161
Articulation defectiveness, severity of	III, 191; III, 303
Articulation proficiency, degree of	VI, 49
Bizarreness, degree of	XII, 246
Breathiness, severity of	XII, 246; XII, 747
Difficulty of listening to compressed speech, degree of	XI, 875
Effeminate voice quality, degree of	IX, 590
Esophageal speech, acceptability of	X, 417
Favorability of description, degree of	X, 339
Force or strain while speaking, degree of	IV, 281
Foreign dialect, degree of	VIII, 43
General merit of speech sample, degree of	IX, 248; IX, 323
Harshness, severity of	I, 155; I, 344; XII, 246
Hoarseness, severity of	XII, 246
Intelligibility, degree of	XII, 246
Language development, level of	X, 41; X, 828
Language usage, intricacy of	XI, 837
Lipreading ability, level of	II, 340
Loudness, level of	XII, 103; XII, 246
Moment of nonfluency, severity of	I, 132
Nasal emission, severity of	XII, 246
Nasality, degree of	I, 383; II, 40; II, 113; IV, 381; V, 103; X, 549; XI, 553; XII, 246
Preference, degree of	I, 86; V, 370
Pitch, level of	XII, 246; XII, 747
Pitch variability, degree of	XII, 747
Quality of EDR audiometric records, level of	IV, 41
Representativeness to intended vowel, degree of	IV, 203
Rhythm pattern, normality of	IV, 281
Roughness, degree of	XII, 330
Sibilant intensity, level of	XII, 747
Similarity, degree of	VI, 239; VII, 310; VIII, 23; X, 225
Social adequacy, degree of	V, 79
Speaking rate, normality of	IV, 281; XII, 246; XII, 747
Stress, normality of	XII, 246
Stuttering severity, degree of	I, 40; I, 61; V, 256; V, 332; VI, 91; VIII, 263; VIII, 401; XIII, 360
Vowel imitation, abruptness of	I, 344

(Roman numerals refer to volumes of the *Journal of Speech and Hearing Research;* Arabic numbers, to the first pages of papers in which the attributes were scaled.)

the fact that psychological scaling methods do not always result in numerals, or ratings, that possess the characteristics they are supposed to possess (i.e., achieve the level of measurement they are supposed to achieve). There are several reasons why this may be the case. One of the commonest is the inability of observers to assign numerals, or rate the stimuli, in the manner in which they are instructed.

To illustrate how psychological scaling methods are used to assign numerals to attributes of events, we will discuss the following six, which are representative, from this frame of reference: paired, or pair, comparisons (Edwards, 1957); rank order, or order of merit (Guilford, 1954); equal-appearing intervals, or category scaling (Edwards, 1957); successive intervals, or successive categories, or graded dichotomies (Edwards, 1957); constant sums (Guilford, 1954); and direct magnitude-estimation (Prather, 1960). These methods, incidently, are the ones that have been used most frequently in speech and hearing research.

Paired (Pair) Comparisons. With this method, which theoretically results in an ordinal scale, all possible pairs of stimuli are compared to an *internally generated standard* (or scale) for the attribute being rated, or scaled, and the stimuli in each pair are ordered on the basis of the amount of the attribute which each is judged to possess. The task is performed by a group, or panel, of observers. Each observer is presented with all possible ordered pairings (i.e., permutations) of the stimuli to be scaled. The number of such pairings that will result from a set of stimuli of a given size (N) can be determined by multiplying the number of stimuli by the number of stimuli minus one, or

$$N(N-1)$$

For a set of 10 stimuli, the number of pairs rated would be

$$N(N-1) = 10(10-1) = 90$$

and for a set of 100 stimuli it would be

$$N(N-1) = 100(100-1) = 9900$$

Note how the number of pairs increases dramatically as the number of stimuli increases.

Observers are told to indicate the stimulus in each pair which possesses the greater amount of the attribute being scaled, or rated. They perform this task by comparing the amount of the target attribute they observe in each of the two stimuli in a pair to their internal standard, or scale, for that attribute. For example, an observer who was presented with speech segments from two persons who have hypernasal speech and was asked to indicate which was most hypernasal would perform this task by comparing the level of hypernasality he perceived in the two segments to his internal standard, or scale, for degree of hypernasality and, on the basis of these comparisons, would indicate which segment is most hypernasal.

Rank Order (Order of Merit). With this method, which theoretically results in an ordinal scale, sets of stimuli are compared to an internally generated standard, or scale, for the attribute being rated, and the stimuli in the set are ordered on the basis of the amount of the target attribute they are judged to possess. The task is performed by a group, or panel, of observers. Each observer is presented with the set of stimuli and is told to rank order them on the basis of the amounts of the target attribute which they possess. He is instructed to indicate the ordering of the stimuli by assigning the numeral to each stimulus which designates its position. The highest numeral assigned (N) is equal to the number of stimuli being ordered. Observers may be instructed to assign either 1 or N to the stimulus possessing the greatest amount of the target attribute. They rank order the stimuli by comparing the amount of the target attribute they perceive in each to their internal standard, or scale, for that attribute. For example, an observer who was presented with speech segments from five persons who have hypernasal speech and was told to order them on the basis of the amount of hypernasality they possess (with 1 designating least hypernasality and 5 designating most) would perform this task by comparing the level of hypernasality he perceived in the five segments to his internal standard, or scale, for degree of hypernasality and on the basis of these comparisons indicate the ordering of the stimuli.

This method can be viewed as an extension of the method of paired comparisons. The only real difference in the judging task is that observers are required to order N rather than two stimuli.

Equal-Appearing Intervals (Category Scaling). With this method, which theoretically results in an interval scale, each of a set of stimuli is compared to an internally generated scale, or continuum, for the attribute being rated, which is *divided into a specified number of equal-size segments* (usually 5, 7, 9, or 11), and the numeral is assigned to it that designates the segment of the internally generated continuum which corresponds to the amount of the attribute it is judged to possess. The task is performed by a group, or panel, or observers. Stimuli are presented to observers one at a time. Observers are instructed to assign the numeral between 1 and the number that corresponds to the number of points on the scale (e.g., 7) to each stimulus that indicates the amount of the target attribute it possesses. They are informed that the scale is one of equal intervals—from 1 to 7 (or some other value)—with 1 representing the least possible amount of the target attribute and 7 (or some other value) representing the greatest possible amount; 4 (or some other median value) represents the midpoint between 1 and 7 with respect to the attribute, with the other numbers falling at *equal distances* along the scale. For example, an observer who was presented with speech segments from five persons who have hypernasal speech and was told to assign a numeral to each on the basis of the amount of hypernasality present (with 1 designating least possible hypernasality, 7 designating most possible hypernasality, and the numbers between falling at equal distances along the scale) would perform this task by comparing the amount of hypernasality he perceived in each speech segment to each of the seven segments of his internal scale for degree of hypernasality and on the basis of these comparisons assign each a numeral between 1 and 7. Observers may assign the same numeral to two or more speech segments. They would rate in such a manner if they felt the degree of hypernasality present in the segments fell within the same segment of their internal scales for hypernasality.

Successive Intervals (Successive Categories; Graded Dichotomies). With this method, which theoretically results in an interval scale, each of a set of stimuli is compared to an internally generated scale, or continuum, for the attribute being rated, which is divided into a specified number of segments (usually, 5, 7, 9, or 11) that are *not necessarily of equal size*, and the numeral is assigned to it that designates the segment of the internally generated continuum that corresponds to the amount of the attribute it is judged to possess. The task is performed by a group, or panel, of observers. Stimuli are presented to observers one at a time. Observers are instructed to assign the numeral between 1 and the number which corresponds to the number of points on the scale (e.g., 7) to each stimulus which indicates the amount of the target attribute it possesses. They are informed that the scale contains a specified number of points which range from 1 to 7 (or some other value). In some instances, each point on the scale is *anchored*, or defined, and in others only the extremes are anchored. A seven-point scale (that could be used for assessing attitudes toward statements) on which each point is anchored is illustrated by the following:

_____	:	_____	:	_____	:	_____	:	_____	:	_____	:	_____
Completely Disagree (1)		Mostly Disagree (2)		Slightly Disagree (3)		Undecided (4)		Slightly Agree (5)		Mostly Agree (6)		Completely Agree (7)

On the other hand, such a scale may have only the extremes anchored:

Strongly Disagree _____	:	_____	:	_____	:	_____	:	_____	:	_____	:	_____ Strongly Agree
	1		2		3		4		5		6	7

For example, an observer who was presented with speech segments from five persons who have hypernasal speech and was asked to assign a numeral between 1 and 7 to each on the basis of the amount of hypernasality exhibited by the speaker with the points on the scale defined as

1. no hypernasality,
2. extremely mild hypernasality,
3. mild hypernasality,
4. moderate hypernasality,
5. moderately severe hypernasality,
6. severe hypernasality, and
7. extremely severe hypernasality,

would perform this task by comparing the amount of hypernasality he perceived in each speech segment to that designated by each of the seven modifiers on his internal scale of hypernasality and on the basis of these comparisons assign each a numeral between 1 and 7. The observer may assign the same numeral to two or more speech segments if he feels the amount of hypernasality present in them is designated by the same modifier.

The primary difference between the methods of equal-appearing intervals and successive intervals is the assumption made regarding the sizes of the segments of the internally generated scale for the attribute. With the method of equal-appearing intervals, these segments are assumed to be of equal size (e.g., the difference in degree of nasality between a speaker assigned the numeral 2 and a speaker assigned the numeral 3 is equal to that between a speaker assigned the numeral 3 and a speaker assigned the numeral 4, etc.). With the method of successive intervals, no assumption is made regarding the relative sizes of segment widths; the segment widths are estimated from the data.

Constant Sums. With this method, which theoretically results in a *ratio* scale, *all possible pairs* of stimuli are compared to an internally generated scale for the attribute being rated, and a judgment is made regarding the relative amount of the attribute possessed by each member of each pair. The proportion of 100 points is then assigned to each of the stimuli in each pair which reflects the relative amount of the attribute possessed by each member of each pair. The points assigned to the stimuli in each pair always total 100. To illustrate this method, suppose that one of the stimuli in a pair was judged to possess twice as much of a target attribute (e.g., nasality) as the other. The former would be assigned 67 points and the latter 33 points.

The task is performed by a group, or panel, of observers. Each observer is presented with all possible ordered pairings (i.e., permutations) of the stimuli to be scaled. The number of such pairings which will result from a set of stimuli of a given size (N) can be determined by multiplying the number of stimuli by the number of stimuli minus one, or

$$N(N-1)$$

Note that the manner of presentation of stimuli to observers is the same as for the method of pair comparisons.

Observers are told to indicate for each pair of stimuli both the stimulus that possesses the greater amount of the target attribute and the *ratio* of the amount of the attribute this stimulus possesses in relation to that possessed by the other stimulus through proportional point assignments to the two stimuli. (Note that the first part of the judging task is the same as for the method of pair comparisons.) They perform this task by comparing the amount of the target attribute they observe in each of the two stimuli in a pair to their internal scale for that attribute. For example, an observer who was presented with speech segments from two persons who have hypernasal speech and was asked to indicate how much more hypernasal the most hypernasal speaker was than the least hypernasal speaker (through a proportional assignment of 100 points) would perform this task by comparing the levels of hypernasality he perceived in the two segments to his internal scale for degree of hypernasality, and on the basis of these comparisons would make the point assignments. Observers could make any point assignments they wished as long as the points totaled 100 and portrayed the ratio of degree of hypernasality exhibited by the two speakers.

Direct Magnitude-Estimation. With this method, which theoretically results in a ratio scale, each of a set of stimuli is compared *to a point* on an internally generated scale, or continuum, for the attribute being rated, and a numeral is assigned to each stimulus which designates the relative amount of the attribute that it possesses as compared to the amount of the attribute at that point on the internally generated scale. If the point on the internally generated scale that is serving as the standard were assigned a value of 100 points, and a stimulus to be rated were judged to possess three times the amount of the attribute as the standard, it would be assigned 300 points. If a stimulus, on the other hand, were judged to possess one-half as much of the attribute as the standard, it would be assigned 50 points.

The rating task is performed by a group, or panel, of observers. Stimuli are presented one at a time. The observers are presented with a stimulus of the type they will be rating to use as a standard, prior to beginning the rating task. The amount of the target attribute present in this stimulus is assigned a value of 100 points. The observers are instructed to assign the number of points to each stimulus which represents the relative amount of the target attribute it possesses with reference to that possessed by the standard stimulus. If, for example, the observers felt a stimulus possessed *twice* the amount of the target attribute as the standard stimulus, they would assign it 200 points. If, on the other hand, they felt it possessed only *half* the amount of the target attribute as the standard, they would assign it 50 points. They can use any point assignment they feel appropriate. They need not limit themselves to even fractions and even multiples of the 100 points assigned to the standard. They can use any point assignment they choose as long as it represents their judgment of the amount of the target attribute possessed by a stimulus in relation to that possessed by the standard. If, for example, observers were presented with speech segments from five persons who have hypernasal speech and were told to assign points to each on the basis of the amount of hypernasality each possesses in relation to that present in the speech segment of a sixth person (standard) which is assigned 100 points, they would perform this task by comparing the amount of hypernasality they perceived in each speech segment they were asked to rate and in the standard segment to their internal scale for degree of hypernasality, and on the basis of these comparisons they would assign each stimulus a number of points. The standard would serve as an *anchor* to align their internal scales of hypernasality. They can assign the same number of points to two or more speech segments if they feel the speakers in these segments exhibit the same amounts of hypernasality.

Considerations in the Choice of a Scaling Method

Six scaling methods were described in the previous section. How do you decide which to use for quantifying a particular attribute of a particular set of stimuli? A number of factors should be considered when making such a decision, including: (1) minimum level of measurement required, (2) number of stimuli to be rated, (3) maximum number of judges available, (4) age and intelligence level of judges, (5) computational ease, (6) maximum length of judging session, (7) necessity that ratings for stimuli scaled at different times be comparable, (8) statistical sophistication of the audience to whom the results are to be reported, (9) duration of individual stimuli, (10) effort involved in preparation of stimuli, and (11) judges' reactions to the scaling task. We will discuss each as it relates to the choice among the six scaling methods that have been described.

Minimum Level of Measurement Required. The question of concern here is whether the minimum acceptable level of measurement for judges' ratings is ordinal, interval, or ratio. This level usually can be inferred from the *kinds of statements* you want to be able to make about the ratings or the *kinds of questions* you want to be able to answer using them. If, for example, you decided to rate "before and after" therapy speech samples for degree of articulation defectiveness and you wanted to make a judgment from these ratings on whether the clients' articulation was *less defective* after therapy than before it, only *ordinal* measurement would be required. On the other hand, if you wanted to be able to make a judgment regarding the *amount of reduction* in articulation defectiveness following therapy (assuming there was such a reduction), *interval* measurement would be required.

Any of the six scaling methods can be used if only *ordinal* measurement is required. They have been empirically demonstrated to order sets of stimuli in the same manner. The orderings of sets of stimuli based on ratings derived through the use of combinations of these six scaling methods have been reported by a number of investigators. References to representative studies in which combinations of the six methods are compared are presented in Table 7.2.

TABLE 7.2. Comparisons between scale values (i.e., average ratings) for sets of stimuli rated by two or more of the following methods: pair comparisons (PC), rank order (RO), equal-appearing intervals (EAI), successive intervals (SI), constant sums (CS), and direct magnitude-estimation (DME).

Methods Compared	References
PC & CS	Senn and Manley, 1966; Sherman and Moodie, 1957.
PC & RO	Barnhart, 1936; Barrett, 1914; Barlett, Heerman, and Rettig, 1960; King and Lau, 1963; Misra and Dutt, 1965.
PC & EAI	Barlett, Heerman, and Rettig, 1960; Crawford, 1965; Hevner, 1930; Hicks and Campbell, 1965; Kelley, *et al*, 1955; Saffir, 1937; Sherman and Moodie, 1957.
PC & SI	Hicks and Campbell, 1965; King and Lau, 1963; Saffir, 1937; Sherman and Moodie, 1957.
PC & DME	Kuennapas and Wikstroem, 1963; Prather, 1960.
CS & EAI	Sherman and Moodie, 1957.
CS & SI	Dudek, 1959; Sherman and Moodie, 1957.
CS & DME	Prather, 1960.
RO & EAI	Bartlett, Heerman, and Rettig, 1960.
RO & SI	King and Lau, 1963.
EAI & SI	Hicks and Campbell, 1965; Saffir, 1937; Sherman and Moodie, 1957; Sherman and Silverman, 1968; Silverman and Sherman, 1967.
EAI & DME	Cullinan, Prather, and Williams, 1963; Eisler, 1962; Eisler, 1963; Ekman and Kunnapas, 1960, 1963; Engen and McBurney, 1964; Galanter, 1962; Galanter and Messick, 1961; Perloe, 1963; Pfeiffer and Siegel, 1966; Prather, 1960; Sherman and Silverman, 1968; Stevens and Galanter, 1957; Stevens and Stone, 1959.
SI & DME	Prather, 1960; Sherman and Silverman, 1968.

If the minimum level of measurement required is *interval*, then equal-appearing intervals, successive intervals, constant sums, or direct magnitude-estimation could be used. If observers perform the rating tasks *as instructed*, these methods should result in ratings that have properties which *approximate* (or come close to achieving) interval level measurement.

If *ratio* measurement is required, either constant sums or direct magnitude-estimation can be used. Both methods should result in ratings with properties approximating those for ratio level measurement *if* the observers perform the rating tasks as instructed.

Number of Stimuli to be Rated. If the number of stimuli to be rated were fewer than 10, this probably would not be an important consideration. However, if this number exceeds 10, three of the scaling methods (i.e., pair comparisons, rank order, and constant sums) may not be practical. The reason for pair comparisons and constant sums is that too many stimulus pairs may have to be rated. As I have already indicated, the number of stimulus pairs that have to be rated when these methods are used is the product of the number of stimuli times this number minus one, or

$$N(N-1)$$

For 20 stimuli, the number of stimulus pairs would be 20(20 − 1), or 380. Obtaining 380 ratings would probably be too time-consuming in many instances. Pair comparisons and constant sums would rarely be practical when the number of stimuli to be scaled exceeded 50.

The method of rank order may not be practical to use when the number of stimuli to be scaled exceeds 10, because it may be quite difficult for an observer to keep in mind the amount of the attribute possessed by each stimulus while ordering them. This is particularly likely to be the case when the stimuli, or events, to be ordered are auditory (e.g., speech segments).

Maximum Number of Judges Available. Some scaling methods require larger panels than others to achieve scale values that possess a given level of reliability. Equal-appearing intervals, for example, tends to require fewer judges to achieve scale values that have a given level of reliability than does direct magnitude-estimation. Also, a variation of direct magnitude-estimation in which an interval rather than a point standard is used (referred to as direct interval-estimation) appears to require fewer raters than direct magnitude-estimation to achieve scale values which have a given level of reliability (Silverman and Johnston, 1975).

Age and Intelligence Level of the Judges. Some rating tasks are more difficult than others. The task associated with the method of pair comparisons probably would be easier for children and for adults with below-normal intelligence than those associated with the other scaling methods.

Computational Ease. Some scaling methods require less computation than others to derive scale values. Equal-appearing interval scale values, for example, require less computation than successive interval scale values. While computational ease probably would not be one of the first considerations in selecting a scaling method, it nevertheless would probably make sense if two or more methods would serve *equally well* to select the one which requires the least amount of computation.

Maximum Length of Judging Session. The number of stimuli that can be rated in a given amount of time is different for different methods. Fewer stimuli can be rated in a given amount of time with pair comparisons and constant sums than with the other methods. Equal-appearing intervals, successive intervals, and direct magnitude-estimation would probably require approximately the same amount of time to rate a given number of stimuli. The time required for rank order is apt to be longer than for equal-appearing intervals, successive intervals, or direct magnitude-estimation, particularly if the number of stimuli to be ranked is relatively large or the differences in the amounts of the target attribute they possess are relatively small.

Necessity that Ratings for Stimuli Scaled at Different Times Be Comparable. With some scaling methods, the rating assigned to a stimulus to indicate the amount of the target attribute it possesses is apt to be influenced by the amount of that attribute present in the other stimuli with which it is rated. This is almost certain to be a problem when the methods of pair comparison, constant sums, and rank order are used. If it is necessary for ratings for stimuli scaled at different times to be comparable, the safest method to use probably would be direct magnitude-estimation (assuming the same standard stimulus is used for rating all stimuli).

Statistical Sophistication of the Audience to Whom the Results Are to Be Communicated. Some scaling methods require a better statistical background to understand intuitively than do others. Equal-appearing intervals, for example, would not require as much statistical sophistication to understand as would successive intervals. While this would not usually be one of the main considerations in the choice of a scaling method, if two or more methods would be equally appropriate for a particular purpose, it would probably make sense to choose the one requiring the least statistical sophistication to understand.

Duration of Individual Stimuli. The duration of individual stimuli may be a relevant consideration in the choice of a scaling method, particularly with regard to the practicality of pair comparisons and constant sums. If their duration is relatively long, the judges may not be able to remember both members of a pair well enough to make a pair comparison or constant sum rating that is adequately reliable. Also, if their duration is relatively long, the number of stimuli that could be rated in a given period of time by these methods may be too few to be practical.

Judges' Reactions to the Scaling Task. Observers' "levels of belief" in their abilities to perform rating tasks is apt not to be a constant. They would probably be more confident of their ability to make pair comparison judgments than direct magnitude-estimation judgments. If they do not believe they can perform the rating task they are asked to perform, they may not try too hard and their ratings may not be adequately reliable.

Preparation of Auditory and Visual Stimuli for Scaling

Once the scaling method has been selected, the next step is to prepare the stimuli for scaling. Since most of the stimuli scaled by speech pathologists and audiologists have been auditory—i.e., speech events or other acoustic signals recorded on audiotape—this discussion will emphasize the preparation of such stimuli for scaling. Most of the comments will be relevant, however, to the preparation of other types of stimuli for scaling, including videotaped stimuli.

A number of factors must be considered in preparing audiotaped stimuli for scaling, including: (1) method of assembling the tape (i.e., splicing versus dubbing), (2) ordering of the stimuli, (3) duration of the "judging interval" between stimuli, (4) selection, frequency of occurrence, and location of the standard stimuli, (5) definition and selection of stimuli, (6) equating stimuli for extraneous attributes, (7) numbering stimuli, (8) acquainting judges with the range of the target attribute present in the stimuli, and (9) determining the number of times each stimulus is to be presented. Comments relevant to each consideration are presented in the paragraphs that follow.

Method of Assembling. Two methods can be used to prepare audiotaped stimuli for scaling. The first is *splicing* together the segments of tape on which the stimuli were recorded. The second is *dubbing* the stimuli on to a master tape. The splicing method obviously cannot be used when a stimulus has to appear more than once on a master tape (as it would for pair comparisons and constant sums). The main limitation of the dubbing process is that some distortion of the signal is introduced by it. In many cases, this distortion would probably not be of sufficient magnitude to influence observers' ratings of the target attribute. While it would be unlikely to influence stuttering severity ratings it may influence voice quality ratings.

Ordering of the Stimuli. The ordering of stimuli on the master tape should be random—i.e., determined by a table of random numbers (see

Appendix B). If there is a possibility of order or sequence effects (see Chapter 5) influencing the ratings, these effects could be controlled for, at least partially, by preparing several randomizations of the stimuli. Since the possibility of order and sequence effects often cannot be ruled out, it is not desirable for all members of a panel to rate a set of stimuli in the same order.

Duration of the "Judging Interval" between Stimuli. This refers to the time interval following the presentation of a stimulus during which it is rated. It must be long enough to permit the judges to make their ratings with adequate levels of validity and reliability, but not so long that it will unnecessarily extend the length of the judging session. An interval duration of approximately 15 seconds appears to be adequate for rating most attributes of audiotaped speech stimuli.

Selection, Frequency of Occurrence, and Location of the Standard Stimuli. Standard stimuli serve as anchor, or reference, points on a scale. They help to reduce intrarater and interrater variability. They usually are used with the method of direct magnitude-estimation. Standard stimuli also are used occasionally with the methods of equal-appearing intervals and successive intervals.

Several decisions must be made if standard stimuli are to be used: (1) which stimulus (for direct magnitude-estimation), or which stimuli (for equal-appearing intervals and successive intervals), to select, (2) how often to present the stimulus, or stimuli, and (3) at what points during the rating session to present the stimulus, or stimuli (i.e., at the beginning only, or at the beginning and periodically during the session). With direct magnitude-estimation, a stimulus is usually selected for the standard in which the amount of the attribute is at the approximate midpoint of the range (based on the judgment of the experimenter or that of a small panel of observers). Theoretically, the "location" of the standard in the range of possible values of the attribute should not influence the characteristics of the scale resulting from its use. As long as the scale is regarded as ordinal, this would probably be a safe assumption to make. However, if it is regarded as having interval or ratio properties, this assumption would be risky to make, since there is some evidence that suggests that the location of the standard used to construct a scale by the method of direct magnitude-estimation influences to some extent the spacings between points on that scale. For this reason, it would probably be most defensible to interpret direct magnitude-estimation scale values as if they had ordinal properties.

In scaling tape-recorded stimuli with the method of direct magnitude-estimation, the standard stimulus usually appears two or three times (one after the other) at the beginning of the tape on which the stimuli are recorded. The standard may also appear on this tape after every third or fourth stimulus. Hence the sequence of stimuli on a tape could be:

1. Standard Stimulus
2. Standard Stimulus
3. Standard Stimulus
4. Stimulus #1
5. Stimulus #2
6. Stimulus #3
7. Standard Stimulus
8. Stimulus #4
9. Stimulus #5
10. Stimulus #6
11. Standard Stimulus
    etc.

The more abstract or vague the target attribute, the more frequently the standard stimulus should be presented.

With the method of equal-appearing intervals and the method of successive intervals, if individual scale points are not defined, two stimuli are selected for the standard which represent the *extremes* of the range of possible values of the target attribute. It is crucial that the amounts of the target attribute present in these stimuli represent the extremes of the continuum. Otherwise, there may be an *end effect*, i.e., a piling up of ratings in one or both of the extreme intervals. Both stimuli that have a value of the target attribute *equal* to that in the standard and *exceeding* that in the standard will be assigned the most extreme ratings. (Such ratings on a seven-point scale would be 1 and 7.) Standard stimuli are often not used with these methods because of the difficulty in identifying stimuli that represent the extremes of the range of possible values of the target attribute. The extremes of the scale in such cases are usually defined verbally, e.g.,

$1 =$ *least* hypernasality and $7 =$ *most* hypernasality

or

$1 =$ *lowest* stuttering severity and $7 =$ *highest* stuttering severity

When standard stimuli are used with these scaling methods, they usually are presented several times at the beginning of the stimulus tape and after every third or fourth stimulus.

Definition and Selection of Stimuli. This is not a problem in many scaling experiments because the events, or stimuli, to be rated have "natural" boundaries. (Examples of events that can be treated as such are phonemes, syllables, and words.) This can present a problem, however, when the events to be rated do not have "natural" boundaries, e.g., conversational speech segments. To illustrate this point, suppose you wished to rate "before and after" therapy conversational speech segments for degree of nasality or degree of stuttering severity. How long a speech segment would be required to obtain ratings which are adequately reliable? Would 20-second segments be adequate? The answers to these questions would depend, in part, on the nature of the attribute being rated. Some attributes could be reliably rated from shorter segments than others. Nasality, for example, could probably be reliably rated from shorter segments than would be required for stuttering severity. Unfortunately, with the exception of a few attributes such as stuttering severity, there are no data in the literature that indicate the shortest segment lengths that can be expected to yield reliable ratings. The only possibly helpful observation from the literature is that in studies where the speech segments rated were 30 seconds in duration, ratings in almost all cases have been reported to be adequately reliable.

After a decision has been made concerning the duration of speech segments, it is then necessary to decide which segments of the available speech samples to rate. This obviously would be of concern only if the available samples were longer in duration than the segment length selected. There are several strategies that can be used for selecting such segments, including the following:

1. Segments are selected by the experimenter. The experimenter chooses segments that he feels are representative. One limitation of this strategy is that the experimenter, without being consciously aware of it, may select segments that instead of being representative would be likely to be rated in a manner consistent with his expectations or hypotheses. (The phenomenon of *experimenter bias* is discussed in several contexts in this book, which may be located by consulting the index.)

2. Segments are selected through the use of a random sampling procedure. The sample could be segmented, for example, into consecutive segments of the length to be rated. (A five-minute sample could be segmented into 10 consecutive, 30-second segments.) These segments would be numbered consecutively, and one or more would be selected by means of a table of random numbers. This sampling strategy is more likely than the first to provide representative samples for rating.

Equating Stimuli for Extraneous Attributes. The stimuli the judges are asked to rate may possess a large number (perhaps, an infinite number) of attributes. The judges are usually instructed to attend to only one such attribute (i.e., the target attribute) when making their ratings. Two strategies have been used to *minimize* the impact of other attributes (i.e., extraneous attributes) on these ratings. The first is to instruct the judges to ignore these attributes when making their ratings, and the second is to equate the stimuli for them. Suppose you did not want judges to be influenced by disfluency level when they were rating speech segments for articulation defectiveness. If you used the first approach, you would tell them to ignore disfluency level when making their ratings. If you used the second approach, you would select speech segments in which no disfluency occurred. (If you were using a random sampling procedure for selecting such segments, you could exclude those containing instances of disfluency.)

Numbering Stimuli (or Stimulus Pairs). Each stimulus (or stimulus pair) to be rated is usually given an identification number. If the stimuli are audiotape-recorded speech segments, a carrier phrase and number is recorded on the stimulus tape preceding each segment, e.g., "sample number one." This carrier phrase-number combination performs two functions. First, it maximizes the odds that the judges will record their ratings at the appropriate places on the response sheet. Secondly, it alerts the judges immediately before the presentation of each stimulus, which maximizes the odds they will attend to it.

Acquainting Judges with the Range of the Target Attribute Present in the Stimuli. With equal-appearing intervals, with successive intervals, and sometimes with direct magnitude-estimation, the judges are acquainted with the range of the target attribute present in the stimuli before beginning the rating task. This may be done by presenting 10 or 15 stimuli to them which represent the range of the attribute. It also may be done by presenting all the stimuli to the judges before they begin to rate them.

Determining the Number of Times Each Stimulus Is to Be Presented. It may sometimes be necessary to present a stimulus more than once before asking judges to rate it. If the duration of individual stimuli is relatively short, such as would be the case for isolated phonemes, judges may be unable to get a sufficiently good impression of the target attribute to rate it reliably after hearing them only once. Suppose you wished to rate isolated vowels for nasality. You might dub each vowel on the stimulus tape three times (with a few seconds between presentations) and have judges listen to the three presentations before assigning it a nasality rating.

Considerations in Writing Instructions to Judges

One of the most important tasks associated with designing a scaling experiment is writing the instructions of the judges. The instructions they are given influence both the validity and reliability of their ratings.

The instructions given the judges in scaling experiments usually provide them with three kinds of information: (1) a description of the attribute to be rated, (2) a description of the scaling task, and (3) descriptions of attributes to be ignored. Two representative sets of instructions are reproduced here which include these three kinds of information. The first is for the method of equal-appearing intervals; the second, for the method of direct magnitude-estimation. Both were used for rating the same attribute, i.e., intricacy of language usage (Sherman and Silverman, 1968).

I

You are asked to judge a series of samples of children's oral language which are presented in written form. You are to judge each sample in relation to a seven-point scale of "intricacy of language usage." Intricacy of language usage, for the purposes of this experiment, is defined as the intricacy of the arrangement of words for the purpose of conveying information. For example, consider the following four sets of words, which without reference to the specific meanings, might be judged to vary with respect to intricacy of language as defined here:

a) two good little boys
b) boys in your school
c) boys who are orphans
d) really very good boys

Although each of the above sets contains four words, it is obvious that they vary with respect to type of arrangement of words for purposes of conveying information.

Make your judgment on the basis of the whole sample. Avoid being influenced by grammatical correctness; for example, "we was" in place of the correct wording "we were." Obviously, the expressions "we was" and "we were" do not differ with respect to the intricacy of word arrangement. Also, do not give a rating based upon a judgment of the extent of vocabulary; for example, "big size" and "extensive area" are equivalent as far as the intricacy of arrangement is concerned, but they probably would not be considered equivalent if judged for the purpose of rating extent of vocabulary usage.

The scale is one of equal intervals—from 1 to 7—with 1 representing *least* intricacy of language usage and 7 representing *most* intricacy; 4 represents the midpoint between 1 and 7 with respect to intricacy, with the other numbers falling at equal distances along the scale. Do not attempt to place samples between any two of the seven points, but only at these points.

Each language sample is preceded by a number. Your task will be to record your judgment on your response sheet to the right of the identifying number of the language sample.

On the following pages there are 50 samples to be rated on a 7-point scale. The experimenter obtained these samples by requesting the children to respond to a picture stimulus. He also encouraged the children to speak by asking them questions and by making comments, as needed. These questions and comments are not included in the material you are to judge. All of the samples are in response to the same picture.

Before you record any judgments, read quickly the first 25 samples to acquaint yourself with the experimental task and to acquaint yourself with the range of samples with respect to the intricacy of language usage which you are requested to judge.

After you have acquainted yourself with the task and the range, make a judgment on every sample. If you are somewhat doubtful, make a guess as to the most suitable scale position.

II

You are asked to judge a series of samples of children's oral language which are presented in written form. You are to judge each sample for *intricacy of language usage*. You are to estimate the relative intricacy of language usage of each language sample in relation to the intricacy of language usage of a standard sample which you will read before making your estimates. Your task will be to assign the number of points you believe represents the relative intricacy of language usage with reference to the standard sample.

Intricacy of language usage, for the purposes of this experiment, is defined as the intricacy of the arrangement of words for the purpose of conveying information. For example, consider the following four sets of words, which without reference to the specific meanings, might be judged to vary with respect to intricacy of language usage as here defined:

a) two good little boys
b) boys in our school
c) boys who are orphans
d) really good little boys

Although each of the above sets contains four words, it is obvious that they vary with respect to type of arrangement of words for purpose of conveying information.

Make your judgment on the basis of the whole sample. Avoid being influenced by grammatical correctness; for example, "we was" in place of the correct wording "we were." Obviously, the expressions "we was" and "we were" do not differ with respect to the intricacy of word arrangement. Also, do not give a rating based upon a judgment of the extent of vocabulary; for example, "big size" and "extensive area" are equivalent as far as the intricacy of arrangement is concerned, but they probably would not be considered equivalent if judged for the purpose of rating extent of vocabulary.

The following sample is to be used as the *standard sample*.

"That's a grandpa lion and he is sitting down in a chair and he is thinking about something. And he is holding a pipe in his hand. And a little mouse is coming out of the mouse hole. Sneak up on the tiger. Cause he is gonna lay on the tiger's head. He would feel up on his head and he'd feel a mouse up on his head and try to catch him. Well, I would get out of there and crawl under the chair and go through there and run. Run away from him. I would run back under the chair and into my mousehole. He couldn't get under the chair."

You will assign *100 points* to this sample. The point assignments you make on the succeeding samples should represent, with reference to the standard, the relative intricacy of language usage of each sample. For example, if you believe that a sample is *twice* as intricate in language usage as the standard sample, you would assign *200 points* to it. On the other hand, if you believe that a sample is *half* as intricate in language usage as the standard, you would assign it *50 points*. You may, of course, use any point assignment you choose to represent your judgment of the intricacy of language usage. You need not limit yourself to even fractions and even multiples of the 100 points assigned to the standard. You might use, for example, 85, or 65, or 20, or even 57, or 112, or 120, or 215, or any other number you choose as long as it represents your judgment of the intricacy of language usage of the sample in relation to the standard sample.

On the following pages there are 50 samples to be judged in relation to the standard sample. The experimenter obtained these samples by requesting the children to respond to a picture stimulus. He also encouraged the children to speak by asking them questions and making comments, as needed. These questions and comments are not included in the material you are to judge. All of the samples are in response to the same picture.

Each experimental sample is preceded by a number. You are to record your judgments on your response sheet to the right of the identification numbers of the samples. Before you record any judgments, read quickly the first 25 samples to acquaint yourself with the experimental task. As you read think about the point assignments you would make if you were recording judgments. Now read the standard sample once again; record your judgments according to the instructions which have been given. Make a judgment on every sample. If you are somewhat doubtful about what number to assign, make a guess.

In the first set of instructions (for the method of equal-appearing intervals), the first paragraph gives a description of the attribute to be rated; the second, the attributes to be ignored; and the remaining paragraphs, a description of the scaling task. In the second set of instructions (for the method of direct magnitude-estimation), the second paragraph gives a description of the attribute to be rated; the third, the attributes to be ignored; and the remaining paragraphs, a description of the scaling task.

These sets of instructions can be modified fairly easily for rating other attributes of speech (or language) segments. Also, the equal-appearing interval instructions can be used for the method of successive intervals, with minor modifications.

Instructions can be presented to judges in oral or written form. An oral mode of presentation can be either tape-recorded or "live." A written mode is usually typed and duplicated (e.g., mimeographed or photo-offset). These presentation modes are often combined. The experimenter reads the instructions aloud while the judges follow along on their copies. This combined mode may be the most satisfactory one (when it is possible to use it) since some judges would probably better comprehend "heard" than "read" instructions, and vice versa.

The judges usually record their ratings on a response sheet. A representative response sheet is reproduced in Figure 7.10. This response sheet

Approaches to Generating Quantitative Data   151

```
Name_____    Date_____
 1____                                     26____
 2____                                     27____
 3____                                     28____
 4____                                     29____
 5____                                     30____
 6____                                     31____
 7____                                     32____
 8____                                     33____
 9____                                     34____
10____                                     35____
11____                                     36____
12____                                     37____
13____                                     38____
14____                                     39____
15____                                     40____
16____                                     41____
17____                                     42____
18____                                     43____
19____                                     44____
20____                                     45____
21____                                     46____
22____                                     47____
23____                                     48____
24____                                     49____
25____                                     50____
```

FIGURE 7.10. Representative Response Sheet

could be used for all the methods discussed, with the exception of constant sums. For the method of pair comparisons, a 1 or 2 would be recorded in the space to the right of each identification number to designate the stimulus in each pair which possessed the greater amount of the target attribute. For the method of rank order, the number recorded to the right of a stimulus identification number would designate the rank of that stimulus in an ordering. For the methods of equal-appearing intervals and successive intervals, this number would be a numeral that designates a point on a scale (having a finite number of points). And for the method of direct magnitude-estimation, this number would be a magnitude estimate.

To make this response sheet usable for the method of constant sums, it would be necessary to have *two* response spaces to the right of each identification number, i.e.,

$$A \quad B$$
1. _____ _____

The point value assigned to the first stimulus in a pair could be recorded in the *A* space and that assigned to the second member in the *B* space.

Considerations in the Selection of a Judging Panel

All scaling methods require a panel of judges, or raters. Several considerations concerning the selection of judges for a panel will be discussed in this section, including: (1) the number to be used, (2) their characteristics, and (3) the procedure by which they are to be selected.

Number of Judges to Be Used in the Panel. If too few judges are used, the scale values for the stimuli may not be sufficiently reliable for the purposes of the experiment. If too many are used, the panel may be unnecessarily "costly." The added cost here includes: (1) judges' time in performing the rating task, (2) experimenter's time in administering the task, and (3) data analysis time and expense.

There is little in the literature to assist the experimenter in deciding how many judges to use, with the possible exception of information pertaining to the magnitude of reliability coefficients reported for scaling experiments in which different numbers of judges were used (e.g., Edwards, 1957, pp. 94–95). Such information has limited usefulness, since the number of judges required to attain a specific level of reliability would be expected to vary as a function of several factors, including: (1) the degree of ambiguity of the attribute being rated, (2) the complexity of the stimuli, and (3) the extent to which the judges are trained to share a common standard. However, in almost all studies reported in which speech segments were scaled by the methods of equal-appearing intervals, successive intervals, or direct magnitude-estimation and panels of approximately 50 judges were used, the investigators concluded that the resulting scale values were adequately reliable for their purposes. Panels of 50 judges, therefore, probably would be sufficiently large for scaling attributes of speech segments for most purposes.

With the approach described, the size of the judging panel is fixed before beginning the rating task, and the reliability of the scale values is permitted to vary. An alternative approach would be to fix the minimum level of reliability desired for the scale values before beginning the rating task and permitting the size of the judging panel to vary. That is, you would gradually increase the number of judges in the panel until the scale values computed from their ratings would possess a predetermined level of reliability. One such approach, based on the principle of sequential sampling, has been described by Silverman (1968).

Definition of the Population from Which the Panel Is to Be Selected. "Organismic" and related variables such as hearing acuity, visual acuity, intelligence, and previous exposure to the attribute being rated can systematically influence the ratings assigned by the members of a panel. A panel consisting of parents of children who stutter may tend to rate segments of disfluent speech as more abnormal than would a panel consisting of parents of children who do not stutter. Also, a panel of speech pathologists may tend to rate speech segments in which the speaker has a lateral lisp as more abnormal than would a panel consisting of laymen.

If it seems possible that a particular attribute might be rated differently by different subgroups of observers, it would be necessary for the experimenters to define the subgroup they wish to use for their panel. The characteristics of the members of this subgroup would be determined, at least in part, by the purpose to which the ratings were to be put. Suppose an investigator wished to determine whether the speech of severe stutterers would be regarded as less defective if they paced their speech with a miniature metronome than if they spoke in their usual manner. Since the ratings of speech pathologists might differ from those of laymen, and since the investigator would probably be interested primarily in how laymen would react to the "metronome" as opposed to the usual speech of such stutterers, the investigator would probably be wise to limit membership in the panel to persons who have not had training in speech pathology.

The more heterogeneous the members of a panel are with regard to organismic variables, the greater the probable dispersion of their ratings and the lower the probable *reliability* of the scale values computed from them (for a given size panel) will be. Also, the more heterogeneous the members of a panel are with regard to such variables, the less *valid* the scale values computed from their ratings are apt to be. If a panel consisted of two or more subgroups who would tend to rate a set of stimuli differently, scale values computed from the ratings of such a panel may not correspond to how the typical member of any subgroup would rate the stimuli. They may be merely "mathematical artifacts." (For a discussion of this point in two somewhat different contexts see Silverman, 1972 and Silverman, 1974.

Selection of the Panel. The panel, strictly speaking, should consist of a random sample of persons from the defined population. Every member of this population should have an equal chance of being selected for the panel. Sometimes it is possible to have such a panel. For instance, suppose the population an investigator wished to sample for a panel consisted of speech pathologists who have been awarded the Certificate of Clinical Competence in Speech Pathology by the American Speech and Hearing Association. A reasonably complete list of such persons could be obtained from the most recent edition of the Association's Membership Directory. Each could be assigned a number, and a panel could be selected by means of a table of random numbers. Such a panel would be practical if the rating task could be mailed.

In some instances it is neither possible nor practical to sample randomly the defined population. Such a population would be adults who are not speech pathologists. All you can do in these instances is to try to select a panel of persons who appear to be representative of the defined population and be cautious when generalizing from their ratings.

Modes of Stimulus Presentation

Once a scaling method has been selected, the stimuli have been prepared, the instructions have been written, and the panel has been selected, the stimuli can be presented to the panel for rating. The primary emphasis in this discussion will be on the presentation of audiotaped stimuli. Many of the comments, however, are relevant for the presentation of other types of stimuli.

A number of decisions have to be made on procedures for presenting audiotaped stimuli for scaling, including the following: (1) individual versus group presentation, (2) head phones versus speakers, (3) loudness level of the stimuli, (4) physical environment, and (5) number of judging sessions.

Individual versus Group Presentation. The issue here is whether the stimuli should be presented to one member of the panel at a time or to several (possibly even the entire panel). The main advantage of group presentation is efficiency. Ordinarily it takes less time to have a set of stimuli rated using a group presentation mode than using an individual one.

The individual presentation mode has several advantages that may outweigh the efficiency advantage of the group mode. First, it ordinarily allows more control to be exerted over the presentation of the stimuli. This permits you to maximize the odds that the stimuli presented to the members of a panel will be similar. They may not be similar if a group presentation mode is used. If, for example, tape-recorded stimuli are presented to a group of judges over a loud speaker, the judges may not "hear" the same stimuli because they are sitting at different distances from the speaker. With an individual presentation mode, judges could be seated the same distance from the speaker.

A second advantage of the individual over the group presentation mode is that it permits order and sequence effects (see Chapter 5) to be minimized. The stimuli can be presented to the members of a panel in different random sequences. This would ordinarily be quite difficult to do if a group presentation mode were used.

A third advantage of the individual over the group presentation mode is that it permits the use of the sequential approach for defining the size of a panel (Silverman, 1968). The main advantage of this approach is that it ensures that the scale values derived from the judges' ratings will possess the required level of reliability and the panel will be no larger than necessary to achieve this end.

Headphones versus Speakers. Two types of transducers can be used to present audiotape stimuli to judges: headphones and loudspeakers. The main advantage of loudspeakers is that they make it relatively easy to present a set of stimuli to more than one rater at a time. Their main disadvantage is that they permit the acoustic properties of the experimental room to interact with the stimuli. This can cause the properties of the stimuli to be distorted for at least some members of a panel. All members may not "hear" the same thing. Headphones (particularly those with a good acoustic seal) minimize the extent to which the stimuli the judges hear are distorted by the acoustical properties of the experimental room.

A second advantage of headphones over speakers is that they make the intensity level at which the stimuli are presented to the raters easier to control since the transducer-to-subject distance is constant. By the same token, headphones also make it relatively simple to compensate at least partially for differences in the hearing thresholds of judges.

Loudness Level of the Stimuli. With audiotape recorded stimuli, it is necessary to define a loudness level for presenting the stimuli to the panel. This level usually is defined by the experimenter (implicitly or explicitly) as one the judges would regard as "comfortable." While such an approach would probably be satisfactory for rating some attributes (e.g., stuttering severity), it may not be satisfactory for others—i.e., those whose magnitudes might vary as a function of the loudness level or levels at which they were presented. For rating attributes that may be of the latter type, it would probably be a good idea to define the loudness level more precisely. One approach would be to determine each panel member's speech reception threshold (SRT) and present the stimuli a given number of decibels above this threshold.

Physical Environment. The environment in which the stimuli are rated can influence the level of reliability of the ratings. As previously indicated, the acoustical properties of the experimental room can interact with those of audiotape recorded stimuli. Such an interaction would tend to increase the dispersion of the ratings and hence reduce their reliability.

The temperature and humidity levels within the experimental room also can influence the reliability of the ratings. If the judges are uncomfortable while rating the stimuli, they may divert some of the attention they should be devoting to the stimuli to their feelings of discomfort. This could reduce the reliability of their ratings.

Number of Judging Sessions. The rating task may be administered at a single session or divided into several sessions. While it is usually most efficient to have all the stimuli rated at a single session, this may not be possible or desirable. If the rating task is relatively long (i.e., longer than an hour), it almost always is desirable to divide the task into several sessions. It would also be desirable to divide the task into several sessions if the task were relatively short, but so demanding that raters would be likely to become fatigued before completing it. Fatigue, of course, can reduce the reliability of the judges' ratings.

Analyses of Judges' Ratings

Once the judges have rated the stimuli, the next task is to analyze their ratings to yield: (1) a scale value for each of the stimuli, (2) an estimate of the reliability of these scale values, and (3) an index of the degree of agreement among the judges in their ratings of individual stimuli. Computational procedures for these three types of analyses are presented in the references cited for the six scaling methods in the section dealing with psychological scaling methods as measuring instruments. Here a general description of each type of analysis will be presented. We will also discuss two related topics: (1) the desirability of eliminating the ratings of judges who did not appear to be following instructions, and (2) the use of multiple regression analysis for inferring the attributes of the stimuli that influenced judges' ratings.

Computation of Scale Values. A stimulus' scale value is a number that designates the amount (relative or absolute) of the attribute rated that it possesses. This number indicates the location of the stimulus on the continuum, or scale, of possible values of this attribute. If a stimulus, for example, had a scale value of 4.0 on a 7-point, equal-appearing interval scale of stuttering severity where 1 designated least possible severity and 7 designated most possible severity, its location on this continuum, or scale, would be at the midpoint.

For the methods of equal-appearing intervals and direct magnitude-estimation, either the mean or median of the ratings assigned to a stimulus can be used as its scale value. Which of these is used may not make too much difference even though mean and median scale values for a stimulus will differ somewhat in magnitude, since both appear to order a set of stimuli in approximately the same manner (Silverman, 1967).

For the methods of pair comparisons, constant sums, rank order, and successive intervals, the computational procedures for deriving scale values are fairly complex. The math involved is not difficult, but it is time consuming. Programs are available at some computer centers for computing scale values from sets of ratings yielded by these methods. If an appropriate computer program is not available, it might be worthwhile to investigate the possibility of having one written.

Estimating Reliability of Scale Values. Before a set of scale values can be interpreted, it is necessary to establish whether they are sufficiently reliable for the purpose they were intended for. If they are not sufficiently reliable for this purpose, they cannot be used to answer the question or questions they were intended to answer. Both intrasubject and intersubject differences and relationships can be obscured.

Suppose you wished to determine whether dysarthrics were less hypernasal after being fitted with some sort of palatal prosthesis. You could have "before and after" treatment speech segments from such persons rated for degree of nasality. If the ratings were not adequately reliable, you could end up concluding the treatment made no difference when, in fact, it did.

What would be the minimum acceptable level of reliability for most purposes? Unless a difference were quite large or a relationship quite strong, you would stand a good chance of failing to detect it if the reliability of your scale values were less than 0.85. A reliability coefficient of 0.90 would probably be adequate except in instances where you were attempting to detect relatively small differences or relatively weak relationships. In such instances, a reliability coefficient of at least 0.95 probably would be necessary. This level probably could be achieved by using a fairly large judging panel—i.e., one with more than 50 judges.

Several approaches have been used for estimating the reliability level of a set of scale values. One such approach that can be used with any scaling method is *test-retest*. With this approach, the panel either rates the entire set of stimuli twice (usually on different days) or a randomly selected sample of the set of stimuli twice (e.g., at the beginning and at the end of the rating session). Two sets of scale values are computed from these ratings and correlated.

Suppose you wished to use the test-retest approach and the number of stimuli you were having rated were 75. You could select from these a sample of 25 by means of a table of random numbers and have them rated twice in different random orders—once at the beginning and once at the end of the rating session. The observers, then, would rate a total of 100 stimuli. Sets of scale values for the 25 stimuli could be computed from the first and second ratings, and these two sets of scale values could be correlated, possibly using a Pearson product-moment correlation coefficient (see Chapter 8). The magnitude of this coefficient would indicate whether the ratings were likely to be adequately reliable.

Another approach that can be used with any scaling method for estimating reliability is the *split-half* method. With this approach, each member of a panel is randomly assigned to one of two groups. Two sets of scale values are computed—one from the ratings of the judges in each group. These sets of scale values are correlated, usually with a Pearson product-moment correlation coefficient. The resulting correlation coefficient can be interpreted as a reliability estimate for a panel *one half* the size of the panel used. This would tend to be a conservative estimate for the entire panel. A more accurate estimate for the entire panel could be obtained by inserting the value of the Pearson product-moment correlation coefficient that was computed into the Spearman-Brown formula (Guilford, 1954, p. 391).

The main disadvantage of the split-half approach is that it is necessary to compute three sets of scale values—two of which are used solely for estimating reliability.

A third approach to estimating the reliability of scale values that can be used with the methods of equal-appearing intervals and direct magnitude-estimation utilizes the *intraclass correlation coefficient for average ratings* (Ebel, 1951). With this approach, the ratings assigned to the stimuli are subjected to an analysis of variance (see Chapter 8). An intraclass correlation coefficient is computed from the resulting mean square values, i.e.,

$$r_{\text{intraclass}} = 1 - \frac{MS_{AS}}{MS_A}$$

One interpretation of this coefficient (which was paraphrased from Winer, 1962) is that if the experiment were to be repeated with another random sample of the same number of judges, but with the same stimuli, the correlation between the *mean* ratings obtained from the two sets of data on the same stimuli would be approximately the value obtained for this coefficient. Because of the close correspondence between mean and median scale values, this coefficient can also be used to estimate the reliability of *median* ratings (Silverman, 1968).

The intraclass correlation coefficient discussed here provides a reliability estimate for the average of the ratings of a *group* of judges. Sometimes it may be necessary to estimate the reliability of the ratings of the *individual* judges in a panel. Ebel (1951) provides formulas for two intraclass correlation coefficients which can be used for this purpose. One provides an estimate of the reliability of single ratings that is adjusted for systematic differences in judges' frames of reference (i.e., internal standards). It is approximately equal to the average intercorrelation between ratings given by all possible pairs of judges (Winer, 1962). This coefficient provides an estimate of how closely judges' ratings order a set of stimuli in the same manner. Suppose three judges rated five speech segments for degree of nasality by the method of direct magnitude-estimation and assigned the following ratings:

Segment	Judge #1	Judge #2	Judge #3
A	150	150	95
B	375	250	165
C	333	200	125
D	400	300	175
E	270	185	115

While the absolute ratings assigned by these judges are quite different, the five segments have been ordered by them in the same manner. For this reason, the magnitude of the intraclass correlation coefficient computed with this formula would be quite high, indicating good interjudge agreement.

Ebel's other formula provides an estimate of the reliability of the *absolute* ratings assigned by individual judges. It indicates how closely the absolute ratings assigned by individual judges agree. This formula could be used for such a purpose as estimating how well speech pathologists agree in their assignment of stutterers to one of the eight points on the Iowa Scale for Rating Severity of Stuttering (Johnson, Darley, and Spriestersbach, 1963, p. 281). If it were applied to the data used to illustrate the other intraclass correlation coefficient for the ratings of individual judges, the formula would yield a coefficient that was considerably lower because of the differences in the absolute magnitudes of the judges' ratings. The magnitude of this coefficient will almost always be lower than that of the other.

One other approach that has been used for estimating the reliability of scale values utilizes the *mean Q value*. This strategy has only been used in conjunction with the method of equal-appearing intervals. The mean Q value is the mean semi-interquartile range (see Chapter 8) of the ratings assigned to each of a set of stimuli. A semi-interquartile range is computed for the ratings assigned to each stimulus in a set, and the mean of these ranges is computed.

The mean Q value is a measure of average interjudge agreement. The smaller the mean Q value, the closer the agreement of the judges in their ratings. And the closer the agreement of the judges in their ratings, the higher the reliability (or stability) of the scale values.

Information on the distribution of mean Q values for stimuli rated on a seven-point, equal-appearing interval scale has been reported (Silverman, 1967). The relative magnitude of an obtained mean Q value can be estimated by locating it in this distribution.

Degree of Agreement among Judges in Their Ratings of Individual Stimuli. Judges do not usually assign identical ratings to stimuli. There is ordinarily some variability in their ratings. It is sometimes useful to be able to describe the degree of agreement among the judges in their ratings of specific stimuli. Such information is useful, for example, in the construction of master scales. Suppose you wished to construct an equal-appearing interval master scale of nasality. You could have a large number of speech segments from persons with cleft palates rated on a seven-point, equal-appearing interval scale of degree of nasality. You would compute from the ratings assigned to each stimulus both a scale value and a measure of dispersion, or spread (e.g., the semi-interquartile range). Next, you would identify segments that had scale values of 1.0, 2.0, 3.0, 4.0, 5.0, 6.0, and 7.0. From the segments having scale values at each of these points, you would select the one on which the judges agreed the best in their ratings—i.e., the one on which the dispersion of their ratings was the smallest. These seven segments ordered on a tape would constitute a seven-point master scale of nasality.

Several measures of dispersion have been used to describe the degree of agreement among the judges in their ratings of individual stimuli, including: (1) the range, (2) the interquartile range, (3) the semi-interquartile range, and (4) the standard deviation. These measures are described in Chapter 8.

Desirability of Eliminating Judges Who Did Not Appear to Follow Instructions. There are a few judges on almost every panel whose ratings are so different from those of the others that it appears likely they failed to follow instructions. Should the ratings of such judges be thrown out? Unfortunately, this isn't an easy question to answer. It is usually quite difficult to discriminate between judges who did not follow instructions and judges who did follow instructions, but reacted to the stimuli differently than the other panel members. Suppose, for example, that a judge who was instructed to rate a set of stimuli by the method of equal-appearing intervals assigned only 1s, 4s, and 7s to the stimuli. While it is likely that he failed to follow instructions, it is possible that all the stimuli fell at one of these three points on his internally generated scale.

If the ratings of only a small proportion of the members of a panel are questionable, the scale values would probably not be influenced very much by including them. There would be no need in such a case to throw them out. If, on the other hand, a relatively high percentage of the members of a panel assigned ratings in a manner that suggested they were not following instructions, it would be important to determine whether this was the case. If it were established that they were not following instructions, it would be justifiable to throw out their ratings.

Use of Multiple Regression for Inferring Characteristics of the Stimuli That Influenced Judges' Ratings. A speech pathologist or audiologist may on occasion wish to answer a question such as the following:

1. What aspects of a stutterer's communicative behavior are apt to influence observers' judgments of his stuttering severity?
2. What aspects of the communicative behavior of an esophageal speaker are apt to influence observers' judgments of the "acceptability" of his speech?

Obviously many aspects of communicative behavior could influence observer judgments such as these. A procedure will be outlined in this section that can be helpful in identifying relevant aspects. This procedure utilizes multiple regression analysis (see Chapter 8). Representative studies from the speech pathology literature in which it has been used include those of Jordan (1960) and Shriner and Sherman (1967).

The procedure can be summarized briefly as follows:

1. A set of stimuli is rated by one of the scaling methods for the attribute the investigator wishes to study. This attribute for the first question would be stuttering severity and for the second question would be acceptability of speech. A scale value is computed from these ratings for each of the stimuli in the set. (These scale values serve as the *dependent variable* in the multiple regression analysis.)

2. Aspects of the stimuli that the investigator feels may have influenced the observers' ratings are measured. One such aspect relevant to the first question could be stuttering frequency; to the second question, speaking rate. (These measures serve as the *independent variables* in the multiple regression analysis.)

3. A coefficient of multiple correlation (see Chapter 8) is computed between the dependent variable (i.e., the scale values) and the composite of the independent variables (i.e., the measures of the aspects of the stimuli the investigator felt may have influenced the observers' ratings). A multiple regression equation (see Chapter 8) is also computed. It is used for predicting the dependent variable from the independent variables.

4. Independent variables that do not appear to be related to the dependent variable are eliminated. Such variables are unlikely to have influenced the observers' ratings. The basic strategy here is to identify the independent variable that is the least related to the observers' ratings and eliminate it. The coefficient of multiple correlation then is recomputed without this variable. If this coefficient is not significantly lower than the original one, the independent variable that is least related to the observers' ratings is identified and eliminated from among the remaining ones. The coefficient of multiple correlation is then recomputed. If it is not significantly (in a statistical sense) lower than the original one, the identification and elimination process is continued until the point is reached where a statistically significant difference exists between a multiple correlation coefficient computed on a reduced set of independent variables and the original multiple correlation coefficient. The independent variables remaining at this point are *hypothesized* to have influenced the observers' ratings. They are not, of course, the only independent variables that could have influenced the observers' ratings. There may have been other aspects of the stimuli which, if measured, would have been found to correlate with the observers' ratings.

REFERENCES

ABBS, J. H., and GILBERT, B. N., Strain gage transduction system for lip and jaw motion in two dimensions: Design criteria and calibration data. *Journal of Speech and Hearing Research*, 16, 248–256 (1973).

BARNHART, E. N., A comparison of scaling methods for affective judgments. *Psychological Review*, 43, 387–395 (1936).

BARRETT, M., A comparison of the order of merit method and the method of paired comparisons. *Psychological Review*, 21, 278–294 (1914).

BARTLETT, C. J., HEERMAN, E., and RETTIG, S., A comparison of six different scaling techniques. *Journal of Social Psychology*, 51, 343–348 (1960).

CARROLL, J., A cinefluorographic technique for the study of velopharyngeal closure. *Journal of Speech and Hearing Disorders*, 17, 224–228 (1952).

CRAWFORD, P. L., Comparison of two attitude scaling methods. *Psychological Reports*, 17, 681–682 (1965).

CULLINAN, W. L., PRATHER, E. M., and WILLIAMS, D. E., Comparison of procedures for scaling severity of stuttering. *Journal of Speech and Hearing Research*, 6, 187–194 (1963).

DEMPSEY, M. E., DRAUGERT, G. L., SISKIND, R. P., and STEER, M. D., The Purdue pitch meter—A direct reading fundamental frequency analyzer. *Journal of Speech and Hearing Disorders*, 15, 135–141 (1950).

DUNN, L. M., *Peabody Picture Vocabulary Test*. Minneapolis: American Guidance Service, Inc. (1959).

EBEL, R., Estimation of the reliability of ratings. *Psychometrika*, 16, 407–424 (1951).

EDWARDS, A. L., *Techniques of Attitude Scale Construction*. New York: Appleton-Century-Crofts (1957).

EISLER, H., Empirical test of a model relating magnitude and category scales. *Scandinavian Journal of Psychology*, 3, 88–96 (1962).

EISLER, H., Magnitude scales, category scales, and Fechnerian integration. *Psychological Review*, 70, 243–253 (1963).

EKMAN, G., and KUNNAPAS, T., A further study of direct and indirect scaling methods. *Scandinavian Journal of Psychology*, 4, 77–80 (1963).

EKMAN, G., and KUNNAPAS, T., Note on direct and indirect scaling methods. *Psychological Reports*, 6, 174 (1960).

ENGEN, T., and MCBURNEY, D. H., Magnitude and category scales of the pleasantness of odors. *Journal of Experimental Psychology*, 68, 435–440 (1964).

FLETCHER, S. G., SHELTON, R. L., JR., SMITH, C. C., and BOSMA, J. F., Radiography in speech pathology. *Journal of Speech and Hearing Disorders*, 25, 135–144 (1960).

GALANTER, E., Contemporary psychophysics. In Brown, R., Galanter, E., Hess, E., and Mandler, G., *New Directions in Psychology I*, New York: Holt, Rinehart and Winston (1962).

GALANTER, E., and MESSICK, S., The relation between category and magnitude scales of loudness. *Psychological Review*, 68, 363–372 (1961).

GAY, T., and HARRIS, K. S., Some recent developments in the use of electromyography in speech research. *Journal of Speech and Hearing Research*, 14, 241–246 (1971).

GUILFORD, J. P., *Psychometric Methods* (2nd Edition). New York: McGraw-Hill Book Company (1954).

HANLEY, T. D., and PETERS, R., The speech and hearing laboratory. In Lee E. Travis (Ed.), *Handbook of Speech Pathology and Audiology*, New York: Appleton-Century-Crofts, 75–140 (1971).

HEVNER, K., An empirical study of three psychophysical methods. *Journal of General Psychology*, 4, 191–212 (1930).

HICKS, J. M., and CAMPBELL, D. T., Zero-point scaling as affected by social object, scaling method, and context. *Journal of Personal and Social Psychology*, 2, 793–808 (1965).

HOSHIKO, M., and HOLLOWAY, G., Radio telemetry for monitoring verbal behavior. *Journal of Speech and Hearing Disorders*, 33, 48–50 (1968).

JOHNSON, W., *People in Quandaries*. New York: Harper and Row (1946).

JOHNSON, W., DARLEY, F. L., and SPRIESTERSBACH, D. C., *Diagnostic Methods in Speech Pathology*. New York: Harper & Row, Publishers (1963).

JORDAN, E. P., Articulation test measures and listener ratings of articulation defectiveness. *Journal of Speech and Hearing Research*, 3, 303–319 (1960).

KELSEY, C. A., MINIFIE, F. D., and HIXON, T. J., Applications of ultrasound in speech research. *Journal of Speech and Hearing Research*, 12, 564–575 (1969).

KELLEY, H. H., HOVLAND, C. I., SCHWARTZ, M., and ABELSON, R. P., The influence of judges' attitudes in three methods of attitude scaling. *Journal of Social Psychology*, 42, 147–158 (1955).

KING, D. J., and LAU, A. W., A comparison of three scaling techniques in estimating the accuracy of written recall. *Journal of General Psychology*, 69, 203–207 (1963).

KUNNAPAS, T., and WIKSTROEM, I., Measurement of occupational preference: A comparison of scaling methods. *Perceptual and Motor Skills*, 17, 611–624 (1963).

LADEFOGED, P., Use of palatography. *Journal of Speech and Hearing Disorders*, 22, 764–774 (1957).

MISRA, R. K., and DUTT, P. K., A comparative study of psychological scaling methods. *Journal of Psychological Researches*, 9, 31–34 (1965).

MOLL, K. L., Cinefluorographic techniques in speech research. *Journal of Speech and Hearing Research*, 3, 227–241 (1960).

MOORE, P. G., WHITE, F. D., and VON LEDEN, H., Ultra high speech photography in laryngeal physiology. *Journal of Speech and Hearing Disorders*, 27, 165–171 (1962).

ORNE, M. T., Demand characteristics and the concept of quasi-controls. In Robert Rosenthal and Ralph L. Rosnow (Eds.), *Artifacts in Behavioral Research*, New York: Academic Press, Inc., 143–179 (1969).

PERLOE, S. I., The relation between category-rating and magnitude-estimation judgments of occupational prestige. *American Journal of Psychology*, 76, 395–403 (1963).

PFEIFFER, M. G., and SIEGEL, A. I., Comparison of category and magnitude scales of technical skills. *Perceptual and Motor Skills*, Monograph Supplement 3, 22, 235–248 (1966).

PRATHER, E. M., Scaling defectiveness of articulation by direct magnitude-estimation. *Journal of Speech and Hearing Research*, 3, 380–392 (1960).

RORSCHACH, H., *Psychodiagnostik Text*. Berne, Switzerland: Verlag Hans Huber (1942). (3rd edition, translated by P. Lemkau and B. Kronenberg.)

ROSENTHAL, R., Interpersonal expectations: Effects of the experimenter's hypothesis. In Robert Rosenthal and Ralph L. Rosnow (Eds.), *Artifacts in Behavioral Research*, New York: Academic Press, Inc., 181–277 (1969).

SAFFIR, M. A., A comparative study of scales constructed by three psycho-physical methods. *Psychometrika*, 2, 179–198 (1937).

SANDERS, L. J., Instrumentation for measurement of lingual strength. *Journal of Speech and Hearing Research*, 11, 189–193 (1968).

SENN, D. J., and MANLEY, M. B., Comparison of scaling methods: Paired comparisons vs. constant sums. *Perceptual and Motor Skills*, 22, 911–918 (1966).

SHERMAN, D., and MOODIE, C. E., Four psychological scaling methods applied to articulation defectiveness. *Journal of Speech and Hearing Disorders*, 22, 698–706 (1957).

SHERMAN, D., and SILVERMAN, F. H., Three psychological scaling methods applied to language development. *Journal of Speech and Hearing Research*, 11, 837–841 (1968).

SHRINER, T. H., and SHERMAN, D., An equation for assessing language development. *Journal of Speech and Hearing Research*, 10, 41–48 (1967).

SILVERMAN, E.-M., Generality of disfluency data collected from preschoolers. *Journal of Speech and Hearing Research*, 15, 84–92 (1972).

SILVERMAN, F. H., An approach to determining the number of judges needed for scaling experiments. *Perceptual and Motor Skills*, 17, 1333–1334 (1968).

SILVERMAN, F. H., Correspondence between mean and median scale values for sets of stimuli scaled by the method of equal-appearing intervals. *Perceptual and Motor Skills*, 25, 727–728 (1967).

SILVERMAN, F. H., Interpretation of mean Q values for sets of stimuli rated on a seven-point, equal-appearing interval scale. *Perceptual and Motor Skills*, 24, 842 (1967).

SILVERMAN, F. H., Intraclass correlation coefficient as an index of reliability of median scale values for sets of stimuli rated by equal-appearing intervals. *Perceptual and Motor Skills*, 26, 878 (1968).

SILVERMAN, F. H., The Porch Index of Communicative Ability: A psychometric problem and its solution. *Journal of Speech and Hearing Disorders*, 39, 225–226 (1974).

SILVERMAN, F. H., and JOHNSTON, R. G., Direct interval-estimation: A ratio scaling method. *Perceptual and Motor Skills*, 41, 464–466 (1975).

SILVERMAN, F. H., and SHERMAN, D., Equal-appearing interval scale values and successive interval scale values derived from the same set of ratings. *Perceptual and Motor Skills*, 25, 226–228 (1967).

SORON, H. I., High speed photography in speech research. *Journal of Speech and Hearing Research*, 10, 768–776 (1967).

STEVENS, S. S., and GALANTER, E. H., Ratio scales and category scales for a dozen perceptual continua. *Journal of Experimental Psychology*, 54, 377–411 (1957).

STEVENS, S. S., and STONE, G., Finger span: Ratio scale, category scale, and JND scale. *Journal of Experimental Psychology*, 57, 91–95 (1959).

STEWART, K. C., A new instrument for detecting galvanic skin response. *Journal of Speech and Hearing Disorders*, 19, 169–173 (1954).

STOUT, M. B., *Basic Electrical Measurements* (2nd Ed.). Englewood Cliffs, N.J.: Prentice-Hall, Inc. (1962).

WINER, B. J., *Statistical Principles in Experimental Design*. New York: McGraw-Hill Book Company (1962).

EIGHT

ORGANIZING DATA FOR ANSWERING QUESTIONS

Once the data have been gathered—whether qualitative or quantitative—they have to be organized, or structured, in a manner that will permit the question or questions posed by the investigator to be answered. Without such organization, the answers derived from the data may not be accurate. You can easily be deceived if you attempt to answer questions merely by skimming through, or eyeballing, the available data. You may, for example, inadvertently give too much weight or too little weight to certain aspects of your data, possibly as a function of experimenter bias (see Chapter 7). Suppose a question you were attempting to answer concerned the effectiveness of a particular therapy, and to answer it you recorded a number of observations (both qualitative and quantitative) before and after administration of the therapy to twenty persons who had a certain communicative disorder. If you skim the available data, you might tend to pay more attention to aspects of it that suggest the treatment was effective than to those that suggest it had little or no effect. Another clinician whose theoretical orientation would give a set not to find the therapy effective might tend to pay more attention to aspects of the data that suggest the treatment had little or no effect. Thus, two persons skimming the same data could arrive at different answers to a question if they had different expectations, or sets.

Another reason why you can be easily deceived if you attempt to answer questions merely by skimming data is that the data needed to answer a particular question may not stand out sufficiently from the other data in the set in which it is included to provide an accurate answer to the question. The problem here can be viewed as one of inadequate separation between figure and background, or between signal and noise. To illustrate this problem, suppose you wished to answer the following question: "How was the communicative behavior of a group of aphasics different following therapy?" If you merely skimmed the pre- and post-therapy observations you had recorded in their folders rather than systematically abstracting, organizing, and summarizing these observations, you might not be able to get a sufficiently good impression of how this behavior was different to answer the question accurately. It would be difficult, if not impossible, to remember all the relevant observations recorded in the folders.

A third reason (which is related to the second) why skimming the data is deceptive is that a large number of observations is likely to be relevant to a particular question. It may not be possible to integrate them sufficiently to arrive at an accurate answer without first organizing and summarizing them.

Several approaches can be used for organizing and summarizing sets of data for answering questions. These include statistical analysis, graphical display, tabular presentation, and narrative description. The first three approaches are the ones customarily used for organizing and summarizing quantitative data. The last two are customarily used for organizing and summarizing qualitative data. This chapter will discuss organizing qualitative and quantitative data through these approaches.

STRATEGIES FOR ORGANIZING QUALITATIVE DATA FOR ANSWERING QUESTIONS

The primary emphasis of this section will be on the organization of qualitative (i.e., verbal descriptive) data for clinical case studies. Such data have been used most frequently by speech pathologists and audiologists in this context.

Observations should be summarized and organized in such a manner that they can be used to answer the question or questions that, implicitly or explicitly, have been posed by the investigator. This involves several processes the first of which is *abstracting* from the available data those relevant for answering each of the questions posed. Suppose you had administered three articulation tests to a child both before and after he had received a particular program of therapy and had transcribed his responses to the test stimuli phonemically. These transcriptions, of course, would be qualitative data. If one of your questions was whether his production of /s/ at the beginnings of words was any different after a period of therapy than preceding it, to answer it you would have to abstract the data on the production of /s/ in the initial position from the remaining articulation test data.

Once the data relevant for answering a question are abstracted, they are summarized and organized. A child's production of /s/ in the initial position in words as sampled before and after a period of therapy by three articulation tests can be summarized and organized by means of a table such as this:

Articulation Test	Before-Therapy Production	After-Therapy Production
I	/θ/	/s/
II	/θ/	/s/
III	/θ/	/s/

After the data have been summarized and organized, they can be used to answer the question. The data in the table indicate that the production of /s/ was different following therapy on all three articulation tests. Specifically, they indicate that /s/ was produced correctly in the initial positions of words following therapy (at least in the situations sampled by these articulation tests).

Abstracting Relevant Data

It is necessary to abstract from the available observations, or data, those that *may* be relevant for answering each of the questions posed. We emphasize "may" to highlight the fact that it may not be possible to determine for certain at this stage of the process exactly which data of those available will be relevant for answering a particular question. If there is any reason to believe an observation may be relevant for answering a question, the observation should be abstracted. It can be deleted if it is found not to be relevant.

One strategy that may assist the abstraction process is recording each observation on a card. These can be either standard file cards or punch cards (i.e., cards in which information can be coded around the edges). For answering a question, you would select those cards from the pile on which you have recorded observations that may be relevant. In most instances this would be a better strategy than reading through the available data and attempting to remember those that may be relevant for answering a particular question.

Organizing and Summarizing Relevant Data

After the observations that may be relevant have been abstracted, they are organized and summarized in a manner which permits the answer to the question to be as evident as the available data allow. Several approaches can be used here. First, the data can be organized in tabular form—i.e., summarized in a table. To illustrate the possibilities for organizing and summarizing qualitative data in tabular form, Table 8.1 presents references to representative tables containing qualitative data from articles published in the *Journal of Speech and Hearing Disorders.*

TABLE 8.1. References to representative tables that have been used to organize and summarize qualitative data in the *Journal of Speech and Hearing Disorders.*

Data Tabulated	Volume	Reference Year	Pages
Phonetic transcriptions of children's utterances	39	1974	24, 27
Survey of earmold manufacturers' nomenclature	38	1973	459–460
Comparison of three children's phonemic errors	37	1972	454
Child's pattern of phonemic change	37	1972	457–460
Summary of speech, language, and hearing findings in three cases of Laurence-Moon-Biedl syndrome	37	1972	411
Description of parent-child interactions	37	1972	224–225
Samples of the utterances of three children	37	1972	70–71
Examples of the sentence repetitions of four children	36	1971	32
Patterns and generalizations found in the articulatory and auditory discrimination behavior of two groups of subjects	35	1970	138–139
Clinical impression vs. cineradiographic evaluation for eight cases of idiopathic hypernasality	35	1970	48
Summary of voice symptoms and associated factors in psychogenic and neurogenic dysphonias	33	1968	229

A second approach for organizing and summarizing is to set down the qualitative observations in narrative form. Speech pathologists and audiologists typically use this approach in evaluation reports for summarizing relevant observations (both formal and informal) made on clients. They also typically use this approach for daily logs of therapy sessions.

This approach is employed in most clinical case studies for summarizing and organizing qualitative observations. The following two paragraphs from case studies published in the *Journal of Speech and Hearing Disorders* illustrate this application:

> Subject 1 in Condition A usually produced touch velopharyngeal closure and his port configuration was oval. . . . Openings lateral to midline palate-poste-

rior pharyngeal wall contact often were observed in this subject. The subject elevated his palate so it usually contacted the posterior pharyngeal wall. The uvula contracted during two trials. Only one lateral pharyngeal wall or palatopharyngeus muscle could be seen at one time, and it moved toward midline only on one trial and then gag was involved. The subject reported gag on three trials. The subject frequently produced a Passavant's ridge. The ridge varied across trials from slight to marked displacement. No other forward movement of the posterior wall of the pharynx was observed. Laryngeal click was usually heard at the end of trials. (Shelton, Paesani, McClelland, and Bradfield, 1975, p. 238)

Once the desired pitch had been obtained, we directed Craig to continue producing phrases. He progressed quickly and by the third therapy session was able to converse using his new voice, which tended to confirm the nonorganic basis of the voice problem. Occasional pitch breaks occurred, however, and the somewhat hoarse quality persisted. Samples of conversational speech and reading were then tape-recorded so he could identify and tabulate instances when he reverted to the old pitch. At that stage both Craig and his mother were pleased with the results of therapy and encouraged. Others had also commented on his improvement. The stabilization phase of therapy continued in the speech clinic and then in various other places where Craig was often accompanied by the clinician. During the last few sessions we observed consistently low pitch and a voice quality that was almost clear of roughness. To evaluate Craig's voice in more stressful situations, one clinician attended his English class; the voice was clear, of natural pitch, and audible to those sitting in the back of the room. With the great satisfaction of Craig and his mother and with our confidence, it was mutually agreed to terminate therapy six weeks after its initiation. An interview two months later revealed that Craig's voice had remained consistently normal. (Yari, 1974, p. 375)

Note the degree of similarity between (1) the first paragraph and an excerpt from an evaluation report, and (2) the second paragraph and an excerpt from a progress note regarding the impact of therapy on a client.

Summarizing and organizing qualitative data involves the assignment of observations to *categories*. This is true regardless of whether the data are to be summarized and organized in tabular or in narrative form.

The categories to which observations are assigned can be categorized in various ways. Some, for example, can be viewed as spatial, some as temporal, some as combinations of these two, and some as neither of these two. An example of a set of *spatial* categories that might be used by a speech pathologist or audiologist to organize qualitative observations would be "right ear" and "left ear." An example of a set of *temporal* categories would be "status prior to receiving therapy" and "status following therapy." An example of a corresponding set of *spatial-temporal* categories would be "status of left ear prior to therapy" and "status of left ear following therapy." And, finally, an example of a set of categories that could be regarded as *neither temporal nor spatial* would be "receptive language" and "expressive language."

The categories to which observations are assigned are determined by, or a function of, the question or questions asked. If you wished to determine, for example, whether a child's speech articulation were any different after a period of therapy than before it, two categories to which you would assign your observations would undoubtedly be "speech articulation prior to therapy" and "speech articulation following therapy." On the other hand, if your question concerned the current status of a child's communicative behavior, several of the categories you might use would be "hearing acuity," "speech articulation," "speech fluency," "language usage," and "voice quality."

A given observation may be assigned to more than one category and used to answer more than one question. Suppose a speech pathologist showed a pencil to a person who had had a stroke and asked this person to name and describe it. Further suppose that the speech pathologist regarded the response as appropriate and all phonemes as correctly articulated. This observation, or judgment, could be assigned to more than one category and could be used to answer more than one question. For example, it could be assigned to the category of "receptive language functioning" and could be used to answer the question: "Does the person exhibit a disturbance in receptive language functioning?" It could also be assigned to the category "dysarthria" and could be used to answer the question: "Does the person exhibit any disturbance in the functioning of the articulators for speech?" Other categories to which this observation could be assigned include "auditory acuity," "auditory perceptual functioning," "conceptual functioning," and "word-finding ability."

The discussion in this section provides only a very general introduction to the organization and analysis of qualitative data. If you wish to pursue this topic further, you may find information in the sociology literature concerning participant observation in field research useful (e.g., Schatzman and Strauss, 1973, pp. 108–127; McCall and Simmons, 1969).

STRATEGIES FOR ORGANIZING QUANTITATIVE DATA FOR ANSWERING QUESTIONS

The remainder of this chapter will be devoted to a discussion of strategies for organizing quantitative data through using: (1) descriptive statistical and graphical procedures, and (2) inferential statistical procedures. The discussion will emphasize when it is appropriate to apply these procedures and how they are interpreted, rather than the mathematical models which underly them. To develop an intuitive understanding of these procedures, however, you must have some experience computing them. A computational appendix has been included to provide such experience (see Appendix A).

The statistical methods included in the computational appendix should be regarded as representative rather than exhaustive. This is particularly true of the inferential statistical methods. While this Appendix contains a test of statistical significance appropriate for almost any set of data, these tests constitute only a small sample of those that have been developed. The tests included were selected because they are the ones that have been used most frequently by speech pathologists and audiologists judging by research reports published in the *Journal of Speech and Hearing Disorders*, the *Journal of Speech and Hearing Research*, and *Language, Speech, and Hearing Services in Schools*.

All statistics in the computational appendix are computed from a single set of data, which consists of frequencies per 100 words spoken of four types of speech disfluency (i.e., interjection of sounds and syllables, part-word repetition, word repetition, and revision-incomplete phrase) for each of 56 elementary-school children. This set of data was selected for inclusion in the Appendix because it can be segmented in ways that make it possible to compute the various statistics included therein. The fact that the frequencies relate to speech disfluencies rather than to some other event of interest to speech pathologists and audiologists, of course, is irrelevant to the statistical analyses made of them. What the frequencies represent has no effect on such analyses—i.e., on the computational procedures used. It does, however, affect the interpretation of the results of such analyses.

The same ordering of topics is used for all statistics in this Appendix. First, the question is presented that the statistic is intended to answer. Second, the computation of the statistic is described, step by step. The computational procedure is described in sufficient detail that you can check yourself on your understanding of it by performing it. Third, the value computed for the statistic is given. Fourth, the question is answered using this value. Fifth, in several instances there is a remark concerning the computation or interpretation of the statistic. And sixth, a computational exercise is presented. In all of these exercises, you are asked to compute the same statistic already computed with different numbers from the data table at the beginning of the Appendix. The question (or questions) you are asked to answer should indicate to you which numbers from the data table you should analyze. You should use the same computational procedure as illustrated in the preceding example; the answer is provided to allow you to check the accuracy of your computations. If your answer differs from the one given (except possibly for a deviation due to rounding error), you should go back through your calculations step by step, checking the computational procedures you used against those in the previous example. Since it is relatively easy to make computational errors (e.g., enter the wrong number into the calculator), it is a good idea to make all calculations twice.

All the calculations in the Appendix can be made with a relatively inexpensive, unsophisticated calculator. The calculations for the examples were made with a miniature electronic slide-rule calculator that cost less than fifty dollars. The only calculator functions essential for these exercises are addition, subtraction, multiplication, division, and square root. Other functions that are useful, but not essential, are x^2, $1/x$, and additive memory.

The material included in the computational appendix is intended to complement the material presented in this chapter. Together they should help you develop an intuitive understanding of: (1) the types of questions given statistics can help answer, (2) how these statistics are computed, and (3) how they are interpreted. This discussion will deal primarily with the first and third points, since the second is discussed in considerable detail in the Appendix. The only instances in which the second point will be discussed in any detail here are those in which statistics not included in the Appendix are described.

Descriptive Statistical Techniques

Descriptive statistics describe an aspect, or attribute, of a set of measures—i.e., of a set of quantitative data. They provide indices for specific attributes of the distribution of the data in such a set. The data tabulated in the computational appendix will be used to illustrate this concept. The frequencies of interjection, part-word repetition, word repetition, and revision-incomplete phrase for the 56 children (a total of 224 measures) presented in this table constitute a set of quantitative data.

If you were to skim read the 224 measures in this table *without looking at the column headings*, they probably would provide little information about the disfluency production of these children. About the only question they would permit you to answer reliably about the children's disfluency production would be: "Were the children homogeneous with regard to the amount of disfluency they produced?" Merely skimming these data would be sufficient to establish that they were relatively heterogeneous with regard to this aspect of their disfluency.

Before these data could be used for answering other questions about these children's disfluency production with an adequate level of reliability, they would have to be organized and summarized. The organization and summarization of quantitative data, like qualitative data, involves the assignment of observations to *categories*. Some such categories have nominal scale characteristics. Others have ordinal, interval, ratio, or logarithmic scale characteristics (see Chapter 6 for a description of these scales of measurement). The assignment of measures to a set of categories results in a *distribution*. To illustrate the concept of distribution, let us again refer to the data table in the computational appendix. The categories "interjection," "part-word repetition," "word repetition," and "revision-incomplete phrase" define a nominal scale; the 56 measures that are assigned to each constitute a distribution. On the other hand, the categories "second grade," "third grade," "fourth grade," "fifth grade," and "sixth grade" define an ordinal scale; the measures that are assigned to each also constitute a distribution. Note that this distribution differs from the first in that the numbers of measures assigned to the categories are different, i.e., 60, 44, 36, 44, and 40 for second- through sixth-grade pupils respectively.

Thus far we have only considered what are referred to as *univariate* distributions. The characteristic of such distributions is that observations are assigned to categories on the basis of only a single attribute of the data. With respect to our illustration, this attribute would be either type of disfluency or grade level of the child producing the disfluency.

In some instances it may be advantageous to categorize observations on the basis of more than one attribute. The resulting distribution would be *multivariate*. The type of multivariate distribution encountered most frequently in speech and hearing research is the *bivariate*. In such distributions, observations are assigned to categories on the basis of two of their attributes. The data table in the computational appendix can be viewed as a bivariate distribution. Each of the 224 measures can be regarded as having been assigned to one of 20 joint categories, or cells. The resulting distribution, or matrix, is illustrated in Table 8.2. The number in each cell indicates how many of the 224 measures were assigned to it.

TABLE 8.2. Data table from the computational appendix viewed as a bivariate distribution.

	I	PW	W	R-IP
Second Grade	15	15	15	15
Third Grade	11	11	11	11
Fourth Grade	9	9	9	9
Fifth Grade	11	11	11	11
Sixth Grade	10	10	10	10

The table in the computational appendix on which Table 8.2 is based provides some information concerning the disfluency production of these children. Merely skimming these data as categorized provides the information necessary to answer at least one question: "Did the children tend to produce more revisions and incomplete phrases than interjections?" A casual inspection of these data suggests that the frequencies for revision-incomplete phrase tend to be higher than those for interjection. On the other hand, merely skimming these data would probably not be sufficient to answer the question: "How much more frequently did the children tend to produce revisions and incomplete phrases than interjections?" To answer this question and most others these data would be appropriate for answering, further organizing and summarizing of the data are necessary. *Descriptive statistics* can be used for this purpose.

What roles do descriptive statistics assume in the organization and summarization of quantitative data? What do they describe? What sorts of questions are they helpful in answering? These questions will be discussed in the three sections which follow. The first concerns measures of central tendency; the second, measures of variability; and the third, measures of association. Following these sections several other types of descriptive statistics that have been occasionally useful in speech and hearing research will be briefly discussed.

Measures of Central Tendency. These indices designate the "average," "typical," or most frequently occurring number in a set of numbers. A number provided by such an index is regarded as *representative* (in some respect) of the numbers in the set from which it was computed.

When the numbers in the set from which indices of central tendency are computed are measures of attributes of persons or of behaviors, they provide information concerning the average, typical, or most frequently occurring amount of an attribute. They designate an amount, or magnitude, of an attribute that in some respect can be regarded as "representative" of that present in the set. If the numbers in a set were scores on a test of articulation proficiency that had been administered to a class of kindergarten children, it would be possible to designate through the use of indices of central tendency: (1) the average score earned by these children, (2) the score earned by the "typical" member of the class, and (3) the score earned most often by the children in the class. Similarly, if the numbers in a set were a given stutterer's stuttering frequencies in fifteen situations, you could designate through the use of these indices: (1) the average rate at which he stuttered in these situations, (2) the rate at which he stuttered that was most typical, and (3) the rate at which he stuttered most often. The values yielded for these three types of "representativeness" are quite similar in some instances and quite dissimilar in others.

There are three commonly used measures of central tendency: the *mean*, the *median*, and the *mode*. Each describes one of the types of representativeness that have been referred to. All are discussed in the computational appendix (see Appendix A).

The *mean* is probably the most commonly used measure of central tendency. One reason for its frequency of use is that it is usually the easiest to compute. The mean is merely an arithmetic average: you total the scores you wish to average and divide by the number of scores totaled.

The mean can be used to answer questions such as these:

1. How many hours of therapy did the average child receive?
2. How long, on the average, was a particular cerebral palsied child able to sustain the vowel /a/ during a series of 10 trials?
3. Did the children tend to be less "nasal" following a particular type of cleft palate surgery than before?

Note that answering the first question requires averaging a single measure (i.e., time) from a number of persons; the second, a number of measures from a single person. The mean can be used as a measure of central tendency for both intersubject and intrasubject measures. The third question was included to indicate that the mean sometimes is used to describe the performance of persons *as a group*. Other measures of central tendency also may be used for this purpose.

Strictly speaking, measures from which a mean is computed must have interval or ratio properties (see Chapter 6). If the properties of such measures do not include equal intervals between scale points, their mean may not be readily interpretable with regard to the magnitude, or amount, of an attribute it represents. Suppose you administered a language test to a group of children on three occasions—i.e., before, halfway through, and after completing a program of therapy—and the means of their scores at these three points were 80, 110, and 120, respectively. If these scores could be assumed to have interval or ratio properties and be *reliable*, the following conclusions would be possible:

1. The children performed better after participating in the therapy program.
2. They exhibited some improvement half way through the program.
3. The amount of improvement they exhibited tended to be greater during the first than the second half of the program.

If, on the other hand, the scores could only be assumed to have ordinal properties (see Chapter 6), the third conclusion would not be possible. Without being able to assume equal intervals between scale points, you would have no way of knowing whether greater improvement occurred during the first or second half of the therapy program. That is, if the scores on this test lacked the equal-interval property, a child would conceivably have to modify his language behavior less to go from 80 to 110 than to go from 110 to 120.

Means, as well as other statistics that require measures to have interval or ratio properties, have been used in speech and hearing research (and in other behavioral science areas) with measures that have been demonstrated to have only *ordinal* properties. The argument against using such statistics with ordinal data can be summarized as follows:

> In developing procedures, mathematical statisticians have assumed that techniques involving numerical scores, orderings, or categorization are to be applied when these numbers or classes are appropriate and meaningful within the experimenter's problem. If the statistical method involves the procedures of arithmetic used on numerical scores, then the numerical answer is formally correct. Even if the numbers are the purest nonsense, having no relation to real magnitudes or the properties of real things, the answers are still right *as numbers*. The difficulty comes with the *interpretation of these numbers back into statements about the real world* [italics added]. If nonsense is put into the mathematical system, nonsense is sure to come out. (Hays, 1963, p. 74)

Thus, while means and other statistics that are appropriate for measures having interval or ratio properties can be computed with numbers having the properties of any measurement scale—even those with nominal properties such as numerals on the backs of football players—they may not lead to accurate answers because of the difficulty of translating them back into statements about the real world.

While the mean is an appropriate measure of central tendency for data having interval or ratio scale properties, it is not necessarily a good index of representativeness for such data. A mean value may not designate the number most representative of a set. In fact, it may designate a number which *never occurs* in the set of which it is supposed to be representative. An example would be the statement that in 1973 the average household contained 3.48 persons (Golenpaul, 1973). I suspect this would not designate the size of a representative household. In instances such as this, where fractional amounts cannot occur, it probably would make most sense to round the mean to a whole number.

A more serious problem can exist when a set of data contains one or more extreme scores. The mean of such a set often is not representative. Suppose the following Language Ages were earned by two groups, each consisting of five children:

	Group I		Group II
	3.5 years		3.5 years
	5.0 years		5.0 years
	6.0 years		6.0 years
	6.5 years		6.5 years
	7.0 years		14.0 years
Mean =	5.6 years	Mean =	7.0 years

The only difference between the groups is the Language Age earned by the fifth child in each. The Language Age earned by the fifth child in Group II is considerably higher than that earned by any of the other children in this group. While the mean Language Age computed for the children in Group I would appear to be representative of those earned by the children in this group, this would not appear to be the case for Group II. The mean Language Age for this group is higher than that earned by four of the five children.

Another artifact that can occur when means are used is that the relationship between means of scores for a group of persons may not be representative of those between such scores for the majority of individuals in the group. Suppose, for example, the following were the percentages of words stuttered by five stutterers before and after a period of therapy:

Stutterer	Percent before Therapy	Percent after Therapy
1	5.2	5.3
2	3.4	3.6
3	7.0	7.0
4	1.1	1.2
5	30.0	12.5
Mean	9.3	5.9

While it would appear from these means that the stutterers tended to be more fluent following therapy, actually only one of the five was more fluent following therapy.

In summary, the mean is a very useful measure of central tendency, but it does have several limitations that you should be aware of both as a user and a consumer of statistics.

The next measure of central tendency that we will consider is the *median*. Except for the mean, it is probably the most frequently used such measure.

The median of a set is that measure which occurs at the midpoint of a set of measures when they are ordered from lowest to highest (or from highest to lowest). The median, for example, of the following set of five measures would be 50.0:

$$25 \quad 26 \quad 50 \quad 60 \quad 200$$

If a set contains an *odd* number of measures, the computation of the median is straightforward. You merely identify the measure that occurs at the midpoint of the ordering. If a set contains an *even* number of measures, the determination of the median is a little more complex, since it involves an interpolation process. To illustrate this process, let us use the following set, which consists of six measures:

$$10 \quad 20 \quad 30 \quad 40 \quad 43 \quad 43$$

The median of this set would be 35, i.e., half the distance between the third and fourth measures.

The median can be used to answer such questions as those listed in the previous section that would be appropriate to answer through the use of the mean. It can also be used to answer questions similar to the following:

1. How many hours of therapy did the "typical" child receive?
2. What score falls at the 50th percentile for six year olds on a particular language test?

Note that to answer the first question it is necessary to identify the measure of the child at the center of the distribution, i.e., the child whose time in therapy is exceeded by that of 50 percent of the children. The second question was included to point out that the median is the 50th percentile and, therefore, the appropriate statistic for answering such questions.

The median can be computed from measures having ordinal, interval, or ratio properties. Thus, one difference between the mean and median is that the latter is appropriate for ordinal data.

The main disadvantage of the median as compared to the mean in instances where both would be appropriate concerns ease of computation. The mean is almost always less time-consuming than the median to compute.

Another variable on which mean and median differ is degree of stability. The mean tends to be a more stable (hence, more reliable) measure of central tendency than the median. A sample mean typically provides a more reliable estimate of a population mean than a sample median does of a population median. Partially for this reason, significance tests for differences between means tend to be more *powerful* than comparable tests between medians, and confidence intervals for means tend to be *narrower* than those for medians (these concepts are discussed later in this chapter). While the mean tends to be a more reliable measure of central tendency than the median, you should keep in mind that the mean may not be as *valid* a measure of central tendency as the median, for reasons that have been cited.

One other possible limitation of the median in comparison to the mean is that it is relatively insensitive to extreme measures. Note that the median of all three of the following sets of measures is the same, i.e., 50:

$$\begin{array}{ccccc} 5 & 19 & 50 & 75 & 80 \\ 15 & 40 & 50 & 55 & 60 \\ 15 & 25 & 50 & 75 & 1{,}000 \end{array}$$

If for some reason you want your index of central tendency to be influenced by extreme measures, the mean probably would be a better choice than the median.

The final measure of central tendency we will consider is the *mode*. The mode of a set, or distribution, is the measure that occurs most frequently. The mode of the following set of 10 measures would be 7 since this is the value which occurs most often:

7   7   7   8   9   10   11   11   12   13

The mode can be used to answer such questions as:

1. What was the most typical (i.e., frequently occurring) response of a person (or group) to a particular test task?
2. Is a stutterer's speech fluency more likely to improve, become worse, or stay the same after receiving a particular therapy?
3. Do persons who have spastic dysarthrias tend to benefit from muscle training?

While the reason the mode would be appropriate for answering the first question should be obvious, it may be less so for the other two. The mode is appropriate for answering such questions as the second—i.e., "probability" questions—because the category most stutterers fall into (the modal category) designates the most probable outcome. The mode is also appropriate for answering such questions as the third—i.e., questions about group tendencies—because the most frequent outcome (assuming there is a most frequent outcome) designates the group tendency.

The mode is appropriate for measures having nominal, ordinal, interval, or ratio properties. It is the only measure of central tendency that can be used with nominal data.

The mode is generally regarded as a less stable (and hence less reliable) measure of central tendency than either the median or the mean. Partially for this reason, significance tests for data treated as nominal tend to be less powerful than those for data treated as ordinal, interval, or ratio (this concept is discussed later in this chapter).

While the mean, median, and mode are the most frequently used measures of central tendency in speech and hearing research, they are not the only such measures. Two others are the geometric mean and the harmonic mean (Campbell, 1974, pp. 73–74). Since these measures have rarely been used in speech and hearing research (or for that matter in research in any behavioral science), they will not be described here.

Measures of Variability. These indices designate the spread, dispersion, homogeneity, or variability of a set of numbers. They indicate how far the numbers in a set deviate from an index of central tendency computed for the set. The more they deviate, the larger the value of the index.

When the numbers in a set are measures of attributes of persons or behaviors, they provide information about the degree of variability of such attributes. In a sense, they provide information about the degree of representativeness of indices of central tendency. The less variable the measures in a set, the more representative would be any index of central tendency. Suppose five children who had a rare neuromuscular disorder earned the following scores on a test of articulation proficiency:

$$75 \quad 77 \quad 78 \quad 78 \quad 80$$

The median score would be 78. Since the other scores deviate little from the median, it would be quite representative of them. If, however, the scores earned by these children had been the following:

$$25 \quad 40 \quad 78 \quad 90 \quad 150$$

the median (which again is 78) would have deviated considerably from several of the scores and hence would not have been particularly representative of them.

There are three commonly used indices of variability: the range, the interquartile (or semi-interquartile) range, and the standard deviation. All are discussed in the computational appendix (see Appendix A).

The *range* is a frequently used measure of variability. It is relatively simple to compute, since it is merely the difference between the highest and lowest measures in a set. In some instances, the highest and lowest measures are reported rather than the difference between them.

The range can be used to answer such questions as:

1. What was the age range of the clients receiving a particular therapy?
2. How variable was a particular client's stuttering frequency on a situational basis?

Note that the range can be used as an index of both intrasubject and intersubject variability.

The range is an appropriate index of variability for measures having ordinal, interval, or ratio properties. As such, it can provide information about the amount of deviation from both the mean and median of a set of measures.

The main advantages of the range are that it is relatively easy to compute and interpret. To compute it you only have to identify the highest and lowest measures in a set. Its interpretation is more straightforward than any of the other indices of variability.

The main disadvantage of the range is that it can make a set of measures appear more variable than they are. A single measure that is relatively large or small compared to the others can increase the magnitude of the range a great deal. Suppose a group of 10 children earned the following scores on a language test:

75   80   80   85   85   85   90   95   95   135

The range of these scores would be 60 points (i.e., 135 − 75). Except for one score (i.e., 135) these measures are not very variable. If it were deleted, the range would only be 20 points (i.e., 95 − 75). Thus, one relatively extreme score resulted in a 300 percent increase in the magnitude of the range.

Because of the susceptibility of the range to distortion by a few extreme measures, various restricted ranges (i.e., ranges in which a certain percentage of the measures are ignored) have been developed. The two such ranges most frequently used in speech and hearing research are the *interquartile range* and the *semi-interquartile range*. Both are based on the middle 50 percent of measures—i.e., the highest 25 percent and lowest 25 percent are ignored. The relationship between them is that the semi-interquartile range is equal to the interquartile range divided by two. For the ten language scores, the interquartile range would be 15 (i.e., 95 − 80); the semi-interquartile range, 7.5.

The interquartile and semi-interquartile ranges can be used to answer questions such as the following:

1. How well do speech pathologists agree when rating speech segments from persons who have cleft palates for degree of nasality?
2. Do children's scores on Form A of a language test tend to be more variable than on Form B?
3. Within what range of scores do the 25th and 75th percentiles fall for six year olds on a particular test of language performance?

Note that both ranges indicate the degree of separation between the 25th and 75th percentiles, i.e., they describe the variability of the middle 50 percent of measures.

The interquartile and semi-interquartile ranges are appropriate indices of variability for measures having ordinal, interval, or ratio properties. In this regard they are similar to the range. They are the most frequently used indices of variability for measures with ordinal properties. As such, they provide an index of the dispersion of measures around the median.

The main advantage of these indices over the range is that they are not susceptible to distortion by a few extreme measures. They are therefore more *stable* indices of variability than the range. Their main disadvantage when compared to the range is that they are not as easily interpretable. While the interpretation of the range is relatively straightforward, even for someone with little or no statistical training, both interquartile and semi-interquartile ranges may be somewhat difficult to interpret even for someone who has had statistical training. This is particularly true of the interpretation of their absolute magnitudes. Their relative magnitudes, however, often can be made readily interpretable. (See Silverman, 1967, for an illustration of how the relative magnitudes of such ranges can be made interpretable.)

Another *possible* limitation of both the interquartile and semi-interquartile ranges is that they do not reflect the variability of all measures in a set, only the middle 50 percent. This is most likely to be a limitation in instances where it is necessary to describe the absolute (as opposed to the relative) variability of the measures in a set.

The final index of variability we will describe here, the *standard deviation*, does not have this limitation. It reflects the variability of all measures in a set. It also has an advantage over the range in that its magnitude is less likely to be distorted by one or more extreme measures. Partially for these reasons, the standard deviation has been the most frequently used measure of variability in speech and hearing research.

The magnitude of a standard deviation indicates the average, absolute deviation of the measures in a set from their mean. It could be computed by determining the absolute deviation of each member of a set from the mean of that set, summing the deviations, and dividing by the number of measures in the set. Suppose we wished to determine the standard deviation of the following set consisting of three measures:

$$3 \quad 5 \quad 7$$

The mean of this set would be 5 [i.e., $(3 + 5 + 7)/3$] and the standard deviation would be 2 [i.e., $(5 - 3) + (5 - 7)/2$]. Note that in the computation of the mean deviation, the signs of individual deviations (i.e., $+$ or $-$) are ignored. If the signs were not ignored and the deviations were summed algebraically, those for measures larger than the mean would have minus signs. Such deviations would tend to cancel those for measures smaller than the mean that would have plus signs. The algebraic sum of the deviations in the illustration would be:

$$(5 - 3) + (5 - 7) = 2 - 2 = 0$$

The deviations above and below the mean here cancel each other and the standard deviation would be 0, indicating no variability (which of course is not the case).

To compute the standard deviation by determining individually the deviation of each measure from the mean would be a tedious process. For this reason, a formula was derived by mathematical statisticians which permits the standard deviation to be computed with considerably less effort. This formula is included in the computational appendix (see Appendix A).

The *magnitude* of a standard deviation indicates the degree of variability of the measures from which it was computed. The larger the standard deviation, the more variable the measures. The smallest possible standard deviation is 0, which, of course, indicates no variability. There is no upper limit on its size, or magnitude.

The *unit* of a standard deviation is the same as that of the measures from which it was computed. If a test has a mean score of 100 points and a standard deviation of 15 points, this indicates that the average (i.e., mean) deviation of the scores from the mean is 15 points.

If the measures in a set are *normally distributed* (which is often the case for scores on standardized tests such as intelligence tests), the percentage, or proportion, of the population which deviates a given number of *standard deviation units* from the mean of that set can be estimated. The normal distribution is a symmetrical bell-shaped curve in which certain relationships hold regarding its height at specified distances from its center (see Figure 8.1). In

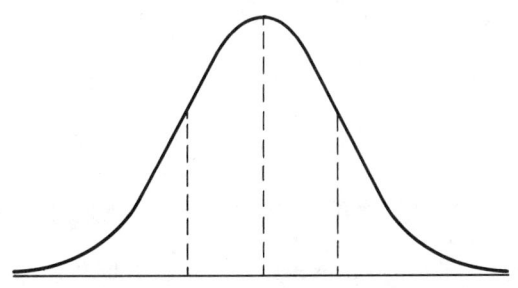

FIGURE 8.1. *The normal curve, or distribution. The vertical line at the center designates the position of the mean, median, and mode, which are identical in this distribution. The other two vertical lines designate positions that are one standard deviation from the mean. Note that approximately 68 percent of the area under the curve falls between these two vertical lines.*

a normal distribution, for example, approximately 68 percent of the measures are within one standard deviation of the mean. If the scores on a test that has a mean of 100 points and a standard deviation of 15 points are normally distributed, approximately 68 percent of persons from the population on which the test was standardized will have scores between 85 and 115.

The standard deviation can be used to answer such questions as:

1. How variable are the scores on a particular diagnostic test?
2. What range of scores would constitute "normal limits" on a particular diagnostic test (assuming that scores on this test are normally distributed)?
3. How far, on the average, did a person's thresholds for a 1000 Hz tone deviate from this mean threshold for this tone? (The assumption is made here that this threshold was measured a number of times. Another way to ask the same question would be: "How representative was a person's mean threshold for a 1000 Hz tone of those that were obtained on repeated testing?")

The first question illustrates the use of the standard deviation as a measure of variability. The second illustrates its use in estimating proportions of the population whose scores (or other measures) fall within certain limits. If you defined the lower boundary of "normal limits" on a particular test as that score that is equaled or exceeded by 90 percent of eight year olds, you could use the standard deviation to estimate that score. The third question illustrates its use in assessing the representativeness of the mean. The smaller the standard deviation (i.e., the less the average deviation of the scores from their mean), the more representative the mean.

The standard deviation is an appropriate index of variability for measures having interval or ratio properties. It is the most frequently used such index for the dispersion of measures around the mean.

The main *advantages* of the standard deviation over other indices of variability are: (1) it reflects the dispersion of all the measures in a set, and (2) it is the most stable index of variability and hence the most reliable such index. Also, if scores (or other measures) are normally distributed, the standard deviation provides more information about them than other indices of variability do.

The main *disadvantage* of the standard deviation as an index of variability is the same as that mentioned for the interquartile and semi-interquartile ranges. Unless measures are normally distributed, the *absolute* magnitude of their standard deviation may be difficult to interpret. To know that a set of measures that are not normally distributed has a standard deviation of 3.5 provides little information regarding their dispersion.

While the absolute magnitudes of standard deviations may be difficult to interpret, their *relative* magnitudes frequently provide useful information. If the means of the scores earned by two groups on a test of language functioning were approximately the same, but the standard deviations of their scores were quite different, this would indicate that the persons in one of the groups were more heterogeneous in their performance on this test than those in the other group.

The range, interquartile range, semi-interquartile range, and standard deviation are the only indices of variability used often enough in speech and hearing research to be worth mentioning.

Measures of Association. These indices are used to describe the *strength* and *direction* of the relationships between sets of measures (these attributes of relationships are described in Chapter 5). They indicate how the attributes described by such sets of measures are related to each other, i.e., correlated. The numbers that are yielded by such indices are referred to as *correlation coefficients.*

Correlation coefficients typically provide several kinds of information about the relationships between the sets of numbers correlated. First, they provide information about the *strength* of the relationship between the attributes measured by such sets. The larger the correlation coefficient (i.e., the closer it is to 1.00), the stronger the relationship. The smaller the correlation coefficient (i.e., the closer it is to 0) the weaker the relationship. (If the correlation coefficient is 0, there is no relationship.)

Suppose you administered a test of auditory discrimination ability and a test of articulation proficiency to a kindergarten class and correlated the two sets of scores earned by the children on these tests. If the resulting correlation coefficient was 0.60, this would suggest that auditory discrimination ability and articulation proficiency were more closely associated, or related, for these children than would have been the case if the resulting correlation coefficient had been, for example, 0.15. The strength of this relationship, however, would *not* have been four times as great if the coefficient had been 0.60 rather than 0.15. Correlation coefficients have *ordinal* properties. Thus, a correlation coefficient of 0.50 indicates a greater degree of association than one of 0.30 and a lesser degree than one of 0.90.

Correlation coefficients may also provide a second kind of information about the relationships between sets of measures: the *direction* of the relationship between attributes measured by pairs of such sets. The direction of this kind of relationship can be either *positive* or *negative*. If it is positive, persons who tend to exhibit relative high (or low) levels of one of the attributes tend to exhibit corresponding levels of the other. Thus, height and weight are positively correlated (i.e., the taller a person is the more he tends to weigh).

If the relationship between two attributes is negative, persons who tend to exhibit relatively high (or low) levels of one of the attributes tend to exhibit opposite levels of the other. Thus, chronological age and number of articulation errors is negatively correlated for elementary-school children (i.e., the older an elementary-school child, the fewer articulation errors he or she is likely to have). If a correlation coefficient is preceded by a minus sign, the relationship between the attributes correlated is negative.

Correlation coefficients typically range between -1.00 and $+1.00$. A correlation coefficient larger than 1.00 is impossible.

The correlation coefficients that are described in detail in this section and dealt with in the computational appendix (i.e., the contingency coefficient, ϕ (phi) coefficient, Spearman rank-order coefficient, and Pearson product-moment correlation coefficient) are for assessing the association between pairs of attributes. While the most frequently used indices of association are of this type, they are not the only ones. Several other types—including multiple correlation and partial correlation—will be dealt with briefly at the end of this section.

The first measure of association we will describe is the *contingency coefficient*. It is an index of the degree of relationship, or association, between two attributes of events that had been assigned on the bases of these attributes to the cells of a contingency table. The contingency table from which the contingency coefficient is computed contains two or more rows and two or more columns. The number of rows and columns does *not* have to be the same. Thus, a contingency table could have two rows and five columns, or five rows and two columns, or five rows and five columns, or two rows and two columns, and so on. (An example of a two-row and two-column contingency table is presented in the Computational Appendix in the section on the contingency coefficient.)

The number of columns (or number of rows) in a contingency table is determined by the number of categories into which the scale for an attribute is divided, or segmented. For the attribute "biological sex," the scale would typically be divided into two categories: male and female. For the attribute "type of speech disorder," the scale could be divided into the following five categories: phonation, articulation, resonance, fluency, and language.

While the scales for attributes mentioned thus far have been nominal, those representing any level of measurement can be used in contingency tables. An example of an attribute with ordinal properties that could be used in such tables would be "grade level." The categories into which the scale for this attribute could be divided would include "first grade," "second grade," "third grade," and so on.

To illustrate the application of contingency tables and contingency coefficients, suppose you wished to determine whether the number of words repeated by elementary-school children tended to be related to their grade level. That is, you wished to determine whether older elementary-school children tended to repeat words less frequently than younger elementary-school children or vice versa. One approach you could use would be to determine the frequency of word repetitions per 100 words spoken by ten first graders and ten sixth graders and then compute the median word repetition frequency for the twenty first and sixth graders combined. Each of the twenty children would then be assigned to one of the four cells of a contingency table (see Table 8.3) on the bases of: (1) whether he or she was a first or sixth grader, and (2) whether his or her word repetition frequency fell at or below the median or above the median. Three possible results from this assignment are depicted in Table 8.3. The configuration of Table A suggests a *strong positive* relationship between word repetition frequency and grade level; the ten sixth graders all had higher word repetition frequencies than the ten first graders. The configuration of Table B suggests *no* relationship between grade level and word repetition frequency; the sixth graders' word repetition frequencies exhibited no tendency to be systematically higher or lower than those of the first graders. The configuration of Table C, on the other hand, suggests a *strong negative* relationship between grade level and word repetition frequency; the ten first graders all had higher word repetition

Organizing Data for Answering Questions 187

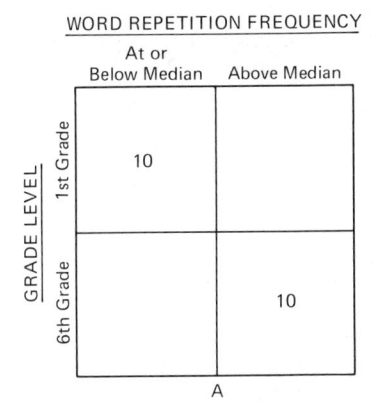

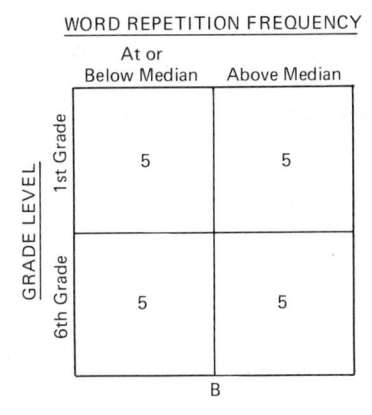

A

WORD REPETITION FREQUENCY

	At or Below Median	Above Median
1st Grade	10	
6th Grade		10

GRADE LEVEL

B

WORD REPETITION FREQUENCY

	At or Below Median	Above Median
1st Grade	5	5
6th Grade	5	5

GRADE LEVEL

C

WORD REPETITION FREQUENCY

	At or Below Median	Above Median
1st Grade		10
6th Grade	10	

GRADE LEVEL

TABLE 8.3. Three possible results from the assignment of twenty children to the cells of a contingency table on the bases of their word repetition frequencies and grade levels.

frequencies than the ten sixth graders. In most "real world" research, the relationships (or lack of them) would not be as clear-cut as those depicted in Table 8.3.

The procedure for computing the contingency coefficient is outlined in the computational appendix (see Appendix A). This procedure is applicable to a contingency table of any size.

The contingency coefficient is zero when no relationship, or association, exists between the two variables. If the relationship between them is perfect (e.g., as depicted in parts A and C of Table 8.3), the value of the contingency coefficient will approach, but not equal, 1.00. How close it will come to 1.00 is a function of the size of the table; the larger the table, the closer it will come to 1.00. For a 2 × 2 table (which is the size of the tables in Table 8.3), the upper limit of the contingency coefficient is 0.71.

The nature of the relationship between the variables in a contingency table (i.e., positive or negative) has to be inferred from the configuration of the table, since it is impossible for a contingency coefficient to have a minus value. Thus, a contingency coefficient of 0.60 can indicate either a positive or a negative relationship between the attributes.

The contingency coefficient can be used to answer such questions as:

1. Is there a relationship between school grade and word repetition frequency for elementary-school children?
2. Is the acceptability of an electrolarynx associated with the socioeconomic level of the person who is laryngectomized?

A contingency table that could be used to answer the first question has already been described (see Table 8.3). One that could be used to answer the second question is presented in Table 8.4. Obviously, socioeconomic status could have been categorized in other ways in this table.

	Acceptable	Unacceptable	Undecided
Upper			
Middle			
Lower			

ACCEPTABILITY OF ELECTROLARYNX / SOCIO-ECONOMIC STATUS

TABLE 8.4. A contingency table for studying the association between acceptability of an electrolarynx and socioeconomic status.

The contingency coefficient can be computed from measures having nominal, ordinal, interval, or ratio properties. It is the only measure of association that can be used with nominal data in contingency tables larger than 2×2.

While the contingency coefficient is a very useful index for assessing degree of association in contingency tables larger than 2×2, it does have several limitations. First, it is somewhat difficult to interpret because its upper limit is less than 1.00. Thus, a contingency coefficient of 0.70 could indicate either a perfect relationship or a fairly strong relationship between the attributes, depending on the size of the contingency table.

A second possible limitation of this index is that contingency coefficients cannot be compared unless they are yielded by tables of the same size, since the upper limits of contingency coefficients are a function of the sizes of tables on which they are computed. Thus, a contingency coefficient of 0.70 for a 2 × 2 table would indicate a higher degree of association between the attributes than one of 0.75 on a 3 × 3 table (the upper limit for a contingency coefficient on such a table would be 0.82).

A third possible limitation of the contingency coefficient as an index of association, or correlation, is that its value is not directly comparable to those yielded by other such indices including the three dealt with in the computational appendix, i.e., the phi coefficient, the Spearman rank-order coefficient, and the Pearson product-moment correlation coefficient.

In summary, the contingency coefficient in spite of its limitations is a useful measure of association (or correlation) for contingency tables, particularly those larger than 2 × 2.

For contingency tables that are 2 × 2, an index of association that ordinarily would be preferable to the contingency coefficient is the ϕ (*phi*) *coefficient*. The phi coefficient has an upper limit of 1.00 (which would indicate a perfect relationship between the attributes), and the nature of the relationship between the attributes (positive or negative) is indicated by the sign of the coefficient. Thus in Table 8.3, the phi coefficient for Table A would be +1.00; for Table B would be 0.00; and for Table C would be −1.00. The phi coefficient is easier to interpret than the contingency coefficient, and its value is directly comparable to those yielded by the Spearman rank-order coefficient and the Pearson product-moment correlation coefficient. The coefficients yielded by these three indices on a given set of data, however, usually are not identical (a demonstration of this is provided in the computational appendix where all three were computed from the same set of data).

The procedure for computing the phi coefficient is outlined in the computational appendix (see Appendix A).

The phi coefficient can be used to answer the same types of questions as the contingency coefficient as long as the data can be cast into a 2 × 2 table.

The phi coefficient (like the contingency coefficient) can be computed from measures having nominal, ordinal, interval, or ratio properties. It is a particularly useful index of correlation between dichotomous attributes. (An example of a dichotomous attribute would be biological sex, which consists of the categories "male" and "female.")

The advantages of the phi coefficient over the contingency coefficient as an index of association for 2 × 2 contingency tables already have been mentioned.

In summary, the phi coefficient is a useful index of association, particularly for measures having nominal properties. The phi coefficient and the contingency coefficient are the only such indices described here that are appropriate for measures having nominal properties.

If the measures of the attributes you wish to determine the relationship between have at least ordinal properties, the *Spearman rank-order coefficient* can be used as an index of association. This coefficient is an index of the extent to which two sets of measures *rank order* a group of persons in the same manner. If both rank order the persons in the identical manner, this would indicate a *perfect positive* relationship between them and the Spearman rank-order coefficient would be +1.00. On the other hand, if they rank order the persons in exactly the opposite manner, this would indicate a *perfect negative* relationship between them and the Spearman rank-order coefficient would be −1.00. Spearman rank-order coefficients for less than perfect relationships fall between −1.00 and +1.00.

The procedure for computing the Spearman rank-order coefficient is outlined in the computational appendix (see Appendix A).

Suppose that in order to determine whether any relationship existed between the degree of recovery exhibited by receptive aphasics and their socioeconomic level, you rank ordered five receptive aphasics both on the basis of the amount of recovery they exhibited and their socioeconomic level. Three possible sets of orderings of the five aphasics on the basis of these attributes are presented in Table 8.5. The Spearman rank-order coefficient for

TABLE 8.5. Three possible sets of orderings of five receptive aphasics based on their socioeconomic levels and the amount of improvement they exhibited. The aphasics are designated by the letters A, B, C, D, and E.

Set I		Set II		Set III	
Socioeconomic Level	Improvement Level	Socioeconomic Level	Improvement Level	Socioeconomic Level	Improvement Level
A	A	A	E	A	E
C	C	C	A	C	D
B	B	B	D	B	B
D	D	D	C	D	C
E	E	E	B	E	A

the first set would be +1.00, for the second approximately 0.00, and for the third −1.00. Thus, the first set would suggest a *strong positive* relationship between improvement level and socioeconomic level, the second essentially *no* relationship between these variables, and the third a *strong negative* relationship between them.

The Spearman rank-order coefficient can be used to answer questions similar to these:

1. Is the amount of recovery exhibited by receptive aphasics related to their socioeconomic level?
2. Do the levels of children's performances on two particular tests of language functioning tend to be similar?
3. How well do two speech pathologists agree in their orderings of clients with regard to degree of improvement following a program of therapy?

Using the Spearman rank-order coefficient to answer the first question has already been described. Answering the second question would involve ordering the children on the bases of the two sets of language scores. And answering the third would involve ordering the clients on the basis of each speech pathologist's ratings of degree of improvement.

The Spearman rank-order coefficient can be computed from measures having ordinal, interval, or ratio properties. It has been one of the most frequently used indices of association for measures having ordinal properties in speech pathology and audiology research.

The Spearman rank-order coefficient provides a satisfactory index of the degree of correspondence (or correlation) between two rank orderings of a group of persons. Thus, it is appropriate for measures having ordinal properties. While it is also appropriate for measures having interval or ratio properties, it has a limitation when used with such measures. This limitation is that the Spearman rank-order coefficient is insensitive to the sizes, or magnitudes, of the differences between measures. It is not possible with this procedure to detect the form of the relationship between a pair of attributes—i.e., whether the form is linear or nonlinear (see Figures 5.1, 5.4, and 5.5 and accompanying text for a description of linear and nonlinear relationships). To answer some questions, you must be able to determine whether the relationship between a pair of attributes is linear or nonlinear; to answer others, this information is not necessary. For answering questions of the second type, the Spearman rank-order coefficient would be satisfactory.

If the measures of the attributes you wish to determine the relationship between have interval or ratio properties and the relationship between them can be assumed to be linear (see Chapter 5), an index of association you can use for assessing this relationship is the *Pearson product-moment correlation coefficient*. This coefficient, which is also known as the *Pearson r*, is probably the most frequently used index of association (or correlation) in speech pathology and audiology research.

The Pearson *r* can be visualized, or interpreted, in several ways. First, it can be viewed as an index of how closely two sets of measures rank order a group of persons. Its magnitude is determined in large part by the extent to which the rank orderings are similar. As long as the relationship between a pair of attributes is not grossly nonlinear, the magnitude of the Pearson *r* will be quite similar to that of the Spearman rank-order coefficient.

The Pearson *r* also can be visualized as an index of the amount of deviation of the points in a scattergram (see Chapter 5) from the straight line from which they would deviate least. The more the points deviate from this line, the smaller will be the value of the Pearson *r*. If the points all lay on the line, the Pearson *r* would be 1.00. If the deviation of the points about such a line looked circular (i.e., if their deviation from this line was considerable), the Pearson *r* would be approximately 0.00. Scattergrams that depict these possibilities are presented in Figures 5.1 and 5.2.

The Pearson *r* is similar to the phi coefficient and Spearman rank-order coefficient in two ways: (1) its possible values fall between -1.00 and $+1.00$, and (2) the closer its value is to $+1.00$, the stronger the association between the attributes.

The procedure for computing the Pearson *r* is outlined in the computational appendix (see Appendix A).

The Pearson *r* can be used to answer questions similar to these:

1. What is the nature of the relationship between preschoolers' auditory discrimination ability and their articulation proficiency?
2. To what extent are first graders' levels of performance on a particular test prior to participating in a therapy program *predictive* of their levels of performance on that test after completing the program?

Note that answering the first question involves assessing the relationship between performances of *different* tasks by a group of persons at the *same* point in time, and answering the second question involves assessing the relationship between performances of the *same* task by a group of persons at different *points* in time.

Strictly speaking, the Pearson *r* is only an appropriate index of association for measures having interval or ratio properties. Nevertheless, in speech pathology and audiology research it has been used a great deal with measures that appear to have ordinal properties. Examples of such measures would be scores on tests of auditory discrimination ability and articulation proficiency. In most instances, probably no great harm is done if the Pearson *r* is used with measures that have ordinal properties. When it is used with such measures, the magnitude of a Pearson *r* can be interpreted as an *approximation* of what the coefficient describing the relationship would have been if the Spearman rank-order coefficient had been used.

To estimate the relative strength of the relationship indicated by a Pearson *r*, the *square* of its value (rather than its value) should be used. Squaring a Pearson *r* results in a reduction in its magnitude (except when its value is 1.00). The extent of this reduction can be surmised from Table 8.6, in which

r^2 magnitudes are presented for selected r values. Note that a Pearson r of at least 0.70 is needed before even 50 percent of the variation observed in a scattergram can be accounted for on the basis of a linear relationship between the attributes. In fact, a Pearson r of 0.50 is needed before even 25 percent of the variation observed in a scattergram can be accounted for on the basis of a linear relationship between the attributes.

TABLE 8.6. r^2 magnitudes for selected Pearson r values.

r	r^2	r	r^2
0.05	0.00	0.55	0.30
0.10	0.01	0.60	0.36
0.15	0.02	0.65	0.42
0.20	0.04	0.70	0.49
0.25	0.06	0.75	0.56
0.30	0.09	0.80	0.64
0.35	0.12	0.85	0.72
0.40	0.16	0.90	0.81
0.45	0.20	0.95	0.90
0.50	0.25	1.00	1.00

How would you describe in words the strength of the relationship depicted by a particular Pearson r? While there is no universality of agreement among statisticians regarding strengths of relationships designated by particular Pearson r values, some rough guidelines exist, with which most statisticians probably would agree, that can be used for making such judgments including the following:

1. Pearson r coefficients of less than 0.30 usually indicate that for most *practical* purposes *no* linear relationship exists between the attributes.
2. Pearson r coefficients between 0.30 and 0.50 usually indicate a *weak* linear relationship between the attributes.
3. Pearson r coefficients between 0.51 and 0.85 usually indicate a *moderate* linear relationship between the attributes.
4. Pearson r coefficients between 0.86 and 0.95 usually indicate a *strong* linear relationship between the attributes.
5. Pearson r coefficients higher than 0.96 usually indicate an *extremely strong* linear relationship between the attributes.

In summary, the Pearson r is an extremely useful index of association between pairs of attributes when the measures of such attributes have interval or ratio properties and the relationship between them is fairly linear. It provides information concerning the strength, direction, and linearity of the relationship between pairs of attributes.

The indices of association described in this section are representative of a fairly large number of indices for assessing relationships between pairs of attributes that have been developed by mathematical statisticians. Descriptions of other such indices can be found in elementary and intermediate statistics texts intended for psychologists and sociologists.

Indices of association are not limited to describing the relationships between pairs of attributes when the relationship between the attributes is presumed to be linear. There are indices of association for other purposes or types of data, including the following:

1. *Indices of association between pairs of attributes where the relationships between the attributes are presumed to be nonlinear.* These indices can be used to answer the same kinds of questions that could be answered by means of a Pearson r if the relationship between the attributes were linear. To determine whether it would be most reasonable to assume that the relationship between two attributes were linear or nonlinear, you can plot the measures you made of them on a scattergram. If the line that best fits the configuration of the points does not appear to be a straight line, it might be safest to assume that the relationship between the attributes is nonlinear (a scattergram in which a nonlinear relationship exists between attributes is presented in Figure 5.4).

These indices assess the goodness of fit of the points plotted in a scattergram to various types of curved lines.

If you feel the relationship between a pair of attributes is nonlinear, show the scattergram to a statistician. He or she should be able to recommend an appropriate nonlinear correlation coefficient.

2. *Indices of association between pairs of attributes with the effects of a third attribute held constant, or eliminated.* Indices used for this purpose are referred to as coefficients of *partial correlation*. Suppose you wished to determine whether a relationship existed between auditory discrimination ability and articulation proficiency for the children in a kindergarten classroom. It is conceivable that there could appear to be a relationship between the two because both are related to mental age. The higher the mental age of a child, the better the child is likely to do on both tasks. You may therefore wish to answer the question: "Would there be any relationship between auditory discrimination ability and articulation proficiency if the effects of mental age were eliminated (i.e., held constant)?" Coefficients of partial correlation can be used to answer this type of question. Since there are several coefficients of partial correlation, a statistician should be consulted for identifying the appropriate one for answering a particular question.

3. *Indices of association between an attribute and the composite of two or more other attributes.* These indices are referred to as coefficients of *multiple correlation*. Suppose you wanted to identify the attributes of speaking behavior which influence judgments of stuttering severity. One approach

would be to have speech samples from a number of stutterers rated for "degree of stuttering severity" by the method of direct magnitude-estimation (see Chapter 7). These samples would also be analyzed to determine the amounts of various attributes each possesses which might influence listeners' impressions of stuttering severity. Such attributes probably would include frequency of stuttering, average duration of moments of stuttering, and speaking rate. The composite of these three attributes would then be correlated with the ratings of stuttering severity by means of a coefficient of multiple correlation. If this coefficient were quite high (i.e., larger than 0.85), this would suggest that these attributes are likely to influence listeners' judgments of stuttering severity. For an illustration of the use of multiple correlation in speech and hearing research, see Young (1961).

Programs for indices of multiple correlation are available at most computer centers. The statistical consultant should be able to advise you about which program is most appropriate for your purpose. The consultant should also be able to help you interpret the results of the computer analysis.

4. *Indices of association between more than two sets of measures.* To answer a question, it is sometimes necessary to assess the degree of association, or agreement, between a number of sets of measures. This need arises most often in speech and hearing research when an investigator wishes to determine how well a group of judges agree in their ratings of a set of stimuli. Suppose you had three speech pathologists rate a group of children for "degree of nasality" by one of the scaling methods described in Chapter 7 and you wanted to determine how well the three agreed in their ratings of the children. Several indices of association could be used for this purpose. The Kendall coefficient of concordance (Siegel, 1956) would be appropriate if the ratings were assumed to be ordinal; the intraclass correlation coefficient (Ebel, 1951) would be appropriate if they were assumed to have interval or ratio properties.

Other Descriptive Statistical Procedures. This section will briefly describe several descriptive statistical procedures which (though complex mathematically) can be useful for answering questions pertaining to communicative disorders. These are factor analysis, discriminant function analysis, and multidimensional scaling. The computations for all three are made on a computer. The necessary programs should be available at most computer centers.

Factor analysis is a procedure for identifying the abilities which underlie the performances of a series of tasks (e.g., psychological or language tests). Suppose you *told* an aphasic to perform the following tasks: (1) point to the objects named, (2) name a series of objects, and (3) protrude his tongue. For his performance to be successful, at least one ability must be relatively intact. This ability could be labeled "language comprehension." If the aphasic were unable to understand the instructions of the tasks, he would probably be unable to perform them. Thus, one general factor, or ability, that underlies the performance of this series of tasks could be labeled "language comprehension."

Factor analysis can be of assistance for answering questions about: (1) general abilities, or factors, that are necessary to perform a series of tasks, and (2) tasks that are heavily weighted for each such factor and hence can be used for evaluating them.

Suppose you wished to develop a comprehensive test for evaluating aphasics. This test would consist of a series of tasks, and a great many tasks could be included. To help you decide which to include, you would want to know: (1) the aspects, or dimensions, of speech and language that are apt to be impaired as a result of the aphasic condition, and (2) the task, or tasks, best for evaluating each such aspect, or dimension. A factor analytic approach that could be used to obtain this information would run as follows:

1. A large number of possible tasks for such a test would be administered to a fairly large group of aphasics. All of the various types of tasks that have been used to evaluate aphasics would be represented.
2. The scores earned by the aphasics on all possible pairs of tasks would be correlated and displayed in a *correlation matrix*. A correlation matrix for five such tasks is depicted in Table 8.7. A correlation coefficient would appear in each square marked with an X. The type of correlation coefficient most often used for factor analysis is the Pearson *r*.

	Task I	Task II	Task III	Task IV	Task V
Task I		X	X	X	X
Task II			X	X	X
Task III				X	X
Task IV					X
Task V					

TABLE 8.7. A correlation matrix for five tasks. Each square marked with an X would contain a correlation coefficient.

3. The correlation matrix would be factor analyzed on a computer. Many programs for factor analyzing a correlation matrix have been developed. A statistician should be consulted to make certain that the most appropriate one available at the computer center is used.

The printout from the computer will contain information about: (1) the number of general factors, or abilities, identified by the program which presumably influenced the aphasics' performances of the tasks, and (2) the specific tasks that had relatively "high loadings" and "low loadings" for each. A task with a "high loading" for a certain factor, or ability, would be good for assessing that factor, or ability. Conversely, a task with a "low loading" for a certain factor, or ability, would not be very good for assessing that factor, or ability. You would probably want to include at least one task in your aphasia test with a relatively high loading for each factor.

How can you identify the ability that each factor represents? The computer does not label the factors. It does provide information, however, that can be used to infer the ability each factor represents. Suppose for a particular factor two tasks had relatively high loadings and three had relatively low loadings. To identify the ability associated with the factor, you would attempt to infer which ability the tasks with high loadings require that is not required of those with low loadings. Obviously, labels assigned to factors by such a reasoning process have to be regarded as tentative. Tasks with relatively high loadings may require more than one ability that is not required of those with relatively low loadings.

In summary, factor analysis can be a useful exploratory procedure for identifying general abilities that underlie the performance of a series of tasks. For further information on this technique, you may find books by Fruchter (1954) and Wolfe (1940) helpful. Though they are relatively old, they provide a good introduction to the subject.

Discriminant function analysis is a statistical procedure used to assign people to categories, usually dichotomous categories. The following are examples of pairs of categories to which discriminant function analysis might be used for assigning persons:

1. "beginning stuttering" versus "normally disfluent speech,"
2. "adequate velopharyngeal closure" versus "inadequate velopharyngeal closure" for speech, and
3. "auditory agnosia" versus "peripheral hearing loss."

Unfortunately, the usefulness of discriminant function analysis for making such diagnostic decisions is uncertain, since the technique has been used very little by speech pathologists and audiologists.

Programs for performing a discriminant function analysis should be available at most college or university computer centers.

The types of questions that discriminant function analysis may be useful for answering include:

1. Is a given four year old exhibiting "beginning stuttering" or "normally disfluent speech?"
2. What variables best differentiate "beginning stuttering" from "normally disfluent speech" for four year olds?
3. Is the velopharyngeal closure of a given child who has a cleft palate "adequate" or "inadequate" to support speech that has normal nasal resonance?
4. What measures best differentiate "adequate" from "inadequate" velopharyngeal closure?
5. Is the auditory comprehension problem of a given two year old due to "auditory agnosia" or a "peripheral hearing loss?"
6. What measures best differentiate "auditory agnosia" from "peripheral hearing loss" for two year olds?

While these questions all involve discriminating between two categories, discriminant function analysis is not limited to the two-category situation. Computer programs are available for discriminating among three or more categories.

The general strategy underlying discriminant function analysis for the two-category case can be summarized as follows:

1. A series of tasks (e.g., tests), which there is some reason to believe might discriminate between persons who fall into the two categories, are administered to two groups. Each consists of persons who fall into one of the categories. For the first question, one group would consist of four year olds who are known to be beginning to stutter and the other would consist of four year olds who have no history of a stuttering problem.
2. A discriminant function analysis is performed on the measures (e.g., test scores). The results of this analysis indicate which task, or combination of tasks, best discriminates between the groups (assuming that both groups did not perform essentially the same on the tasks).
3. The task, or combination of tasks, identified by the analysis can be used for determining the category, or group, to assign a person when the group to which he or she should be assigned is unknown. The analysis provides an equation for this purpose. In this equation, the person's score on each task (S) is multiplied by a weight (W) that is determined by the program and the products of these multiplications are summed algebraically. The form of a typical such equation would be similar to:

$$X = S_1 W_1 + S_2 W_2$$

In words, you would multiply the person's score on task one by the weight assigned to that task and add this to his score on task two multiplied by the weight assigned to task two.

The value of X would indicate the category to which the person should be assigned. If it exceeds one given in the computer printout, the person would be assigned to one category; if it is smaller than this value, the person would be assigned to the other category. The computer printout also provides information on the likelihood of category assignments being incorrect.

The procedure for a discriminant function analysis involving more than two categories is essentially the same as that outlined here.

In summary, discriminant function analysis can be a useful procedure for: (1) identifying the way, or ways, in which the members of a group differ and (2) identifying the categories, or groups, to which people belong.

Multidimensional scaling is a procedure for identifying the attributes of stimuli (or events) to which people attend, i.e., the attributes which they abstract. Suppose you wanted to identify the attributes of moments of stuttering to which people attend. To do this, you could collect "moments of stuttering" from a number of stutterers on videotape. You would then have these taped moments of stuttering rated for *degree of similarity* by a fairly large number of observers. The similarity ratings could be made in several ways. The one that appears to be used most often can be called the "method of triads." With this method, all possible combinations of the moments of stuttering taken *three* at a time would be formed. Observers would be asked to indicate the two moments of stuttering in each group of three that are most similar. The resulting similarity ratings would be subjected to several computer analyses, including a factor analysis. The attributes of the stimuli to which the observers consciously or unconsciously attended while making their similarity ratings can be inferred from the factors identified by the factor analysis.

Multidimensional scaling is a relatively new technique that probably would be useful to speech pathologists and audiologists for answering certain questions. Information about the technique can be obtained from a number of sources, including books by Torgerson (1963) and Green and Carmone (1970).

Two-Dimensional Graphical Displays. Such displays are frequently used by speech pathologists and audiologists for organizing quantitative data. In these displays, the scale for one attribute is presented on the horizontal axis and the scale for the second on the vertical axis (see Figure 8.2). Each event is plotted at the point that would correspond to its value for the attributes. If its value for the first attribute were 3 and for the second, 2, it would be plotted at the point indicated in Figure 8.2.

Several types of two-dimensional graphical displays are often used by speech pathologists and audiologists. One of these, the *scattergram*, already has been described in considerable detail (see Chapter 5). Another used both

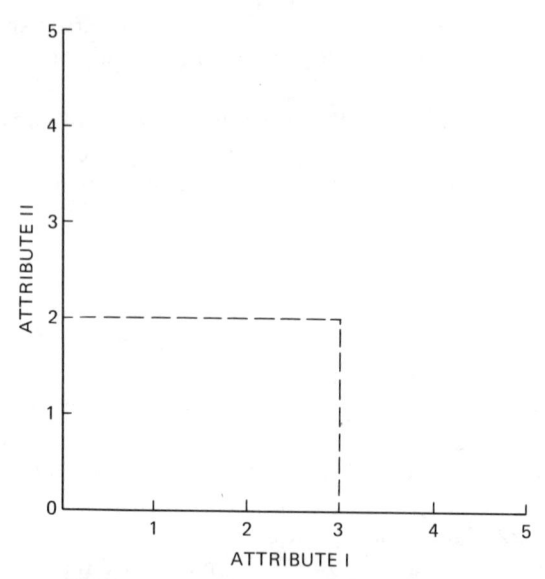

FIGURE 8.2. *A two-dimensional graphical display.*

by speech pathologists and audiologists is the *pure-tone audiogram*. A third, which is frequently used by behaviorally oriented clinicians (particularly those who utilize operant conditioning), plots the frequency of occurrence of a specified behavior (or behaviors) over time. In Figure 8.2, *Attribute I* would be a time measure (e.g., seconds, minutes, hours, days, or weeks), and *Attribute II* would be frequency of occurrence (on a specified task or during a specified time period). Numerous examples of two-dimensional graphical displays can be found in almost any volume of the *Journal of Speech and Hearing Disorders* or the *Journal of Speech and Hearing Research*.

Two-dimensional graphical displays can be used to answer such questions as:

1. What is the nature of the relationship between number of articulation errors and chronological age?
2. What are a person's thresholds for pure tones of various frequencies?
3. What is the effect of response-contingent reinforcement on a particular behavior over a period of time?

The types of graphical displays that could be used for answering questions one through three respectively would be a scattergram, a pure-tone audiogram, and a behavior chart.

Two-dimensional graphical displays can be used for organizing measures with ordinal, interval, ratio, or logarithmic properties.

Inferential Statistical Techniques

The statistical techniques discussed thus far are intended for summarizing, organizing, or describing aspects of a set of measures. They allow you to make statements and answer questions about a set of measures *you have obtained*. Strictly speaking, they do not allow you to make statements or answer questions about a set of measures *you might have obtained*. That is, they do not provide the information you need to *generalize beyond* your set of data or sample of subjects. Inferential statistical techniques provide this information.

Inferential statistical techniques allow you to answer several kinds of questions about a set of data that go beyond the analyses that were made of it. One such category of questions pertains to the *reliability* of differences or relationships observed in a set of data. Suppose you found that a group of children, on the average, made fewer articulation errors after participating in an experimental therapy program than before participating in it. This finding would allow you to answer the question: "Did the children in the experimental therapy program improve?" It would not by itself, however, permit you to answer the question: "If some other children similar to these children went through this experimental program, is it likely they also would improve?" The reason you could not answer this question is that the reliability of the difference between pre- and post-therapy measures would be uncertain. These measures would be unlikely to be identical even if the program had no effect. In fact, assuming the therapy had no effect, the children would stand a 50 percent chance of having the difference between their pre- and post-therapy measures suggest that it had an effect merely on the basis of "chance," or random fluctuation. Before concluding, therefore, that an observed difference between pre- and post-therapy measures could have resulted from participating in a therapy program, it would be necessary to determine the likelihood that it could have resulted from random fluctuation. *Significance tests*, which are an aspect of statistical inference, can be used to estimate the probability that observed differences between means or medians (or other descriptive statistics) resulted from chance, or random fluctuation. Such tests do not tell you whether an observed difference arose from this source, only the probability that it did.

Significance tests also can be used to assess the reliability of observed *relationships* between attributes. Specifically, they can be used to estimate the probability that a correlation coefficient indicating a relationship between the attributes correlated resulted from chance, or random fluctuation.

Another type of question that inferential statistical techniques allow you to answer concerns the *generality* of differences and relationships you observe in a set of data. Specifically, they allow you to answer the question:

"How likely is it that the differences or relationships (or both) that I have observed in the sample of persons I've studied also are present in the *population* from which these persons were selected?" Suppose you developed a therapy program that seemed to be very effective for modifying some aspect of the communicative behavior of persons in your caseload, based on differences between the means (or medians) of measures made of this aspect of their communicative behavior both before and after they participated in the program. While the difference you observed would permit you to conclude that the program appeared to be effective for the average or typical person in your caseload on which it was used, it would not permit you to conclude it also would be effective for persons like them not in your caseload. Significance tests provide you with a way of estimating how safe you would be in concluding that differences or relationships you observed in a *sample* of persons also are present in the *population* to which these persons belong (assuming that your sample was *randomly selected* from this population). It should be noted, however, that such tests only indicate the likelihood that *a* difference or relationship observed in a sample is present in the population from which it comes. They do *not* provide an estimate of the *magnitude* of the difference or relationship in the population. You *cannot* assume that the magnitude of a difference or relationship present in a sample is a good estimate of that in the population from which the sample comes. This magnitude in the population may be considerably smaller or larger than that in the sample.

While significance tests do not permit you to estimate the magnitudes of differences and relationships (i.e., correlations) in a population from those in a sample, there are inferential statistical methods known as *confidence intervals* which do permit you to estimate such magnitudes. These methods will be described next.

A third type of question that inferential statistical techniques allow you to answer pertains to estimating population values, or magnitudes, of descriptive statistics and of differences between descriptive statistics. Once you have established by means of a significance test that a difference or relationship in your sample is likely to be present in the population to which your sample belongs, you may wish to estimate the magnitude of this difference or the strength of this relationship in the population. Also, you may wish to estimate indices of central tendency and variability for the population. Confidence intervals allow you to make such estimates. They will be described in some detail later in this chapter.

Inferential statistical techniques, as I have indicated, fall into two broad categories: significance tests and confidence intervals. Representative examples of each type can be found in the computational appendix (see Appendix A). The remainder of the chapter will be devoted to a discussion of these types of statistical methods.

Significance Tests. These statistics can be used for answering the following question: "How likely is it that a difference or relationship observed in a set of data is the result of chance, or random fluctuation?" The differences referred to could be between almost any types of measures including means, medians, modes, frequencies, percentages, proportions, standard deviations, and correlation coefficients. The relationships referred to involve correlation coefficients.

What does the chance, or random fluctuation, estimated by significance tests refer to? The most direct way to answer this question is through the use of probability theory. The basic point here is that measures that are not different or related can appear to be different or related. Suppose you had a stutterer perform a speaking task in two situations, and she stuttered on 10 percent of the words she spoke in Situation I and 13 percent of those she spoke in Situation II. Would it be safe to conclude that she tends to stutter more frequently in Situation II than in Situation I? The answer to this question would be "no," because this outcome would occur by chance approximately 50 percent of the time. (We use the word "approximately" here because the two stuttering frequencies would be identical by chance a small percentage of the time.) For probability, the situation is analogous to tossing a coin. If you tossed a penny many times, approximately 50 percent of the time it would come up heads and approximately 50 percent of the time it would come up tails. A small percentage of the time it may stand on edge, which would be analogous in our illustration to the two stuttering frequencies being identical.

Suppose you had the stutterer perform the speaking task a second time under the two conditions and the results were the same as the first time—i.e., she stuttered more frequently in Situation II than in Situation I. Would you then be able to conclude that she tends to stutter more frequently in Situation II than in Situation I? The approximate probability of this outcome being due to chance would be:

$$\tfrac{1}{2} \times \tfrac{1}{2} = \tfrac{1}{4}$$

While you would probably feel more confident concluding now than you would have after the first trial that she stutters more frequently in Situation II than in Situation I, the probability is still relatively high (i.e., 25 percent) that the observed effect was due to chance, or random fluctuation. Most investigators would be unwilling to conclude that an observed effect (e.g., tending to stutter more frequently in one situation than another) was a "real" one unless the probability of its being due to chance was *five percent or less*. The probability that the observed difference between situations in our illustration was due to chance would be less than five percent if the stutterer stuttered more frequently in Situation II than in Situation I on five consecutive repetitions of the experimental task (i.e., speaking in two situations):

$$\tfrac{1}{2} \times \tfrac{1}{2} \times \tfrac{1}{2} \times \tfrac{1}{2} \times \tfrac{1}{2} = \tfrac{1}{32}$$

This outcome would only occur by chance approximately three percent of the time.

To determine whether the probability that an outcome which was due to chance, or random fluctuation, is adequately small, a significance test can be used to assess the viability of a *null hypothesis*. Null hypotheses state that observed differences or relationships are due to chance, or random fluctuation. They state that if it were not for chance, or random fluctuation, the differences between the measures or the magnitudes of the correlation coefficients would have been 0.00. All significance tests have a single function: to determine the probability that null hypotheses are true. If the probability of a null hypothesis being true were relatively small, it would be *rejected*. The investigator decides before the significance test is made how small the probability of a null hypothesis being true has to be before it is rejected. The levels that are used most frequently for this purpose are 0.05 (5 percent probability of a null hypothesis being true) and 0.01 (1 percent probability of a null hypothesis being true). Obviously, the 0.01 level is more conservative than the 0.05 level, since it requires stronger evidence that an observed difference or relationship isn't the result of chance, or random fluctuation, before a null hypothesis can be rejected.

In the statistical literature, the 1 percent level is referred to as the *0.01 level of confidence*, and the 5 percent level as the *0.05 level of confidence*. Thus, if a null hypothesis were rejected at the 0.01 level of confidence, it would be approximately 99 percent certain that the observed difference or relationship was not the result of chance, or random fluctuation.

Rejection of a null hypothesis only means that an observed difference or relationship is unlikely to have resulted from chance, or random fluctuation. It does not mean that it was due to the reason suggested by the experimenter in his *research hypothesis*. Usually more than one explanation can be posited for an observed difference or relationship other than chance, or random fluctuation. Rejection of a null hypothesis provides no information about which of these explanations is most viable. It only indicates that chance, or random fluctuation, is unlikely to be the explanation.

How do you decide on an explanation for an observed difference or relationship? Two approaches can be used: logical and logical-empirical. With a logical approach, you specify the possible explanations for a difference or relationship and, on the basis of the information that is available to you, decide which explanation (or combination of explanations) is the most plausible. One obvious limitation of this approach is that the "real" explanation (or explanations) may not have occurred to you and thus would not have been among those you considered. Under this circumstance, the most plausible explanation would not be the most plausible explanation.

The logical-empirical approach goes one step beyond the logical approach. After the explanation for a difference or relationship that appears to be the most plausible is identified by a reasoning process, an experiment or a series of experiments is conducted to assess its viability. If the findings of the experiment or experiments are consistent with the explanation, you could have more confidence in its viability than if it were arrived at by a reasoning process alone.

Failure to reject a null hypothesis does *not* necessarily mean that the difference or relationship observed was the result of chance, or random fluctuation. There are at least two other possible explanations:

1. The difference or relationship was a real one, but because its magnitude was relatively small, the significance test was not *powerful* enough to detect it. The smaller a difference or the weaker a relationship, the larger the number of subjects or observations needed to detect it, i.e., cause the null hypothesis to be rejected. While a significance test on the difference between the means of two groups, each consisting of ten persons, may not lead to rejection of the null hypothesis, the same significance test on the difference between the same means could lead to this outcome if the groups consisted of twenty-five persons.

2. The "real" difference or relationship (i.e., the one in the population) is larger in magnitude than the observed difference or relationship. By chance, subjects representing the extremes of the population distribution (or distributions) were not adequately represented in the sample. If the sample had been more representative, the difference between the means would have been larger, or the relationship stronger, and the null hypothesis would have been rejected.

Failure to reject a null hypothesis when it should be rejected is known as a *Type II error*. This is one of the two types of error that can occur in a decision on a null hypothesis. The other, a *Type I error*, occurs when a null hypothesis is rejected when it should not have been rejected—i.e., when the observed difference or relationship really was the result of chance, or random fluctuation.

A Type I error can occur for several reasons. First, on the basis of random fluctuation you will occasionally obtain a difference large enough, or a relationship strong enough, for a null hypothesis to be rejected. Thus, if a significance test were run at a 5 percent alpha level (i.e., a 0.05 level of confidence), the probability of the null hypothesis being rejected on the basis of chance alone would be 5 percent. You would expect 5 percent of the null hypotheses you test to be rejected when they should not be rejected—i.e., when they are true.

A Type I error may also occur because the measures on which a significance test is performed are biased. One of the most common sources of such bias is the investigator's expectations regarding the results of the research. Such expectations can consciously or unconsciously influence measurements. This is particularly apt to happen in therapy outcome research. Clinicians may feel such a strong need for their therapy to appear effective that they may unconsciously manipulate pre- and post-therapy measures so that the magnitude of the difference between them is increased. This could cause a true null hypothesis to be rejected.

Suppose that in order to assess the impact of a therapy program on a group of stutterers, you measured twenty-five aspects of their behavior both before and after participating in the program and that you tested the reliability of the difference between the means of each of these twenty-five pairs of measures at the 5 percent (i.e., 0.05) level of confidence. Suppose, further, that the difference between only one of these twenty-five sets of pre- and post-therapy means was *statistically significant*—i.e., was large enough for the null hypothesis to be rejected. Could you conclude that the behavior this measure measured had changed? The answer to this question is "no," because you would expect approximately one out of every twenty true null hypotheses tested at the 0.05 level of confidence to be rejected. The probability of a Type I error having occurred when this null hypothesis was rejected is *not* 5 percent (the probability if only one null hypothesis had been tested), but *close to 100 percent*. It is necessary to consider the *experiment-wise* error rate then, when interpreting the results of studies in which more than one null hypothesis is tested. The level of confidence at which a given null hypothesis is tested applies only if a single null hypothesis is tested. Otherwise, it is higher.

Many types of significance tests have been developed for testing null hypotheses. A representative sample of such tests is presented in Table 8.8 and the computational appendix (see Appendix A). There is a test in this sample that would be appropriate for most occasions when a speech pathologist or audiologist wished to assess the statistical significance of differences between sample means or medians.

How do you identify an appropriate significance test? To do this, you need several pieces of information about the data on which the significance test is to be performed:

1. the level of measurement of the measures,
2. whether the measures are independent or related, and
3. the number of means, medians, or other measures you wish to test the differences between.

With this information, you can probably locate an appropriate significance test in Table 8.8.

The level of measurement of the measures refers to whether they possess nominal, ordinal, interval, or ratio properties (see Chapter 6). There are different significance tests for nominal, ordinal, and interval-ratio measures

TABLE 8.8. Significance tests categorized on the bases of: (1) their level of measurement, (2) whether they are intended for independent or related samples, and (3) whether they are intended for the two-sample case or for the more than two-sample case.

Level of Measurement	Two-Sample Case		More than Two-Sample Case	
	Related Samples	Independent Samples	Related Samples	Independent Samples
Nominal		Chi square		Chi square
Ordinal	Sign test	Mann-Whitney U test	Friedman two-way analysis of variance	Kruskal-Wallis one-way analysis of variance
Interval and Ratio	t-Test for related measures	t-Test for independent measures	One-way analysis of variance for dependent measures	One-way analysis of variance for independent measures

(see Table 8.8). While it is permissible to use a significance test appropriate for a lower level of measurement than that present in the data, this is usually not done, because such a test would probably be less *powerful* than one appropriate for the level of measurement present in the data. (Nominal would be a lower level of measurement than ordinal, ordinal would be a lower level of measurement than interval, and so on.) One consequence of using a less powerful test is that more subjects (i.e., larger groups) are needed to detect differences between means, medians, or other measures of a given size—i.e., cause a false null hypothesis to be rejected at a given significance, or confidence, level. The less powerful the test you use, the more likely you are to commit a Type II error (i.e., retain a false null hypothesis).

Another piece of information you need about the data to select an appropriate significance test is whether the sets of measures which you wish to assess the difference (or differences) between are independent or related. If the sets of measures were made on the same persons, they are *related*. Thus, if you wished to assess the difference between measures made on a group of persons before and after participating in a therapy program, you would have to use a significance test appropriate for related measures.

If the sets of measures were made on different persons, they *usually* would be regarded as *independent*. Thus, if you wished to compare a group of persons who had spastic dysarthria to a group of persons who did not have spastic dysarthria on some measure, ordinarily you would have to use a significance test appropriate for independent measures. We use the qualifier "ordinarily" here because there is one circumstance when this would not be true. If the persons on whom the sets of measures were made were *very closely matched* for all relevant variables, the sets of measures would be treated as related. About the only time you can be reasonably confident that this level of matching has been achieved is when the persons in the groups are identical twins (where one twin from each set would be in each group). If there is any doubt about whether groups are closely matched, it probably would be safest to treat them as independent.

The third piece of information you need to select an appropriate significance test is the *number* of means, medians, or other summary measures you wish to assess differences between. If this number is *two*, one set of significance tests is appropriate; if it is *more than two*, a second set is appropriate.

With these three pieces of information, you may enter Table 8.8 to identify an appropriate significance test. To illustrate how to use this table, let us suppose you administered a picture vocabulary test to a group of children twice, once preceding and once following their participation in a therapy program. Most likely you would wish to determine whether a difference you observed between the medians of the two sets of scores were large enough for chance, or random fluctuation, to be unlikely as an explanation. It would probably be safest to assume that the scores on such a vocabulary test have *ordinal* properties. The sets of measures would be *related* because they were made on the same persons, and the number of sets would be *two*. The significance test in Table 8.8 appropriate for two sets of measures having ordinal properties is the *sign test*.

Table 8.8 does not present any tests for sets of related measures having nominal properties. There appear to be no commonly used tests for such measures in speech and hearing research. Significance tests have, however, been developed for such measures—i.e., the McNemar test for the significance of change (Siegel, 1956)—and a statistician should be consulted to help identify the most appropriate for a given instance.

Table 8.8 also does not include tests appropriate for relatively complex comparisons between means or medians. Such tests would be required to answer questions similar to this one: "Was the effect of a speech improvement program that was administered to a group of kindergarten children different for boys than for girls?" If a difference did exist, it would probably be inadvisable to combine outcome data from boys and girls. A complex analysis-of-variance design could be used to assess the likelihood that the program affects boys and girls differently (i.e., to test the null hypothesis that differences between boys and girls arose from chance, or random fluctuation). You should consult a statistician if the comparisons you wish to make are relatively complex.

All of the significance tests dealt with thus far have been for *differences* between means, medians, and other descriptive statistics. As indicated earlier, there are also significance tests for assessing the likelihood that observed *relationships* (as designated by non-zero correlation coefficients) arose from chance, or random fluctuation. A test of this type appropriate for Pearson product-moment correlation coefficients is included in the computational appendix (see Appendix A). For tests of this type appropriate for other correlation coefficients, consult a statistician.

After the statistic for a significance test has been computed, it is necessary to determine whether the probability of its occurrence, if the observed difference or relationship were due to chance, or random fluctuation, is smaller than the alpha level, or level of confidence, selected. If the value of this statistic (e.g., x^2, x, z, t, or F) is such that the probability of its occurrence as a result of random fluctuation is less than the alpha level, the null hypothesis is rejected. Otherwise, it is retained.

How do you determine whether the value you computed for a significance test statistic has a small enough probability of occurrence under the null hypothesis that it can be rejected? To accomplish this, you use a *table* in which you can locate either: (1) the probability that a difference or relationship was due to chance fluctuation, or (2) the value the test statistic would have to *exceed* before you could conclude that the probability of a difference or relationship being due to chance fluctuation was equal to or less than the alpha level (i.e., level of confidence) selected. The tables in Appendix A for the binomial distribution (Table A.3) and the normal distribution (Table A.4) provide probability values, and those for the chi square distribution (Table A.2), the t-distribution (Table A.5), and the F-distribution (Table A.6) provide values that have to be exceeded.

You are likely to need several pieces of information before you can enter a table to determine if the outcome of a statistical test permits the null hypothesis to be rejected. Those required most often include:

1. the appropriate distribution to use,
2. the alpha level, or level of confidence, at which the null hypothesis is being tested,
3. the degrees of freedom (df),
4. whether the test is to be one-tailed or two-tailed, and
5. the value computed for the test statistic.

The first thing you need to know before you can determine if the outcome of a statistical test permits the null hypothesis to be rejected is what distribution to use. The appropriate distribution, or table, for a particular test statistic is usually indicated in the description of that statistic. Tables containing the most frequently used distributions are presented at the end of Appendix A.

A second piece of information you will almost always need is the alpha level, or level of confidence, at which the null hypothesis is being tested. Though any level 0.05 or smaller is considered acceptable by the editors of scientific and professional journals, most investigators limit themselves to the 0.05 and 0.01 levels. The tabled distributions at the end of Appendix A can all be entered at these two alpha levels.

A third piece of information you may need to enter a table is the number of degrees of freedom (df) in your data. Tables that require this information to enter them (e.g., x^2, t, and F) contain a *number* of distributions, one for each df value designated in them. The df value for a set of data designates the distribution in a table that contains the *critical value* of the statistic for testing the null hypothesis. The critical value is the value of the statistic that the one computed on the data must *exceed* before the null hypothesis can be rejected. With one exception (contingency tables), the number of degrees of freedom is related to the number of subjects whose data are being assessed by the significance test.

For contingency tables, df values are based on the numbers of rows and columns in a table rather than the numbers of subjects contained in them.

The procedure for determining the df value for a particular test is indicated in the description of the computational procedure for that test. (Such procedures are indicated in Appendix A for all significance tests that require df values.) Note that the table for the F distribution (Table A.6) requires two df values rather than one to locate critical values of the statistic.

A fourth piece of information sometimes necessary to determine if the outcome of a statistical test permits the null hypothesis to be rejected is whether the test is *one-tailed* or *two-tailed*. If, to answer a question, you must only be able to detect a difference in one direction, a one-tailed test can be used. The following are representative questions that can be answered with a one-tailed test:

1. Are stutterers more anxious than nonstutterers in a particular situation?
2. Do children evince fewer articulation errors after participating in a particular therapy program?

To answer the first question, it would not be necessary to determine whether nonstutterers are more anxious than stutterers. To answer the second question, it would not be necessary to determine whether children exhibit more articulation errors after participating in the therapy program.

If you must be able to detect a difference in either direction to answer a question, you must use a two-tailed test. The following are representative questions that can be answered with a two-tailed test:

1. Do stutterers and nonstutterers *differ* with regard to their anxiety levels in a particular situation?
2. Do children's stuttering severities tend to be *different* two years after they terminate a particular therapy program from the time of the termination of the program?

To answer these questions, it would be necessary to be able to detect differences in both directions. Stutterers would differ from nonstutterers if their anxiety levels were either higher or lower in the situation tested. Also, the children's stuttering severity levels two years following termination of treatment would be different, whether they were higher or lower, than at termination.

If you wish to use a one-tailed test (or tests) for assessing group or treatment differences in your data, you are required by the assumptions underlying statistical inference to decide on the direction in which you are interested in being able to detect a difference before you begin to collect data. It is not legitimate to change your mind or decide on the direction after you have seen your data. If you do either, the probability of a Type I error will be higher than the level of confidence would indicate.

There is a direct way of entering some tabled distributions for two-tailed tests. For other such tables, there is no direct way. In these instances, critical values for two-tailed tests can be obtained by adjusting the alpha level, or level of confidence. For a two-tailed test at the 0.05 level, you would enter the table at the 0.025 level. For a two-tailed test at the 0.01 level, you would enter the table at the 0.005 level. Note that larger values of a test statistic are necessary to reject a null hypothesis if a two-tailed test rather than a one-tailed test is used.

A final piece of information that may be necessary to determine if the outcome of a statistical test permits the null hypothesis to be rejected is the value computed for the test statistic. This information is required to enter the normal distribution (Table A.4) and the binomial distribution (Table A.3).

Once you have the necessary information to enter the appropriate distribution table for a test statistic, you can determine whether the null hypothesis should be rejected. The procedure for entering each distribution table in Appendix A is as follows:

1. *Chi Square Distribution (Table A.2).* Enter this table with the appropriate *df* value for your data and the level of confidence at which the null hypothesis is to be tested. The *df* values are indicated in the first column and levels of confidence in the top row. To identify the critical value of chi square for testing the null hypothesis, you first locate the row containing the appropriate *df* value and then the column for the level of confidence you wish to use. The value of chi square that appears at the intersection of this row and column is the critical value for testing the null hypothesis. If the value you computed is larger, the null hypothesis can be rejected. The levels of confidence are for one-tailed tests. Two-tailed tests are rarely, if ever, used for contingency tables. Rejection of the null hypothesis permits you to conclude that the configuration of frequencies in a contingency table is unlikely to have resulted from chance, or random fluctuation.

2. *Binomial Test* (*Table A.3*). Enter this table with the value of x for your data (see sign test in Appendix A) and the number of subjects (N) whose data are being tested for statistical significance. Numbers of subjects are indicated in the first column and x values are indicated in the top row. To determine the *probability* that a value of x resulted from chance, or random fluctuation, you locate the row for the appropriate number of subjects and the column for the obtained x value. The probability value that appears at the intersection of this row and column is the probability that the obtained value of x resulted from chance, or random fluctuation. If this probability is smaller than the level of confidence you selected, the null hypothesis should be rejected. These probability values can be used for either one-tailed or two-tailed tests.

3. *Normal Distribution* (*Table A.4*). Enter this table with the value you compute for z. Note that z values to one decimal place are indicated in the first column and those to two decimal places in the top row. The numbers in the table are probabilities that given z values resulted from chance, or random fluctuation. For a one-tailed test at the 0.05 level, if the probability associated with a given z is less than 0.05, the null hypothesis is rejected. For a two-tailed test at the 0.05 level, if the probability associated with a given z is less than 0.025, the null hypothesis is rejected.

4. *t-Distribution* (*Table A.5*). Enter this table with the appropriate df value for your data and the level of confidence at which the null hypothesis is to be tested. The df values appear in the first column. The levels of significance, or confidence, for one-tailed tests appear in the top row and those for two-tailed tests in the second row. To identify the critical value of t for testing the null hypothesis, you locate the row containing the appropriate df value and the column for the level of confidence you wish to use. (Note that different columns are used for one-tailed and two-tailed tests.) The value of t that appears at the intersection of the row and column is the critical value for testing the null hypothesis. If the value you computed is larger, the null hypothesis should be rejected.

5. *F-Distribution* (*Table A.6*). Enter this table with two df values: df_1 is the degrees of freedom for columns (or between group or treatment variation) and df_2 is the degrees of freedom for row (or within group or treatment variation). The set of numbers which appears at the intersection of the df_1 column and df_2 row are critical values of F for selected levels of confidence, including 1 percent and 5 percent levels. If the value you compute is larger than that in the table for the level of confidence you are using, the null hypothesis should be rejected.

Confidence Intervals. Thus far, we have dealt with the use of statistical inference for assessing the reliability and generality of differences and relationships. This section will describe the use of statistical inference for estimating population values of descriptive statistics and the differences between such statistics. The *confidence interval* is the type of inferential statistic used for this purpose.

Why might you want to use a confidence interval? There are several reasons. First, you may need to estimate the population value of a descriptive statistic. The following are representative of questions requiring such an estimate to answer:

1. By what age do 50 percent of children perform a particular task correctly?
2. What percentage of persons with a particular communicative disorder derive benefit from a particular therapy program?
3. How predictive is a person's score on a test before he or she participates in a therapy program of what it will be after he or she participates in the program?

To answer the first question, you have to estimate a *population median;* to answer the second, a *population percentage;* and to answer the third, a *population correlation coefficient* (between the scores of a group of persons before and after participating in the program).

A second reason to use a confidence interval is to estimate the population value of a difference between descriptive statistics. Once a null hypothesis has been rejected, indicating that an observed difference is likely to be a real one, it *may* be important to estimate the magnitude of the difference. Such an estimate may be useful in assessing its significance, or importance—i.e., for determining whether it is a difference that should affect clinical practice. Aphasics may make gains if they participate in a particular intensive therapy program (judging by the results of a significance test on the difference between pre- and post-therapy scores), but the magnitudes of these gains may not be sufficient to effect any real improvement in their ability to communicate. To determine if this were likely to be the case, the magnitude of the difference between pre- and post-therapy scores could be estimated by means of a confidence interval (assuming that the results of a test of the difference between pre- and post-therapy measures resulted in rejection of the null hypothesis). Unless the null hypothesis were rejected, indicating that the observed difference is likely to be a real one, it would make no sense to estimate the magnitude of the difference.

The following are representative of questions about differences between descriptive statistics that could be answered by means of a confidence interval:

1. How much of a reduction in the severity of a particular communicative disorder could be expected to result from participation in a particular therapy program?
2. How much of a difference is there apt to be between persons who have a particular communicative disorder and those who do not have it in their performance of a particular task?

Both questions can be answered by a confidence interval for the difference between the mean (or median) performances of the groups.

What are confidence intervals? These are intervals designated by two values (a lower limit and an upper limit) between which we can be a given percent certain (usually 95 percent or 99 percent) that a population value falls. Thus, based on confidence intervals, we might conclude it is 95 percent certain that the mean IQ for a population falls between 90 and 100 points, or it is 99 percent certain that the difference between pre- and post-therapy mean stuttering frequencies for a particular therapy program falls between 10 and 21 instances of stuttering per 100 words spoken.

The two most frequently used confidence levels for confidence intervals are 95 percent and 99 percent. With the first, you can be 95 percent certain that the population value falls between the specified limits, and with the second, you can be 99 percent certain that it falls between these limits. These interpretations, of course, would only be valid if the subjects in the sample on whose data the confidence interval was computed were representative of those in the population to which it was desired to infer—i.e., if they were a reasonably random sample from this population.

A 95 percent confidence interval always would be *narrower* than a 99 percent confidence interval. The *higher* the degree of confidence that the population value lies within the interval, the *wider* it will be.

Another factor that influences the widths of confidence intervals is *sample size*. The larger the number of subjects in the sample, the narrower the confidence interval.

The narrower a confidence interval, the more useful the information it provides. Knowing that the mean IQ for children in a population (e.g., those who have cleft palates) is probably somewhere between 90 and 95 is likely to provide more useful information than knowing it is somewhere between 80 and 105.

What can you do to ensure that the width of a confidence interval will be minimized? One way would be to use a 95 rather than a 99 percent confidence level and another would be to use as many subjects (i.e., as large an N) as possible.

Confidence intervals can be computed from measures having ordinal, interval, or ratio properties. The confidence interval for the median (see Appendix A) is one that can be computed from measures having ordinal properties. Those for the mean and difference between means (see Appendix A) can be computed from measures having interval or ratio properties.

It is possible to compute a confidence interval for almost any descriptive statistic and for the differences between almost any descriptive statistics. A statistician should be able to provide the necessary formulas.

Significance tests and confidence intervals are not the only aspects of statistical inference. There are several others, including Bayesian decision theory (Hayes, 1963) and game theory (Davis, 1970; Rapoport, 1966). While these have not been used extensively in speech pathology and audiology research, they could probably be useful for answering some questions relevant to evaluation and therapy.

REFERENCES

CAMPBELL, S. K., *Flaws and Fallacies in Statistical Thinking.* Englewood Cliffs, N.J.: Prentice-Hall, Inc. (1974).
DAVIS, M. D., *Game Theory: A Nontechnical Introduction.* New York: Basic Books (1970).
EBEL, R., Estimation of the reliability of ratings. *Psychometrika,* 16, 407–424 (1951).
FRUCHTER, B., *Introduction to Factor Analysis.* New York: Van Nostrand Reinhold Company (1954).
GOLENPAUL, D. (Ed.), *Information Please Almanac, Atlas, and Yearbook 1974.* New York: Simon and Schuster, Inc. (1973).
GREEN, P. E., and CARMONE, F. J., *Multidimensional Scaling and Related Techniques in Marketing Analysis.* Boston: Allyn and Bacon, Inc. (1970).
HAYS, W. L., *Statistics for Psychologists.* New York: Holt, Rinehart, and Winston (1963).
MCCALL, G. J., and SIMMONS, J. L., *Issues in Participant Observation: A Text and Reader.* Reading, Mass.: Addison-Wesley Publishing Company, Inc. (1969).
RAPOPORT, A., *Two-Person Game Theory: The Essential Ideas.* Ann Arbor: University of Michigan Press (1966).
SCHATZMAN, L., and STRAUSS, A. L., *Field Research.* Englewood Cliffs, N.J.: Prentice-Hall, Inc. (1973).
SHELTON, R. L., PAESANI, A., MCCLELLAND, K. D., and BRADFIELD, S. S., Panendoscopic feedback in the study of voluntary velopharyngeal movements. *Journal of Speech and Hearing Disorders,* 40, 232–244 (1975).
SIEGEL, S., *Nonparametric Statistics for the Behavioral Sciences.* New York: McGraw-Hill Book Company (1956).
SILVERMAN, F. H., Interpretation of mean Q values for sets of stimuli rated on a seven-point equal-appearing interval scale. *Perceptual and Motor Skills,* 24, 842 (1967).
TORGERSON, W. S., *Theory and Methods of Scaling.* New York: John Wiley & Sons, Inc. (1963).
WOLFE, D., *Factor Analysis to 1940.* Chicago: The University of Chicago Press (1940).
YAIRI, E., A sudden onset of high-pitched voice associated with unilateral vocal fold paralysis: A case report. *Journal of Speech and Hearing Disorders,* 39, 373–375 (1974).
YOUNG, M. A., Predicting ratings of severity of stuttering. *Journal of Speech and Hearing Disorders,* Monograph Supplement 7, 31–54 (1961).

NINE

CONSIDERATIONS IN INTERPRETING ANSWERS TO QUESTIONS

This chapter deals with interpreting answers to questions—relating them to, or incorporating them into, the existing body of knowledge. Specifically, it indicates a number of factors that must be considered when interpreting, or evaluating, answers to questions. These considerations are relevant both to consumers and to producers of research.

Consumers of research have to be able to evaluate the adequacy of findings (i.e., answers to questions) reported in journal literature as well as the cogency of interpretations made of them and generalizations made from them. It is not safe to assume that the findings reported in a journal article permit the questions asked to be answered in the ways they were answered, or the answers to be interpreted in the ways they were interpreted, merely because the study was published. Even though most journals subject submitted manuscripts to a careful review process, and many are rejected as a consequence of this process, papers are nevertheless published in which the answers to the questions asked or the interpretations made of these answers are either not appropriate or are not the only possible answers or interpretations. Sometimes when readers detect an error in authors' answers or interpretations, they write a letter to the editor in which they indicate alternative answers or interpretations. (Letters to the editor appear at the ends of most issues of the *Journal of Speech and Hearing Disorders* and the *Journal of Speech and Hearing Research*.) However, this is not always done. One reason is that most journals permit an author to reply to a letter critical of his paper, and this rebuttal is printed along with the letter to the editor. In his or her rebuttal, the author can appear to answer the points raised in the letter to the editor and thus suggest implicitly or explicitly that the criticisms are not valid. Since the writer of the letter to the editor usually is not given an opportunity to respond to the author's rebuttal, it can appear that the author answered the points raised adequately when in fact he or she did not. Such a situation would obviously discourage some persons from writing letters to the editor. For this as well as other reasons, there are instances in which answers to questions are incorrect and interpretations are inappropriate that are never pointed out to consumers of the research.

It is necessary to approach published research with an attitude of *healthy skepticism*. Your *presumption*, or set, should be that the answers reported may be incorrect and the interpretations that are made of them may be inappropriate. If insufficient information is reported to evaluate the accuracy of an answer, it should be regarded as suspect and obviously should not be utilized with a high degree of confidence. If the interpretations offered do not appear to be the appropriate or the most plausible ones, they also should be regarded as suspect and should not be utilized with a high degree of confidence.

An attitude of healthy skepticism, of course, is particularly important when you are reading studies the results of which could influence your clinical practice—i.e., your approach to evaluation or therapy. If you approach such studies with this attitude, you will probably be less likely to modify your clinical approaches in a manner that would tend to reduce their effectiveness.

Criteria for interpreting, or evaluating, answers to questions are also relevant for *producers* of research. Once an investigator has answered a question, he or she usually attempts to relate the answer to the existing body of knowledge in the area of research. The investigator may use it to fill a gap or gaps in this body of knowledge, or to question the accuracy of certain information contained in it, or for both purposes.

DIMENSIONS TO CONSIDER WHEN EVALUATING ANSWERS

What dimensions should you consider when you are evaluating answers so that you can determine the interpretations and generalizations that can be made from them? The three most important dimensions are probably *validity*, *reliability*, and *generality*.

Validity

The validity of observations refers to their *appropriateness* for answering the questions they are used to answer. If they are not appropriate, the answers they yield *may* be inaccurate and the interpretations made of them *may* be inappropriate.

Because the observations used to answer a question are invalid does not necessarily mean that the answer will be inaccurate or that the interpretations of it will be inappropriate. An investigator will occasionally arrive at the right answer for the wrong reason—i.e., through the use of invalid observations. A classic example previously mentioned (see Chapter 3) is Gall's conclusion, on the basis of a friend's eyes being widely separated, that the anterior portion of the brain is important for motor speech (Head, 1963).

If the observations used to answer a question appear to be invalid, it probably would make most sense to regard the question as *not having been answered* (at least as far as the observations reported are concerned). It would *not* be appropriate to regard the question as having been incorrectly answered, since a certain percentage of the time an investigator will arrive at a correct answer from invalid observations. As a matter of fact, if a question could only be answered in two ways (e.g., yes or no), you could arrive at a correct answer *without even knowing the question* approximately 50 percent of the time. An example of such a question would be: "Do most stutterers tend to become more fluent following administration of a particular therapy?"

The probability of a correct answer by chance would be the reciprocal of the number of ways a question could be answered. If a question could be answered in three ways, the probability of a correct answer by chance would be $\frac{1}{3}$ or 0.33.

In summary, if the observations used to answer a question seem valid, the odds probably will be *greater than chance* that the answer reported is correct. On the other hand, if the observations used to answer a question do not seem valid, the odds probably will be approximately *equal to chance* that the answer reported is correct.

Reliability

The reliability of the observations used to answer questions refers to their *repeatability*. The more repeatable (or replicable) a set of observations, the greater will be their reliability.

The extent to which observations can be repeated, or replicated, is a function of how similarly a *given observer* would describe them on *different* occasions, or how similarly a *group of observers* would describe them on a *given occasion* (or occasions). The description could be qualitative, quantitative, or a combination of the two. The more similar the descriptions, the more reliable the observations.

The more reliable the observations used to answer a question, the more likely it is that the answer to the question is accurate. How reliable the observations have to be for the odds to be reasonably good that an answer to a question is accurate depends on the question. Some questions require more reliable observations than others to answer, so that you can have the degree of confidence you feel you need in the accuracy of the answer. For questions concerning *differences* (e.g., "Were the language formulation abilities of a group of children better on the average after participating in a particular therapy program than prior to participating in it?"), more reliable observations are required before you can have a given degree of confidence in the accuracy of an answer, if a difference is relatively small rather than relatively large. Similarly, for questions concerning *relationships* (e.g., "Is there a relationship between the scores earned by a group of persons who have a particular type of communicative disorder on two tests of auditory functioning?"), more reliable observations are required before you can have a given degree of confidence in the accuracy of an answer, if a relationship is relatively weak rather than relatively strong.

Because the observations used to answer a question do not seem sufficiently reliable does not necessarily mean that the answer to the question is incorrect. The answer can be correct by chance alone. As I indicated in the discussion of validity, the probability of an answer to a question being correct by chance is the reciprocal of the number of ways the question could be answered. Also, the observations may be more reliable than they appear to be. Some types of observations typically tend to be viewed as less reliable than in fact they are. An example would be ratings obtained through the application of psychological scaling methods. Many persons who have not had much experience with these methods tend to feel intuitively that ratings resulting from them could not be very reliable. It has been demonstrated in a large number of studies, however, that in most instances such ratings are highly reliable (see Chapter 7).

As previously indicated, one consequence of observations not being adequately reliable is a relatively high probability of a Type II error (see Chapter 8). Briefly, this means concluding that there is no real difference or relationship when there is. Usually, when an investigator fails to reject a null hypothesis, he does not indicate how likely it was that this failure was due to some sort of "error"—e.g., not using measures that were sufficiently reliable to detect a difference or relationship of the magnitude present. One reason, then, why an investigator might answer a question in a manner that indicates that no difference or relationship exists is that the measures used were not sufficiently reliable to detect the difference or relationship present.

It is quite likely that in a relatively high percentage of instances in the speech pathology and audiology literature where the null hypothesis was not rejected, the reason was a Type II error that may have been caused by measures that were not adequately reliable.

In summary, the impact of the reliability of the observations used to answer a question on the answer obtained may not be clear-cut. Observations that do not appear to be very reliable can yield both correct and incorrect answers. Evaluations of the accuracy of answers to questions, therefore, should be regarded as quite tentative until the answers have been replicated (preferably by other investigators at other institutions).

Generality

A third factor to be considered when evaluating answers to questions and interpretations made from them is the *generality* of the observations used to answer the questions. This refers to the extent to which the persons or events observed are representative of those in the population designated by the question. The more representative of this population they are, the more viable will be the generalizations made from them.

The persons or events observed to answer a question are most likely to be representative of those in the designated population if they constitute a *random sample* from that population. The only way you can be reasonably certain they constitute such a sample is if they were selected from the population by a table of random numbers (see Appendix B) or by a series of random digits generated by a computer. If they were not selected in this manner, their generality would be uncertain *to some degree*. Of course, even if they were selected by a random process, it still would be possible they would not be representative because of sampling error.

The persons and events observed in speech pathology and audiology research usually do not constitute a random sample from any "meaningful" population. A meaningful population is one to which an investigator would wish to generalize. While the population to which the investigator may wish to generalize consists of *all persons* who have a particular communicative disorder, the population sampled may consist of *all persons available to the investigator* who have that communicative disorder.

If an investigator wishes to limit generalizations to the *subpopulation* of persons who have a particular communicative disorder from which he sampled (e.g., a caseload), then so long as the sample were randomly selected from this subpopulation, the generalizations made should be viable. There are instances, of course, when it would be meaningful to generalize to such a subpopulation. One such instance would be when you wished to assess the impact of participation in a treatment program on a group of persons at your own institution. Rather than assessing the impact of the program on all participants, it may be more economical and efficient to limit the assessment to a random sample. Inferences could be made about the impact of the program on all participants from observations made on this sample. With the probable continuing interest of administrators of clinical speech and hearing programs in "accountability," such inferences could be quite useful for demonstrating the efficacy of given programs.

If you do not want to limit your generalizations to the subpopulation from which your sample was drawn, or if your sample was not randomly selected from the population to which you wish to generalize, the cogency of your generalizations will be uncertain. To have a reasonable degree of confidence in the viability of such generalizations, you have to be willing to assume that the persons observed constitute a *representative*, or random, sample from the population to which you wish to generalize. In some instances, this assumption will seem reasonable; in others, it will not seem reasonable; in still others, insufficient information will be presented about the sample observed for any judgment to be made regarding its reasonableness. Knowing, for example, that the persons observed were being seen for therapy at a particular school or rehabilitation center without knowing the attributes (i.e., physical, intellectual, emotional, socioeconomic, etc.) of persons who receive therapy at that school or center is apt to leave you uncertain regarding their representativeness.

Can generalizations legitimately be made from observations of persons who were not randomly selected from a meaningful population? The answer to this question would be "yes" if: (1) an individual subject design were used, and (2) you were willing to assume that it is highly unlikely that the only person (or persons) in the population who would perform as your subject (or subjects) performed under the experimental condition or conditions is (or are) your subject (or subjects). If you are willing to make this assumption, it would seem reasonable for you to conclude that the performance of your subject or subjects is representative of the performance of a *segment* of the population from which he, she, or they were selected. While it wouldn't be possible to specify the proportion of persons in this population who would have responded similarly to your subject or subjects under the experimental conditions, it would seem reasonable to conclude that his, her, or their performance is representative of the performance of a segment of this population.

Because the interpretations and generalizations made by an author from his data seem inappropriate does not necessarily mean they are incorrect. An author can arrive at a correct conclusion for the wrong reasons. An interpretation that does not seem plausible can be correct. An inference about a population made from a sample that was not randomly selected from it can be accurate. In fact, an accurate interpretation or generalization can be arrived at by chance alone.

CRITERIA FOR EVALUATING RELIABILITY, VALIDITY, AND GENERALITY

Now that we have commented upon the relevance of validity, reliability, and generality for assessing accuracy, we will suggest several questions that should be asked when evaluating these dimensions. The answers to these questions provide a basis for evaluating the accuracy of answers to research questions as well as to interpretations and generalizations made from them.

Validity

A necessary question to answer when you wish to assess the validity of the observations used to answer a question is: *Were the observations made appropriate for answering the question asked*? That is, did the investigator observe and describe the attribute (or attributes) of the events that he wished to observe and describe? If the investigator did, the observations will be valid to some degree. If the investigator did not, they will be invalid.

An investigator may not observe the necessary attribute or attributes needed to answer a question because the filter used to isolate it for observation and description (see Chapter 1) may not isolate it. This can result from using an inappropriate or inappropriately calibrated instrument or by giving oneself an inappropriate set. An inappropriate instrument in this context would be one that would not permit the investigator to isolate the attribute he wished to observe and describe. Such an instrument could be part of an electronic instrumentation measurement scheme, or it could be a psychological or educational performance test or task (see Chapter 7). An example of using inappropriate electronic instrumentation to isolate a target attribute would be using an electromyographic (EMG) recorder with *surface electrodes* to study the differential activity of the internal and external intercostal muscles during breathing for speech. (*Needle electrodes* would be needed at least at some sites to study the differential activity of these muscles.) An example of an inappropriate application of educational or psychological tests for isolating and describing a target attribute would be using articulation test performance to infer intelligence level. (While both are related in a general way to overall development, articulation test performance does not appear to be a particularly valid index of intelligence level.)

An *inappropriately calibrated* instrument in this context would be one which properly adjusted, or calibrated, would permit the investigator to isolate the attribute he wished to observe and describe. If the target attribute was "thresholds for pure tones" and the audiometer used was not properly calibrated, the investigator would be unable to describe this attribute validly on the basis of the thresholds obtained. The investigator would, of course, be able to describe the attribute with this type of instrumentation if it were properly calibrated.

An *inappropriate set* in this context would be one an observer possesses that does not permit the isolation of the attribute he wishes to observe and describe. On psychological scaling tasks (see Chapter 7), for example, where observers are asked to rate a series of speech segments for two attributes *separately* (e.g., degree of "articulation defectiveness" and degree of "nasality") they may be unable to assume the appropriate sets. That is, they may be unable to ignore one of the attributes (e.g., nasality) while rating the speech segments for the other (e.g., articulation defectiveness). Their ratings would be contaminated and *possibly* invalid. Their ratings may not be invalid because what the judges did rate was highly, positively correlated (see Chapters 5 and 8) with the attribute they were instructed to rate. Degree of nasality and degree of articulation defectiveness, for example, appear to be highly, positively correlated for persons who have cleft palates (Spriestersbach and Sherman, 1968).

Reliability

A necessary question to answer when assessing the reliability of observations is: *Were the observations made sufficiently free from random and systematic measurement error (including experimenter bias) to answer reliably the question asked?* The sources from which both types of error arise have already been discussed (see Chapter 7). If the answer to this question is "yes," the observations are likely to be sufficiently free of error to answer reliably the question asked. If, on the other hand, it appears to be "no," the answer should be regarded as suspect.

Impact of Random Measurement Error on Reliability. Random measurement error can influence the accuracy of answers to questions on differences and relationships (and hence the interpretations made of them) by increasing the probability of a Type II error—i.e., the probability of not rejecting the null hypothesis when it should be rejected (see Chapter 8). Obviously, if the null hypothesis is rejected, this source of error could not have influenced the accuracy of the answer. If the null hypotheses is retained, however, random measurement error could have been responsible. That is, rather than retaining the null hypothesis, which indicates that an observed difference or relationship probably resulted from chance, or random fluctuation, it merely may indicate that the level of random error was too high to detect a difference or relationship of the magnitude present with the number of subjects used. If more subjects had been used, the null hypothesis might have been rejected. (The larger the sample size, the less likely you are to retain a false null hypothesis because of random error.) For this reason, whenever you are interpreting an answer to a question that was based on failure to reject the null hypothesis, one possibility you must always consider is a Type II error. (A statistician should be able to provide you with the appropriate formula for estimating this probability for a given significance test.) Unfortunately, most journals don't require authors to specify the probability of a Type II error when they fail to reject the null hypothesis.

A Type II error is particularly likely to explain retaining the null hypothesis if at least two of the following three statements apply:

1. The sample size was relatively small.
2. The observed difference or correlation was relatively small.
3. The alpha level (i.e., level of confidence) used was relatively small (e.g., 0.01).

In summary, unless it were possible to demonstrate the probability of a Type II error was acceptably small (i.e., 0.05 or smaller), it would be inappropriate to interpret failure to reject the null hypothesis as evidence that an observed difference or relationship was due to chance, or random fluctuation.

Impact of Systematic Measurement Error on Reliability. Systematic measurement error can influence the accuracy of answers to questions (and hence the interpretations made of them) by biasing the observations used to answer them. Systematic measurement error can make it appear that a difference or relationship exists where there is none, or that no difference or relationship exists where there is one. This type of error, then, can have a *profound* effect on qualitative observations as well as descriptive and inferential statistics, and hence on the accuracy of answers to questions.

Therapy outcome research is particularly vulnerable to systematic measurement error (e.g., Beasley and Manning, 1973; Meitus, Ringel, House, and Hotchkiss, 1973). This is particularly likely to be the case when the person or persons doing the evaluating have an ego investment in the outcome of the research (e.g., Rosenthal, 1963, 1966, 1969). An investigator may strongly desire a therapy to be found effective, or vice versa. This is especially true in studies where an investigator is comparing several therapy approaches, one of which he or she has emotionally identified with and hopes (or expects) to be the most effective. Human nature being what it is, it would not seem reasonable to expect an investigator who is comparing the effectiveness of a therapy approach in which he or she has an ego investment with that of one or more other approaches to be completely unbiased. The bias may be subtle, and the investigator may not be conscious of it.

How might an investigator bias the results of therapy outcome research? One way is that the investigator may only make (or report) observations and data analyses that are likely to make the approach in which he or she has an ego investment seem superior to those to which it is being compared. Suppose, for example, an investigator was comparing the impact of a stuttering therapy program he or she helped to develop to the impact of another one. The investigator might use as a criterion measure stuttering frequency before and after participating in a program. The results may indicate that the stutterers who participated in the investigator's program had a greater reduction in stuttering frequency than those who participated in the other program. Therefore, based on a stuttering frequency criterion measure, it would seem reasonable to conclude that the investigator's program was more effective than the other one. However, if a different criterion measure or design had been used, the conclusion quite possibly might have been different. Another criterion measure that could have been used is "avoidance of speaking when stuttering is anticipated." Perhaps the other therapy would have been more effective in treating this aspect of the stuttering problem. Also, if the stuttering frequency criterion measure had been used with a different design—e.g., one that included a two-year follow-up—the other therapy could have appeared more effective (i.e., the amount of relapse for the stuttering therapy program which resulted in the greatest reduction in stuttering frequency at the point therapy was terminated could have been sufficient to make it no longer appear to be the more effective of the two).

An investigator can bias the results of therapy outcome research in other ways as well. If he or she attempted to evaluate retrospectively the effectiveness of a therapy program, several types of distortion could bias the evaluation. The investigator may be more successful, for example, in remembering factors that suggest the therapy was effective than factors that suggest it was ineffective, or vice versa. Or the investigator could conclude that a reduction in the severity of a person's communicative disorder has occurred because the investigator has "adapted" to it (e.g., Trotter and Kools, 1955). A person with a severe articulation problem could seem more intelligible to his clinician following a period of therapy because the clinician has learned the lawful ways in which the person's articulation differs from the standard. And a stutterer's stuttering could seem less severe to his clinician after a period of therapy because the clinician has grown accustomed to it.

Another way an investigator can bias the results of therapy outcome research is by the criteria he or she uses for selecting persons on whom to report the effects of a therapy program. This is not a potential source of bias if the effects of the program on all persons on whom it was tried are reported. It may be a potential source of bias, however, if failures are not reported along with successes. While it is sometimes justifiable (and indeed necessary) to exclude clients from reports of therapy outcome because the therapy was not administered to them in the prescribed manner, such exclusion should be done only when absolutely necessary—i.e., when not excluding them would *almost certainly* lead to a biased evaluation. Unfortunately, it is usually relatively easy to rationalize the elimination of any client from a study of therapy outcome who does not respond to the therapy as the investigator desires.

Therapy outcome research also can be biased when the findings are interpreted. Data pertaining to the effectiveness of therapy can often be interpreted in more than one way. In fact, a given finding can often be interpreted *both* to support the conclusion that a therapy was effective and to support the conclusion that it was ineffective. It depends on whether one wishes to view the proverbial cup as half full or half empty. Suppose a particular stuttering therapy was found to reduce stuttering frequency by 15 percent. This could be used both to support the conclusion that the therapy was effective (i.e., it reduced stuttering frequency) and to support the conclusion that it was ineffective (i.e., it didn't produce enough of a reduction in stuttering frequency to make a meaningful difference in the severity of a stuttering problem). Both interpretations are defensible. It is therefore particularly important, when you are reading and evaluating therapy outcome research (as well as other research), to seek out the data on which conclusions, or interpretations, are based.

Generality

A question you must answer when you wish to assess the generality of observations is: *Did the subjects observed at least approximate a random sample from the population to which the question refers?* If the subjects observed were chosen by a table of random numbers (see Appendix B) from the population to which a question refers, it is highly likely (but not certain) that they constitute a random sample from that population. It would therefore be appropriate to use them to make inferences about this population. Significance tests and confidence intervals could be used for this purpose if observations are described quantitatively.

If subjects were selected other than randomly from the population to which a question refers, it would be *uncertain* whether they constitute a random sample from that population. Any inferences or conclusions made from observations of such subjects would have to be regarded as *quite tentative*. Almost all significance test results and confidence intervals are not readily interpretable if they are computed from numerical descriptions of such observations. Inferential statistics require that the subjects observed be a random sample from the population about which you wish to make inferences. If they do not constitute such a sample, the probability values associated with significance test results, as well as the upper and lower limits of confidence intervals, are more likely to be inaccurate than accurate.

REFERENCES

BEASLEY, D. S., and MANNING, J. I., Experimenter bias and speech pathologists' evaluation of children's language skills. *Journal of Communication Disorders*, 6, 93–101 (1973).
HEAD, H., *Aphasia and Kindred Disorders of Speech*, Volume 1. New York: Hafner Publishing Company (1963).
MEITUS, I. J., RINGEL, R. L., HOUSE, A. S., and HOTCHKISS, J. C., Clinical bias in evaluating speech proficiency. *British Journal of Disorders of Communication*, 8, 146–151 (1973).
ROSENTHAL, R., *Experimenter Bias in Behavioral Research*. New York: Appleton-Century-Crofts (1966).
ROSENTHAL, R., Interpersonal expectations: Effects of the experimenter's hypothesis. In Robert Rosenthal and Ralph Rosnow (Eds.), *Artifacts in Behavioral Research*, New York: Academic Press, Inc., 182–277 (1969).
ROSENTHAL, R., On the social psychology of the psychological experiment: The experimenter's hypothesis as unintended determinant of experimental results. *American Scientist*, 51, 268–283 (1963).
SPRIESTERSBACH, D. C., and SHERMAN, D. (Eds.), *Cleft Palate and Communication*. New York: Academic Press, Inc. (1968).
TROTTER, W. D., and KOOLS, J. A., Listener adaptation to the severity of stuttering. *Journal of Speech and Hearing Disorders*, 20, 385–387 (1955).

TEN

COMMUNICATING QUESTIONS AND ANSWERS

Once a question has been formulated and answered and the answer has been interpreted, the next step is to communicate the question, answer, and interpretation to potential consumers of the information. This is the final step in the research process. If your findings are not formally communicated, their impact probably will be limited to your caseload and those of your colleagues with whom you communicate informally. This, of course, would be undersirable.

MODES FOR DISSEMINATING RESEARCH FINDINGS

There are two main modes for disseminating research findings: written reports and oral presentations. Written reports usually consist of papers published in journals and books. Oral presentations usually consist of talks and exhibits (including poster sessions) at local, state, national, and international meetings. Other modes for disseminating research findings include audiotapes, videotapes, and motion picture films.

Written Reports

Written reports are the most frequently used mode for disseminating research findings in speech pathology and audiology. They are published in a variety of journals, including those of state speech and hearing associations, the American Speech and Hearing Association, and educational, psychological, medical, physics, speech communication, and linguistics associations. (To identify journals that have published, and presumably will continue to publish, papers dealing with certain aspects of communicative disorders, look up the aspects of interest in the indices of several recent volumes of *dsh Abstracts* and note the journals in which papers concerned with them have been published.)

Written reports can range in length from less than a page to more than 100 pages. Most are between six and twelve journal pages in length. They may be classified as articles, reports, clinical exchange reports, case reports, points of view, or letters to the editor.

Journals that classify papers as articles and reports usually distinguish between these two categories on the basis of length—longer papers are classified as articles. The magnitude of the research reported also may be a consideration. Papers that report a single study may tend to be classified as reports and those that report a series of related studies as articles. Organization is the same for both types of papers.

Clinical exchange contributions tend to be relatively short reports that are clinically relevant—i.e., deal with diagnostic or therapy procedures. They are published by several journals, including the *Journal of Speech and Hearing Disorders* and *Language, Speech, and Hearing Services in the Schools*.

Case reports (i.e., case studies) are descriptions of individuals who are noteworthy for some reason. The symptomatology or etiology of their communicative disorder may be unusual in some respect; they may have responded in an unexpected manner to a diagnostic or therapeutic procedure; or an unusual diagnostic or therapeutic procedure may have been administered to them. Such papers may contain a single case study or several related case studies.

Point-of-view papers are not intended primarily for the dissemination of research findings. They are sometimes included, however, as support for the contentions, or points of view, presented.

Letters to the editor are occasionally used to disseminate research findings. They are particularly likely to be used for this purpose when an investigator has data to report that are relevant to a question answered in a published paper. The investigator may write a letter to the editor of the journal that published the paper reporting data that either replicate those used to answer the question or suggest a different answer to the question. Letters to the editor are sometimes also used to disseminate research findings unrelated to any that have been reported when such findings can be presented in a few paragraphs.

Oral Presentations

Oral presentations are the second most frequently used mode for disseminating research findings in speech pathology and audiology. They can be made in a variety of settings, including state speech and hearing association and American Speech and Hearing Association conventions. The three most common types are talks, poster presentations, and exhibits.

The typical oral convention presentation consists of a fifteen-minute talk and a five-minute question and answer period. The organization of this kind of talk is similar to that of a written report; however, the language is usually less formal and more conversational, and the presentation is less detailed and more redundant, than that of a written report.

The poster presentation is a relatively recent addition to convention programs. Each presenter is assigned to a poster board for an hour to an hour and a half. The presenter mounts research findings on this board in graphical, tabular, photographic, or narrative form and then stands beside this "poster" for the period assigned and answers questions about it.

Scientific exhibits, such as those at American Speech and Hearing Association conventions, can be used to disseminate research findings. They are generally similar to poster presentations. However, scientific exhibits can be larger and more elaborate and last a longer period of time than poster presentations.

Other Approaches to Disseminating Research Findings

While written reports and oral presentations are the most frequently used modes for disseminating research findings in speech pathology and audiology, they are not the only ones. Others include motion picture films, audiotapes, and videotapes.

Motion picture films have been used by speech pathologists and audiologists to disseminate research findings for a relatively long period of time. Reading the descriptions of films published by the American Speech and Hearing Association in its *Film Bibliography for Speech Pathology and Audiology* will give you an impression of the potential of this medium for this purpose.

Audiotapes and videotapes have been used by speech pathologists and audiologists for disseminating research findings. Such audiotapes are distributed by book publishers (e.g., Aronson, 1973). Videotapes on topics relevant to communicative disorders are distributed by several organizations, including the Amercan Speech and Hearing Association.

OBJECTIVES OF SCIENTIFIC COMMUNICATION

Regardless of the mode used, certain types of information should be communicated in disseminating research findings. These types of information will be discussed in the context of the objectives of scientific communication.

Overall Purpose of Scientific Communication

Before indicating the specific objectives of scientific communication as they relate to research, let us briefly consider its overall purpose, i.e., *communication*. Scientific communication should provide information on questions, answers, and interpretations as unambiguously as possible. Anything that facilitates communication is desirable, anything that impedes communication is undesirable.

What factors can influence the adequacy of scientific communication? The answer to this question would be partially dependent on the mode of communication used. Factors likely to impede communication in oral presentations differ somewhat from those likely to exert such an influence in written reports or motion picture films.

While the factors that can influence the adequacy of scientific communication are to some extent specific to the medium, several can exert an influence in almost any medium. One is *organization*. If the information to be disseminated is not organized in a manner that can be easily comprehended, the adequacy of the communication will be reduced. For this reason, the organization (or structure) of both written and oral research reports has been standardized to a degree to facilitate communication. (This organization will be described later in the chapter.)

Another factor that can influence to some extent the adequacy of scientific communication in almost any medium is *language*. Accurate, detailed verbal "maps" facilitate communication, and inaccurate or vague ones impede it (see Chapter 6 for a discussion of map-territory relationships).

Specific Objectives of Scientific Communication

To be effective, scientific communication requires satisfying these conditions:

1. stating each question to be answered as unambiguously as possible,
2. demonstrating the importance of answering each question and thereby establishing scientific justification,
3. describing how the observations were made to answer each question,

4. reporting the observations made to answer each question (i.e., answering each question), and
5. suggesting the impact of the answer to each question on the total body of knowledge.

Let us briefly indicate the contribution made by each of these conditions to the communication of research findings.

One of the most important requirements of scientific communication is that each question to be answered be stated as unambiguously as possible. If potential consumers of the research reported do not know what questions were being asked, they would probably be unable to understand the answers (or findings) reported and the conclusions and generalizations made from them. It is desirable, therefore, that the questions that were asked be stated as clearly as possible at the beginning of a research report, regardless of the mode of communication used.

A second requirement is that the importance of answering each question be made explicit. This involves providing cogent answers for the "so what" or "who cares" questions—i.e., establishing scientific justification for the research. If potential consumers of the research reported feel, rightly or wrongly, that an answer to a particular question does not affect them, they will probably pay little, if any, attention to the answer. This, of course, would impair the communication process. It is risky to assume that your audience will see the importance of answering particular questions without its being pointed out to them. The more explicitly scientific justification is established, the more likely they are to attend to and utilize the findings presented, regardless of the communication mode used.

A third requirement is a description of how the observations were made to answer each question which is sufficiently detailed so that someone else could replicate the process. Basic to the scientific method is *intersubjective testability* (see Chapter 3), the requirement that the observations used to answer questions be verifiable by other investigators. For this to be possible, adequate descriptions of both the subjects observed and the procedures used to observe them must be present.

A detailed description of methodology is also necessary to permit consumers of the research reported to assess the validity, reliability, and generality of the observations made (see Chapter 9).

A fourth requirement is reporting the observations made to answer each question as clearly, or unambiguously, as possible. The observations relevant to answering a particular question should be organized for reporting in such a manner that the reason or reasons for the answer given are obvious (see Chapter 8).

Finally, a fifth requirement is an indication of possible implications of the answer to each question for the existing body of knowledge. Where possible, both theoretical and clinical implications should be suggested. It is usually not safe to assume that consumers of the research reported will see the implications of the findings without their being pointed out. And, of course, if your audience is unaware of the implications of the findings, these findings are unlikely to have any impact on theory or clinical practice.

ORGANIZATION OF WRITTEN REPORTS

We will now describe the organization of the two most commonly used modes of scientific communication: written and oral reports. The information presented in such reports is usually organized in the manner described here to facilitate communication. There are several reasons why this kind of organization tends to facilitate communication. First, the sequence in which the topics are presented is a logical one. It begins with the questions and the reasons for seeking to answer them. The sequence then moves to a description of how the observations were made to answer each question. Next, is the presentation of the observations that answer each question. Last, possible theoretical and clinical implications of the answers are suggested.

There is a reason besides logical sequence why the organization we will describe facilitates communication. With this organization, a reader will know where to locate desired information within the report. Information on the subjects observed, for example, would almost always be presented in methodology.

The traditional research report has most, if not all, of the following parts:

1. title,
2. abstract (or summary),
3. introduction,
4. methodology,
5. results,
6. discussion,
7. acknowledgments,
8. references, and
9. appendices.

The purpose and content of each part is described in the following sections.

Title

The title given to a research report is very important. If the information presented in a research report is not indicated by its title, the report may not reach potential consumers, for several reasons. First, the title is the main source of information used for indexing articles in most computerized information retrieval systems. Papers dealing with communicative disorders are indexed in a number of such systems, including some in the fields of linguistics, biology, physics, engineering, education, psychology, and medicine. If the title does not clearly indicate the content of an article, it is likely to be indexed improperly.

A title is also important because people scan titles (in bibliographies, tables of content, and so forth) to identify papers they wish to read. Because of the large numbers of articles relevant to communicative disorders currently being published, speech pathologists and audiologists must be selective in what they read. If the content of a paper is not evident from its title, the paper may not be read by potential consumers of the information presented in it.

What factors should be considered when you are composing a title for your paper? First, the wording should indicate as explicitly as possible the content of the paper—i.e., the questions dealt with. It should indicate both the specific population or populations studied (e.g., adults over the age of fifty who have cerebellar ataxia) and what was studied (e.g., the outcome of a particular therapy.) Both types of information can be combined to form a title such as:

> Therapy X: Impact on Adults over the Age of Fifty with Cerebellar Ataxia

Second, be as concise as possible when you are writing a title. All unnecessary words should be eliminated. Consider this title:

> A Study of the Impact of Therapy X on Adults over the Age of Fifty with Cerebellar Ataxia

The first four words ("A Study of the...") can probably be eliminated without altering the information communicated by the title.

Third, consider the ordering of the words of your title. The first word (or words) should at least partially define the topic. Consider the two titles suggested for a study of the impact of a therapy on persons over the age of fifty who have cerebellar ataxia. Even if the first four words of the second were eliminated, the first would probably be regarded as better than the second because it begins with a word that is more important to the content of the paper—i.e., the name of the therapy.

Abstract

The abstract (or summary) is also an important part of a research report. It provides the reader (usually in less than 150 words) with concise information about the question or questions asked, the procedures used to answer them, the answers obtained, and how the answers were interpreted.

In most journals, the abstract appears below the title and provides an overview of the material presented in the paper. Its most important function, however, is to indicate the content of the article to users of abstract journals such as *dsh Abstracts, Language and Language Behavior Abstracts,* and *Psychological Abstracts*. The titles and abstracts of almost all published papers relevant to communicative disorders are reproduced in these journals. An investigator doing a search of the communicative disorders literature ordinarily uses these journals. If the title and abstract of a paper do not accurately or completely indicate its content, the information in the paper may be lost to potential users.

There are two basic types of abstracts. The first (and most commonly used) *summarizes* the content of the paper—i.e., the question or questions asked, the observational procedures, the observations made, the answers to the questions, and the interpretations made. Here is a representative abstract of this type:

> The purpose of the study was to ascertain whether nonstutterers, like stutterers, become more fluent when pacing their speech with a metronome. Each of 20 adult male nonstutterers read four different passages. Two of the passages were read at their normal rate and two were read with a metronome at one word per beat. Based on the number of disfluencies observed in each condition, it appears not only that nonstutterers become more fluent when pacing their speech with a metronome, but also that the degree to which they become more fluent is within the range which has been reported for stutterers. This finding provides additional support for the argument recently advanced by several investigators that the effect of the metronome on stuttering is not primarily a result of distraction, at least in the way distraction has been traditionally defined. (Silverman, 1971, p. 350)

The second type of abstract *describes* the content of the paper. It indicates the topics dealt with in the paper. This type of abstract is most often used for relatively long papers where the content cannot be summarized in the number of words allowed. Here is a representative abstract of this type:

> This paper describes a dimension of the stuttering problem of elementary-school children—less frequent revision of reading errors than their nonstuttering peers. (Silverman and Williams, 1973, p. 584)

What factors should you consider when you are writing an abstract (or summary)? The primary consideration is that it must indicate the contents of the paper as accurately and completely as possible within the length (i.e., word) limit imposed by the journal. The writing must be as concise as possible. The most appropriate (e.g., descriptive, concrete) words for conveying what you wish to convey should be used. All unnecessary words should be eliminated. You may find it helpful to read a number of abstracts (e.g., all those in several issues of the *Journal of Speech and Hearing Disorders*) one after the other. This intensive reading should help you develop an intuitive feeling for how they are written.

Introduction

In the introduction to a paper you indicate *what* you were trying to do and *why* you were trying to do it. That is, you indicate the questions you attempted to answer and why you felt it important to attempt to answer each. Stating the importance of answering each question establishes the *scientific justification* for the study.

It is very important to demonstrate as explicitly as possible the relevance of the research you are reporting—i.e., the questions you are answering. You should indicate as many *cogent* theoretical and clinical implications of possible answers to your questions as you can. Lead your readers to the point where they would agree that the questions you sought to answer were worth answering. As mentioned previously, it is not safe to assume that readers will understand the implications of answers to questions without having these implications pointed out to them.

In the introduction you also review the literature that is *relevant to the questions you were attempting to answer*. Specifically, you indicate any data you are aware of that directly or indirectly suggest an answer to these questions. These data, of course, may suggest different answers to given questions (which would make any answer to them equivocal). An investigator usually attempts to indicate in the literature review why the available data only permit the questions asked to be partially answered and why it is important to gather additional data so that they can be answered unequivocally. If, based on a careful review of relevant literature, it appears that no data have been reported that suggest an answer to the questions asked, this finding should be indicated.

Before you attempt to write an introduction, you might find it helpful to read a number of them, one after the other, in articles published in the *Journal of Speech and Hearing Disorders* or the *Journal of Speech and Hearing Research*. This intensive reading should give you some feeling for how they are structured.

Methodology

In the methods section of a research report you indicate *who* you observed and *how* you observed them. That is, you describe the subjects who were observed and the procedures followed in observing them. Both should be described in enough detail that another investigator could replicate your observations, but not in so much detail that this section would become unnecessarily long and confusing.

How do you decide what information should be included in a methods section? The sole criterion for any bit of information is whether it is necessary to someone who wished to replicate your observations. If you feel a given piece of information is likely to be necessary for this purpose, it should be included. If you do not feel it is necessary for this purpose, you can probably safely exclude it. If you are uncertain whether it is necessary, however, it should be included.

Before you attempt to write a methods section, you may find it helpful to scan a number of methodology sections, one after the other, paying particular attention to how they are organized.

Results

In the results section of a research report you describe *what* was observed—i.e., the observations that were made to answer each question. You organize these observations in a manner that should make the answer to each question fairly obvious to most readers. In this section you answer each question and report the data upon which your answers are based.

Interpretations of the data are usually made not in this section, but in the discussion. There are instances, however, when it is desirable to interpret the data while they are being presented. A combined results and discussion section can be used in these cases.

Discussion

In the discussion section of a research report you indicate *possible implications*—*both* theoretical and clinical—of the answers you obtained. You indicate both the ways in which your answers appear to be consistent with existing theory and clinical practice and the ways in which they raise questions concerning the validity of aspects of existing theory and clinical practice.

It is particularly important, in the discussion section, to deal with the possible implications of the research mentioned in the introduction to establish scientific justification. You should summarize the answers to the questions and indicate their implications for these aspects of theory and clinical practice.

Questions for future research are sometimes suggested in the discussion section. A study may raise more questions than it answers. By mentioning such questions and indicating why each would be important to answer, you can help an investigator who wishes to attempt to answer them establish scientific justification. He or she can cite your arguments as part of a scientific justification.

Acknowledgments

The primary purpose of an acknowledgments section is to credit and recognize the financial and other support of individuals and organizations you received while doing the research and preparing the research report. Any financial assistance should be acknowledged, as should any persons who significantly contributed to the research by performing such functions as locating subjects, administering the experimental treatments, or assisting in the process of data analysis. Other persons you may wish to acknowledge are consultants, investigators who provided you with unpublished data, administrators who in some manner facilitated the research process, and persons who read the manuscript critically and offered suggestions for improvement.

Another type of information presented in an acknowledgment section is the author's current institutional affiliation if it differs from that given at the beginning of the article.

Some journals also include the name and address of the person to whom requests for reprints should be directed in the acknowledgment section.

References

All papers and books mentioned in the paper should be listed here. Since there is no standard reference style, you should acquaint yourself with the style used by the journal to which you plan to submit the paper before preparing this section.

Appendices

Included in an appendix or appendices would be various documents related to the research reported that are unpublished. An example would be an unpublished test or other assessment instrument that was used in gathering the data reported.

ORGANIZATION OF ORAL PRESENTATIONS

The organization described for written reports is generally suitable for oral presentations. The two main ways in which oral reports differ from written ones are *length* and *style*. Because an investigator is usually permitted only a short period of time at most conventions and other professional meetings to report the research, he or she must summarize methodology and results briefly rather than describing them in detail.

A second difference is that the style of oral reports is usually less formal and more redundant than the style of written reports. The language of an oral report should be as conversational as possible, because the goal is to communicate with the audience. If the language of a paper read aloud is similar to that of a formal, written research report, at least some members of the audience will not pay attention and communication will be impeded.

To communicate effectively, an oral report must be more repetitious than a written one. If you do not understand something in a written report, you can reread it. This is not possible with an oral presentation, unless it is on audiotape or videotape. One strategy that is helpful for providing the necessary redundancy in oral reports is beginning by summarizing what you are going to say, then saying it, and ending by summarizing what you have said.

PREPARATION OF WRITTEN AND ORAL REPORTS

Besides reading a number of already published reports for organization and wording, you can learn how to prepare reports by consulting references on scientific writing. There are several relevant books and articles you may find helpful for this purpose. The *Publications Manual for the American Psychological Association* (1974) is a highly useful source of such information. Other publications you might wish to consult are those of Forscher and Wertz (1970), Jerger (1972), King and Roland (1970), Moore (1969), Strunk (1972), Trelease (1969), and Woodford (1967).

Before preparing a written report that you intend to submit for publication, you should read the information to contributors provided by the journal you plan to submit it to. Some journals (e.g., the *Journal of Speech and Hearing Research*) publish this information in every issue; others publish it at regular intervals (e.g., one issue a year); still others do not publish it, but send copies on request. The information usually provided in the section on information to contributors includes:

1. types of papers the journal prints (e.g., research reports, review papers) and their topics (e.g., hearing problems, cleft lip and palate),
2. instructions for preparing tables and figures and for typing the manuscript,
3. maximum length for the abstract,
4. reference style,
5. number of copies that should be submitted, and
6. name of the editor to whom the copies of the manuscript should be submitted.

LOCATING OUTLETS FOR SPEECH PATHOLOGY AND AUDIOLOGY RESEARCH

Your final task in the research process is disseminating your questions, answers, and interpretations where they are likely to reach potential consumers of the information. This process usually involves either locating a journal to which to submit a written report or locating a professional meeting (e.g., a convention of an organization) at which to present an oral report (or both, since many papers presented at professional meetings are later published).

The outlets probably most often used by speech pathologists and audiologists for disseminating research findings are the publications and convention programs of the American Speech and Hearing Association (A.S.H.A.). The A.S.H.A. journals include:

Journal of Speech and Hearing Disorders
Journal of Speech and Hearing Research
Language, Speech, and Hearing Services in Schools
Asha
ASHA Monographs
ASHA Reports

Each issue of these journals contains a statement of the types of research reports it will consider. One advantage of publishing in A.S.H.A. journals is that you are quite likely to reach most speech pathologists and audiologists who would be potential consumers of your research.

More than 500 research reports dealing with all aspects of speech pathology and audiology are usually included in the program of the annual convention of the American Speech and Hearing Association. For a research report to be considered for inclusion in the convention program, a summary and abstract of the research have to be submitted to the program committee. Additional information can be found in the annual "Call for Papers," which is usually published in the January issue of *Asha*.

State speech and hearing association publications and convention programs are also outlets for disseminating research findings. Their main limitation is that the audience you can reach through them is geographically limited.

A number of other associations publish research relevant to speech pathology or audiology in their journals and include such reports in their convention programs. The following is a representative, not an inclusive, list of such organizations:

American Psychological Association
American Cleft Palate Association
Acoustical Society of America
Academy of Aphasia
Academy of Cerebral Palsy
International Association of Logopedics and Phoniatrics
Canadian Speech and Hearing Association
College of Speech Therapists (London)
Council of Exceptional Children
Alexander Graham Bell Association

Finally, several journals not published by scientific and professional associations can serve as outlets for speech pathology and audiology research. Two examples would be the *Journal of Communication Disorders* and *Perceptual and Motor Skills*.

Perhaps the best strategy for identifying possible journals to submit a particular research report to is to scan abstracts dealing with the same topic in *dsh Abstracts* and note the journals in which the papers have been published.

EDITORIAL PROCESSING OF MANUSCRIPTS

How is a manuscript processed after it has been submitted to a journal to be considered for publication? After receiving the copies of the manuscript, the editor usually sends a form letter to the author indicating that the manuscript has been received and that the decision concerning it will be relayed as soon as the manuscript has been reviewed. The editor sends copies of the manuscript to at least two editorial consultants, or reviewers, who the editor feels are competent to assess the suitability of the manuscript for publication. The editor asks them for a recommendation on the disposition of the manuscript (accept as is, accept if revised according to instructions, reject, etc.), the reason or reasons for their recommendation, and suggestions for improving the manuscript. After receiving the reviewers' recommendations and reading the manuscript, the editor decides on the disposition of the manuscript and informs the author of the decision and the reason or reasons for it. If the editor feels that parts of the manuscript need to be rewritten before it is suitable for publication, he or she will indicate to the author the parts that have to be rewritten and may offer some suggestions for rewriting them. (Almost all manuscripts, incidentally, require some rewriting.) The review process can take anywhere from a few weeks to more than a year; in most cases, it takes between one and four months.

What should you do if a manuscript you write is rejected by a journal? Few people enjoy being rejected; and if a manuscript you write is rejected, it can hurt your ego. Since some journals have rejection rates of more than 75 percent, most (if not all) investigators are going to have papers rejected sooner or later. What you should do with such a manuscript depends on the reason or reasons for its rejection (as well as this can be determined from the editor's and reviewers' comments). Among the reasons for a manuscript being rejected are these:

1. the author failed to establish scientific justification for the study (i.e., the reviewers regarded it as trivial);
2. the observational procedures used would probably not permit the question or questions to be answered with an adequate level of validity, reliability, and generality;
3. the data analyses procedures were inappropriate;
4. the writing did not meet minimum standards for publication;
5. the content of the manuscript was inappropriate for the journal; and
6. the reviewers did not like the question or questions the author asked or how he interpreted his findings.

If your manuscript is rejected because you failed to establish adequate scientific justification for the study reported in it, you should attempt to rewrite the introduction to demonstrate the relevance of the study. Assuming this was the *only* reason why the manuscript appeared to have been rejected, and you feel that you have established adequate scientific justification for the study in your rewrite of the introduction, you may wish to resubmit the manuscript to the journal with a note indicating how it has been revised. Or you may wish to submit it to some other journal.

If your manuscript is rejected because something was wrong with the methodology used to make the observations, and you agree that the reviewers' criticisms are valid, you may want to rerun the study using observational procedures that were modified as recommended. However, if you feel that the reviewers' criticisms are not valid, you may wish to send a rebuttal to the editor indicating why you felt your methodology was adequate and requesting that the editor reconsider the manuscript. Or you may wish to submit the manuscript to another journal.

If your manuscript is rejected because something was wrong with how the data were analyzed, you should reanalyze the data and either resubmit the corrected manuscript to the journal or submit it to some other journal. If you feel, however, that the data have been appropriately analyzed, you may wish to write the editor indicating why you feel your analyses were appropriate, including, if possible, supporting statements from one or more statisticians.

If your manuscript is rejected because it was badly written, it should be rewritten (with particular consideration given to relevant comments by reviewers) and either resubmitted to the journal or submitted to some other journal. Hopefully, some person at your institution experienced in writing research reports could assist you with the rewriting.

If your manuscript is rejected because the content was inappropriate for the journal to which it was submitted, it should be submitted to a journal for which the content would be appropriate. You should be able to identify such a journal by scanning several volumes of *dsh Abstracts* for papers with similar content.

Occasionally, a manuscript is rejected by a journal because the reviewers did not like the questions the author asked or the interpretation of the findings. This is particularly likely to occur when an author's findings challenge accepted theory or clinical practice. An author who feels a manuscript has been rejected on this basis should submit it to another journal.

REFERENCES

ARONSON, A. E., *Psychogenic Voice Disorders* (Audio Seminars in Speech Pathology). Philadelphia: W. B. Saunders Company (1973).

FORSCHER, B. K., and WERTZ, R. T., Organizing the scientific paper. *Asha*, 12, 494–497 (1970).

JERGER, J., Scientific writing can be readable. *Asha*, 4, 101–104 (1962).

KING, L. S., and ROLAND, C. G., *Scientific Writing*. Chicago: American Medical Association (1970).

MOORE, M. V., Pathological writing. *Asha*, 11, 535–538 (1969).

Publications Manual for the American Psychological Association, 1974 Revision. Washington, D.C.: American Psychological Association (1974).

SILVERMAN, F. H., The effect of rhythmic auditory stimulation on the disfluency of nonstutterers. *Journal of Speech and Hearing Research*, 14, 350–355 (1971).

SILVERMAN, F. H., and WILLIAMS, D. E., Use of revision by elementary-school stutterers and nonstutterers during oral reading. *Journal of Speech and Hearing Research*, 16, 584–585 (1973).

STRUNK, W., Jr., *The Elements of Style* (2nd ed.). New York: The Macmillan Company (1972).

TRELEASE, S. F., *How to Write Scientific and Technical Papers*. Cambridge, Mass.: M.I.T. Press (1969).

WOODFORD, F. P., Sounder thinking through clearer writing. *Science*, 156, 743–745 (1967).

part III

Clinical Research Considerations

ELEVEN

ASSESSING THE EFFECTS OF THERAPIES

To continue to grow as clinicians, we must continually evaluate the effects of our therapies—both positive and negative—upon our clients. Without the information such an evaluation gives, we are apt to use either a small number of approaches (or strategies) over and over again or continuously seek out the "newest" approaches. Our reason for adopting or rejecting a given therapy is likely to be its acceptance or rejection by an "authority," such as the author of a textbook we are familiar with, rather than its impact upon our client's behaviors, particularly their communicative behaviors. We will have no way to improve systematically the effectiveness of our repertoire of therapy strategies without constant reevaluation.

CHOICE OF PRESUMPTION

This discussion will briefly consider the choice of presumption concerning the impact of a therapy upon behaviors contributing to a client's communicative disorder. There are two choices here: (1) to consider a therapy effective until it is proven ineffective, or (2) to consider a therapy ineffective until it has been proven effective. The choice between these presumptions is somewhat analogous to considering a person innocent until proven guilty in law as opposed to considering him guilty until proven innocent.

What are the *consequences* of choosing each presumption? There are two types of consequence: clinical and logical. A *clinical* consequence is one related to the impact of the choice upon the treatment received by the client. Each presumption has associated with it a type of treatment error. That is, considering a therapy effective until there is reasonable evidence that it is ineffective exposes the client to a therapy that could have no effect, or an undesirable effect, upon him. On the other hand, considering a therapy ineffective until there is reasonable evidence that it is effective exposes the client to the possibility of not receiving a therapy that could benefit him.

The type of treatment error, hence the presumption, most likely to lead to undesirable consequences for a client would not be the same in all instances. To illustrate this point, let us consider two instances in which we might be tempted to try a therapy that seems sound theoretically but has not yet been proven effective. In instance A, at least one other therapy has been proven effective; in instance B, no therapies have been proven effective. The consequences of *using* the new approach in instance A and finding it ineffective are likely to be more undesirable than not using it when it would have been effective. On the other hand, the consequences of *not using* this approach in instance B when it may have been effective are likely to be more undesirable to the client than using it and finding it ineffective. Thus, from the clinical point of view, neither of these presumptions would always be the most desirable.

The second type of consequence can be referred to as *logical*. A logical consequence is one related to the choice of research design, particularly statistical inference. If our presumption is that a therapy is ineffective until it is proven effective, we can use traditional statistical hypothesis testing procedures to determine the likelihood that it has been effective. Recall that the null hypothesis—the hypothesis tested by all traditional statistical significance tests—states that a treatment has produced no difference, i.e., has had no effect. For determining whether a therapy has influenced behavior, the null hypothesis would state that any effects the therapy appears to have had are not real but the result of chance fluctuation or sampling error. Stated slightly differently, differences in behavior after receiving a therapy are not sufficiently *reliable* to be attributed to that therapy.

Rejecting the null hypothesis provides some support for the alternative, or research hypothesis, that the therapy has been effective—i.e., has resulted in behavioral change. However, it is necessary to keep constantly in mind that rejecting a null hypothesis or null hypotheses only indicates that any behavioral changes observed following therapy are unlikely to have been the result of chance fluctuation or sampling error. It does not establish that such changes resulted from the therapy. Other events occurring while a client was receiving therapy could be responsible for the observed behavioral change. Examples of such events would be: (1) maturation (particularly of concern in the evaluation of articulation therapies), (2) improved self-concept (particularly of concern in the evaluation of therapies for stuttering and voice disorders), (3) spontaneous recovery (of concern in the evaluation of therapies for aphasia, agnosia, apraxia, and dysarthria), and (4) events, other than those directly related to the therapy being evaluated, resulting from the interaction between the client and the clinician, or the client and the environment, or both. One of the author's clients, a university student who stuttered, illustrates the second and fourth of these possibilities. During the period he worked with her, her stuttering reduced considerably in severity. However, approximately a month after he began seeing her, she participated in an encounter group. As a result of this experience, she apparently realized that what she had to say was: (1) more important than how she said it, (2) of interest to others, and (3) could influence others. In this case, then, the change observed in the client's behavior is more likely to have been the result of the "something else" that occurred during the period she was receiving therapy than of the therapy per se.

We will now consider the logical consequences of the alternative presumption—i.e., considering a therapy effective until it is proven ineffective. Here, failure to reject a null hypothesis could be interpreted as support for a therapy's effectiveness. As you may recall from our previous discussion of the null hypothesis, it is usually considered inappropriate to interpret failure to reject a null hypothesis as support for a research hypothesis (in this case, that a therapy was effective). This would be particularly inappropriate if the probability of making a Type II error were either relatively high (i.e., exceeded 5 percent) or unspecified. In the context of the present discussion, this would be the probability of not finding a therapy ineffective when it is ineffective. We are again becoming concerned about " ... the effects of an investigator's expectancy or hypothesis on the results of his research ...." (Rosenthal, 1969, p. 182). It is relatively easy "subconsciously" to design an experiment to assess the effects of a therapy in which the probability of making a Type II error is considerably higher than the 5 percent limit usually considered tolerable. This can be done by: (1) keeping the sample size relatively small, and (2) setting the probability of a Type I error—the probability of finding a therapy effective when it is ineffective—at a relatively conservative level (e.g., 0.01). Unfortunately, in most reports of significance tests in therapy outcome research, the probabilities of Type II errors are not specified.

In most instances considering a therapy ineffective until there is reasonable evidence that it is effective would probably be more defensible than the alternative presumption, i.e., considering it effective until there is reasonable evidence it is ineffective.

QUESTIONS TO CONSIDER WHEN EVALUATING A THERAPY

A basic premise of this book is that research can be viewed as a process of answering "answerable" questions. Systematic research to assess the effects of a therapy upon persons who have a communicative disorder should provide answers to a series of such questions, including the following:

1. *What are the effects of the therapy upon specific behaviors that contribute to a client's communicative disorder at given points in space-time?* Here "specific behaviors" include what are traditionally called "attitudes" and "feelings." We become aware of attitudes and feelings by observing behavior —that is, attitudes and feelings are *explanations* of behavior. "Points in space-time" refers to how the effects of a therapy upon specific behaviors vary, over a period of time and according to situation. "Space-time" is hyphenated to indicate (as Einstein and others have pointed out) that time cannot be separated from space but provides the fourth dimension necessary to specify the location, or coordinates, of an event.

2. *What are the effects of the therapy upon other attributes of a client's communicative behavior at given points in space-time?* A therapy with a desirable effect on behaviors that contribute to a client's communicative disorder may have an undesirable effect on other attributes of the client's communicative behavior. Other attributes affected might include: (1) speaking rate, (2) auditory acuity, (3) speech rhythm, (4) speech articulation, (5) voice intensity, (6) voice quality, (7) language formulation, (8) verbal output, (9) spontaneity, and (10) credibility as a communicator. If, for example, a stutterer is taught to monitor his speech for moments of stuttering and voluntarily reduce their severity, this may not only result in a reduction in his stuttering severity but in his speaking rate, spontaneity, and inflection as well. If a client's communicative behavior after receiving a therapy called more adverse attention to itself than it did before receiving that therapy, this would obviously raise questions concerning the value of the therapy.

3. *What are the effects of the therapy upon a client other than those directly related to communicative behavior at given points in space-time?* The intent of this question is similar to the second, since it is concerned with identifying negative side effects of the therapy. The side effects we are concerned with here would include: (1) a poorer self-concept, (2) reduced peer acceptance, (3) disturbed biological rhythms, and (4) increased anxiety. A client given an instrumental aid (such as an electrolarynx or a miniature metronome with which to pace his speech) might be able to communicate better with the device, but might also feel there is something wrong with him for having to rely on it rather than being able to overcome the problem by "force of will."

4. *What are the client's attitudes toward the therapy and its effects upon his communicative and other behaviors at given points in space-time?* A client's attitudes toward a therapy and its effects upon his or her behavior can influence (reduce or enhance) the effectiveness of the therapy. If, for example, a person with a hearing loss refused to wear a hearing aid, the use of this therapy could not be effective in reducing the severity of the communicative disorder (unless, of course, the person's attitude could be changed). On the other hand, a client with strong belief that a therapy could benefit him or her would invest more time and energy in the therapy program which, in turn, would enhance the therapy's effectiveness.

5. *What are the attitudes of a client's clinician, family, friends, and others toward the therapy and toward its effects upon the client's communicative behavior and other attributes of behavior at given points in space-time?* The attitudes of persons with whom a client interacts toward a therapy the client is receiving and toward its effects on his or her behavior can influence the probable success of that therapy. A clinician who does not believe that a therapy will be effective is likely to communicate this attitude to the client and thereby reduce the odds that the client will benefit from that therapy. If, for example, a clinician were directly or indirectly to communicate to a client who had a laryngectomy and could benefit from a mechanical larynx that he or she considered the use of such a device a last resort, the clinician might reduce the odds that the client would use the device and thereby benefit from it.

6. *What investment is required of client and clinician at given points in space-time?* Several types of investment can be required, including: (1) financial, (2) time and energy, and (3) willingness to be uncomfortable, i.e., to do things one does not wish to do (things that tend to make a person uncomfortable or increase one's anxiety level). A therapy may be effective but may be too demanding in cost or time to be practical for many clients. An example of such a therapy would be traditional psychoanalysis, in which the client may be required to be seen by the psychoanalyst daily for a period of several years. Also, a therapy may be effective but may cause clients to be so uncomfortable that few would be willing to make the necessary investment. One such therapy would be voluntary stuttering—"fake" stuttering—outside the clinic situation. Many stutterers find this activity extremely noxious and refuse to do it when asked by their clinician.

7. *What is the probability of relapse following termination of the therapy?* Persons with communicative disorders, particularly stutterers, may relapse to some degree when they stop seeing their clinicians on a regular basis. While a person exposed to almost any therapy approach can relapse, the probability of relapse tends to be higher for some approaches than for others. If the positive effects of a therapy were quite likely to wear off after termination, that therapy would be of questionable value. It is important, then, when evaluating a therapy, to take the probability of relapse into consideration.

RESEARCH DESIGN CONSIDERATIONS FOR ASSESSING THE EFFECTS OF THERAPIES

This section will discuss considerations in designing research to answer the questions raised in the preceding section. Most of the topics we have already examined, particularly descriptive statistics, inferential statistics, and measurement, are relevant when you are attempting to answer such questions. Our comments here will be almost completely limited to topics not previously discussed.

While little methodological research has been reported that concerns assessing the effects of therapies on persons who have communicative disorders, considerable relevant methodological research has been published in education, clinical psychology, and psychiatry journals. Since the problems involved in assessing the effects of teaching methods and psychotherapies are much the same as those involved in assessing the effects of therapies for communicative disorders, this methodological information can be utilized for designing research to assess the outcome of therapy on communicative disorders. Some of this information has been incorporated into the discussion.

What Are the Effects of the Therapy upon Specific Behaviors That Contribute to a Client's Communicative Disorder at Given Points in Space-Time?

A number of considerations must be taken into account when we wish to assess systematically the effects of a therapy upon behaviors contributing to a client's communicative disorder, including the following:

1. choosing a criterion measure or measures,
2. establishing a baseline,
3. establishing a measurement interval,
4. selecting criteria for deciding whether a therapy has been effective,
5. identifying viable alternatives to the hypothesis that a therapy was responsible for an effect, if an effect is observed,
6. reducing the effects of the experimenter's expectations and theoretical biases on the data,
7. identifying relevant organismic variables,
8. identifying relevant therapist variables, and
9. controlling positive and negative placebo effect contamination.

Let us now consider each of these factors.

Choosing a Criterion Measure or Measures. The choice of a criterion measure or measures is one of the most important considerations when you are designing research to assess the effects of therapies on persons with communicative disorders. If a criterion measure selected is not sufficiently reliable and valid, it can make an effective therapy appear ineffective. That is, the use of such a criterion measure can increase the probability of a Type II error.

One way to maximize the probability that an effective therapy will be judged effective (and hence reduce the probability of a Type II error) is to use more than one criterion measure. If, for example, we wish to determine whether a therapy for an articulation error is effective, we might use as criterion measures the percent correct production of the "error" phoneme on several types of speaking tasks. The reliability of a composite measure (e.g., the mean of several measures) will tend to be higher than that of the individual measures that contribute to it. A composite measure, therefore, is less likely than individual measures to result in a Type II error. The effects of a therapy on individual criterion measures also can be evaluated.

If a criterion measure is invalid—if it does not measure what it is supposed to measure—it will obviously be useless for evaluating the effects of therapies. Indeed, if a valid criterion measure of a behavior is not available, attempting to assess the effects of therapies on that behavior would probably be futile.

Establishing a Baseline. To determine if a given therapy has been effective, a client's behavior after being exposed to the therapy is compared to his or her behavior before being exposed to it. The measures to which the behavior following therapy are compared constitute the baseline. The simplest baseline would consist of a single criterion measure made once before beginning therapy. More complex baselines would consist of: (1) a single criterion measure made more than once, (2) multiple criterion measures made once, or (3) multiple criterion measures made more than once. Graphic representations of these baselines are presented in Table 11.1. In this table and through-

TABLE 11.1. Graphic representations of baselines.

Single criterion measure made once	O
Single criterion measure made more than once	$O_{11} \ O_{12} \ \ldots \ O_{1n}$
Multiple criterion measures made once	O_{11} O_{21} $\cdot$ $\cdot$ $\cdot$ O_{j1}
Multiple criterion measures made more than once	$O_{11} \ O_{12} \ \ldots \ O_{1n}$ $O_{21} \ O_{22} \ \ldots \ O_{2n}$ $\cdot \quad \cdot \quad \quad \cdot$ $\cdot \quad \cdot \quad \quad \cdot$ $O_{j1} \ O_{j2} \ \ldots \ O_{jn}$

out this chapter, Campbell and Stanley's code for representing research designs graphically was used (Campbell and Stanley, 1963, p. 6). In the graphic representations of research designs,

> An X will represent the exposure of a group [or an individual] to an experimental variable or event [or therapy], the effects of which are to be measured; O will refer to some process of observation or measurement; the Xs and Os in a given row are applied to the same specific persons. The left-to-right dimension indicates the temporal order, and the Xs and Os vertical to one another are simultaneous.

The subscript in the graphic representations is that of a standard two-dimensional table. The first digit identifies the criterion measure; the second, the number of the administration. Thus, O_{12} would be the second administration of the first criterion measure, and O_{1n} would be the nth administration of the first criterion measure, and O_{jn} would be the nth administration of criterion measure j.

Of what advantage is a baseline where each criterion measure is made more than once? The main advantage of such a baseline is increased *stability*. The more times a criterion measure is made under a baseline condition (i.e., before therapy), the more stable the baseline, hence the lower the probability of a Type II error (i.e., concluding a therapy was ineffective when it was effective). This is because, as mentioned previously, the more times a measure is made, the less its fluctuation as a result of random measurement error will be.

What benefits would derive from using a multiple baseline, i.e., a baseline consisting of more than one criterion measure? One benefit is that a multiple baseline permits you to assess the effects of a therapy on more than one of the behaviors contributing to a client's communicative disorder. With such a baseline, for example, you could assess the effect of a speech improvement program on the production of more than one phoneme. A separate criterion measure would be used for each phoneme. (For an illustration of the use of a multiple baseline to assess the effects of an articulation therapy, see the paper by M. Elbert, R. Shelton, and W. Arndt cited at the end of this chapter.)

Establishing a Measurement Interval. One consideration in designing therapy outcome research is how frequently to make the criterion measure. The measurement interval probably used most frequently in therapy outcome research can be graphically represented in the following manner:

$$O_1 \quad X \quad O_2$$

This is the traditional *pretest-posttest* design. The criterion measure is made twice: once preceding a period of therapy (O_1), and once following it (O_2).

This design is not a particularly good one for several reasons. First, it is more likely than most designs to result in a Type II error, since relatively high levels of random measurement error are possible when comparisons are made between single measures. Second, it is more difficult to interpret than most others. If a client's communicative disorder is less severe at point O_2 than at point O_1, there may be plausible explanations for this difference other than its resulting from the therapy. Among the classes of extraneous variables that could account for such a difference, according to Campbell (1963, p. 215), are the following:

> 1. *History:* the other specific events occurring between the first and the second measurement in addition to the experimental variable [i.e., the therapy].
> 2. *Maturation:* processes within the respondents [clients] operating as a function of the passage of time *per se* (not specific to the particular events), including growing older, growing hungrier, growing more tired, and the like.
> 3. *Testing:* the effects of taking a test upon the scores of a second testing.
> 4. *Instrumentation:* changes in the calibration of a measuring instrument or changes in the observers or scorers which may produce changes in the obtained measurements.
> 5. *Statistical regression:* regression operating when groups have been selected on the basis of their extreme scores.
> 6. The *reactive* or *interactive effect of testing*, in which a pretest might increase or decrease the respondent's sensitivity or responsiveness to the experimental variable and thus make the results obtained for a pretested population unrepresentative of the effects of the experimental variable for the unpretested universe from which the experimental respondents were selected.

The effects of three of these classes—maturation, testing, and statistical regression—can be at least partially controlled by substituting a *time series* design such as the one illustrated for a pretest-posttest design:

$$O_1 \quad O_2 \quad O_3 \quad O_4 \quad X \quad O_5 \quad O_6 \quad O_7 \quad O_8$$

With this design, the criterion measure is made a predetermined number of times (in the above example, eight) at a set time interval. The duration of the interval between measures would be approximately equal to the duration of the therapy being evaluated. The clients receive the therapy during the interval between two measures (in the example, they would receive it between measures four and five). The criterion measures are then plotted, and the pattern of the resulting trendline is interpreted to indicate whether the therapy has had an effect (see Figure 11.1). This design is most practical for therapies of relatively short duration.

A treatment does not have to occur at the midpoint of a time series. It could occur toward the beginning:

$$O_1 \quad O_2 \quad X \quad O_3 \quad O_4 \quad O_5 \quad O_6 \quad O_7 \quad O_8$$

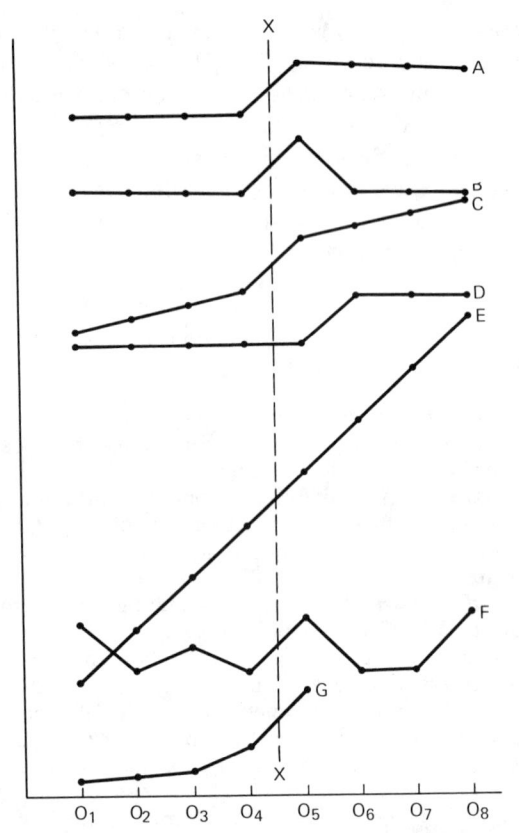

FIGURE 11.1 *Some possible outcome patterns from the introduction of an experimental variable at point X into a time series of measurements, O_1–O_8. Except for D, the O_4–O_5 gain is the same for all time series, while the legitimacy of inferring an effect varies widely, being strongest in A and B and totally unjustified in E, F, and G.*

(From Campbell, D. T., From description to experimentation: Interpreting trends in quasi-experiments. In Chester W. Harris (Ed.), *Problems in Measuring Change*. Madison: University of Wisconsin Press, 1963).

Such a design could be useful for assessing the long-term effects of a therapy.

A variation of the time series design, the *multiple time series* (Campbell, 1963, p. 232), is even more effective in controlling for the effects of extraneous variables. Such a design is illustrated graphically by the following:

GROUP A O_1 O_2 O_3 O_4 X O_5 O_6 O_7 O_8

GROUP B O_1 O_2 O_3 O_4 O_5 O_6 O_7 O_8

This design controls at least partially for five of the six classes of extraneous variables to which the pretest-posttest design is sensitive—history, maturation, testing, instrumentation, and statistical regression.

With a multiple time series design, the measures made on the members of a group who receive a therapy (in the example, Group A) are compared to those made on the members of a comparable group who do not receive that therapy (in the example, Group B). The measures are made on both groups at the same time intervals. The measures made on the control group provide a secondary baseline against which to assess those made on the experimental group. The primary baseline is the same as for the pretest-posttest and single time series designs, i.e., the measures made before a client has received therapy.

The control, or secondary, baseline can be helpful in interpreting several of the outcome patterns in Figure 11.1. If, for example, the eight measures made on the members of a control group were approximately equal (i.e., the control baseline was relatively flat), Pattern D would indicate that the therapy had been effective.

One limitation of the multiple time series design is the need for a control group. We would probably have reservations about withholding therapy from a group of clients who need it. There are circumstances, however, when this ethical consideration would not occur. One would be when enough people are on a waiting list who: (1) have the same type of communicative disorder as the members of the experimental group, and (2) do not differ systematically from them in relevant organismic variables such as age and intellectual level. A second circumstance would be when a therapy is of relatively short duration. Delaying beginning therapy in this instance would probably do no harm.

The three designs described here are obviously not the only possible ones for assessing the effects of therapies on communicative disorders. For descriptions of other designs, see Campbell (1963) and Campbell and Stanley (1963).

Selecting Criteria for Deciding whether the Therapy Has Been Effective. Before concluding that a therapy has been effective, it is necessary to demonstrate a difference between pre- and post-therapy measures that: (1) is unlikely to have resulted from random, or chance, fluctuation, and (2) is more likely to have resulted from the therapy than from extraneous variables. Demonstrating the first requires the use of statistical inference, specifically tests of the null hypothesis that no difference exists between clients' pre- and post-therapy measures that is unlikely to have been the result of random, or chance, fluctuation. Considerations in selecting and interpreting such tests are discussed in Chapter 8. One point that must be stressed again is the importance of specifying and keeping relatively low the probability of a Type II error. In therapy outcome research, the size of the experimental group (and of the control group, if one is used) is apt to be relatively small and hence the probability of a Type II error is apt to be relatively high.

If a null hypothesis is rejected, the next step is to demonstrate that the observed difference between pre- and post-therapy measures is more likely to have resulted from the therapy than from extraneous variables. The ease with which it is possible to accomplish this objective is partially a function of the measurement interval used. It would be much simpler to accomplish, for example, with a time series than with a pretest-posttest design. With a pretest-posttest design, it is doubtful that you could be reasonably certain that an observed difference was the result of a therapy rather than of extraneous variables.

Identifying Viable Alternatives to the Hypothesis That a Therapy Was Responsible for the Effect, if an Effect Is Observed. The identification of viable alternative hypotheses is not, strictly speaking, a problem of research design or statistics. To identify factors that could explain an observed difference other than the therapy being evaluated, an investigator must do a careful search of relevant literature.

Reducing the Effects of the Experimenter's Expectations and Theoretical Biases on the Data. A number of investigations have demonstrated that an experimenter's expectations and biases can influence the results (Rosenthal and Rosnow, 1969). The nature of this influence is such that the investigator may not be consciously aware of it. While it is probably not possible in most instances to eliminate these effects completely from therapy outcome research, there are ways to reduce their influence, including the following:

1. Have someone *other than the experimenter* conduct the therapy and make and interpret the criterion measures. Ideally, the person who performs these tasks should be relatively neutral in expectation concerning the effectiveness of the therapy.
2. Whenever possible, the person who makes and interprets criterion measures should not know whether he or she is dealing with pre- or post-therapy material. This can be done when the criterion measures are ratings of audiotapes or videotapes. The observers rating the tapes should not know whether any given tape was recorded prior to or following therapy. This approach also can be used when the criterion measures are from physiological data readouts and psychological test protocols.
3. If the design used has both experimental and control group subjects—i.e., both subjects who receive and do not receive the therapy—the person who makes and interprets the measures should not know in any given instance which group a subject belongs to.
4. In studies of the relative effectiveness of several therapies, it would be best if the same clinician did not administer all therapies. A clinician may expect certain ones to be more effective than others, which could influence the data on their relative effectiveness.

Identifying Relevant Organismic Variables. Organismic variables are properties or attributes of the individual (Edwards and Cronbach, 1966). Examples are sex, chronological age, socioeconomic status, intellectual level, and educational level. The degree of effectiveness of a therapy may be influenced by such variables. A particular stuttering therapy, for example, may be more effective with adults than with children.

There are at least two reasons for identifying relevant organismic variables in therapy outcome research. First, organismic variables may help define the subpopulation for which a given therapy is (or is not) effective. If there are no relevant organismic variables, a therapy that is effective with some persons who have a given communicative disorder would be expected to be effective with most persons who had that disorder (assuming etiology were held constant). On the other hand, if organismic variables did influence the effectiveness of a therapy, that therapy probably would be effective with only a subset of the population. This subset would consist of persons who fall into a specific category (e.g., male or female), or categories, with respect to each relevant organismic variable.

A second reason for identifying relevant organismic variables is concerned with the meaningfulness of combining subjects into groups. The effects of a therapy can be cancelled by combining data from subjects who differ with respect to relevant organismic variables. If a therapy were effective with children but not with adults, for example, combining data from children and adults could make it appear to have been ineffective (particularly if there were more adults than children in the sample).

Identifying Relevant Therapist Variables. A therapy administered by one therapist may not have the same effect as the same therapy administered by a second therapist. Certain attitudes and attributes of therapists can enhance or reduce the effectiveness of therapies. One such attribute is amount of clinical experience. A therapy administered by a clinician with considerable experience may be more effective than the same therapy administered by a beginning clinician. Also, a clinician who expects a therapy to be effective may get a different result from one who expects it to be ineffective. Other therapist variables that could influence the effectiveness of a therapy are sex, chronological age, socioeconomic status, degree of confidence in self, ability to communicate, and professional title (Dr. versus Mr., Ms., Miss, or Mrs.).

If the effectiveness of a therapy is at least partially a function of therapist variables, this has several implications. First, it limits the generality of research findings on the effectiveness of that therapy. Perhaps a therapy would only be recommended for clinicians with considerable experience or for those with considerable confidence in its effectiveness. Second, it may not be possible to combine, or "lump," data from different clinicians. If such data are combined, a therapy that is effective for certain clinicians may appear to be ineffective, particularly if it is ineffective for the majority of clinicians.

Controlling Positive and Negative Placebo Effect Contamination. A placebo is

> ... any therapeutic procedure (or that component of any therapeutic procedure) which is given deliberately to have an effect, or unknowingly has an effect on a patient, symptom, syndrome, or disease, but which is objectively without *specific* activity for the condition being treated. The therapeutic procedure may be given with or without conscious knowledge that the procedure is a placebo, may be an active (non-inert) or nonactive (inert) procedure, and include, therefore, all medical procedures no matter how specific—oral and parenteral medication, topical preparations, inhalants, and mechanical, surgical, and psychotherapeutic procedures. The placebo must be differentiated from the placebo effect which may or may not occur and which may be favorable or unfavorable. The placebo effect is defined as the changes produced by placebos (Shapiro, 1964, p. 75).

Thus, the placebo effect can either enhance or reduce the effectiveness of a therapy. That is, the placebo effect can make a therapy appear more effective or less effective than it really is. In therapy outcome research, therefore, one should recognize the possibility of, and control for, the placebo effect whenever possible.

What factors may be responsible for a placebo effect? According to Shapiro (1964), any of the following can result in a placebo effect:

1. The client's faith in the ability of the clinician, the therapy, or both, to help him. This can result in either a positive or negative placebo effect.
2. The clinician's attitude toward the therapy—his or her faith or confidence in the effectiveness of the therapy. This also can result in either a positive or negative placebo effect.
3. The clinician's relationship to the client. The interested clinician "... who imparts confidence, who performs a thorough examination, and who is not anxious, conflicted, or guilty about the patient or his treatment is more likely to elicit positive placebo reactions. Negative placebo reactions are more likely when the doctor [or clinician] is angry, rejecting, and contemptuous toward patients or seriously preoccupied with his own problems" (Shapiro, 1964, p. 77).

How can a placebo effect be distinguished from an effect resulting from a therapy? One approach would be to replicate the therapy with a client and clinician who are relatively neutral in their expectations concerning the effectiveness of the therapy. If the therapy was ineffective when replicated, this would suggest (not prove) that the previous positive results were a function of something other than the therapy. On the other hand, if the same results were obtained, this would provide additional support for the hypothesis that the therapy is effective.

What Are the Effects of the Therapy upon Other Attributes of a Client's Communicative Behavior at Given Points in Space-Time?

What Are the Effects of the Therapy upon a Client other than Those Directly Related to Communicative Behavior at Given Points in Space-Time?

The considerations in designing research to assess systematically the effects of a therapy on attributes of a client's communicative disorder other than those being studied are the same as for assessing the effects of a therapy on behaviors that contribute directly to a client's communicative disorder. The same would be true for designing research to assess systematically the effects of a therapy on a client other than those related directly to communicative behavior.

What Are the Client's Attitudes toward the Therapy and Its Effects upon His Communicative and Other Behaviors at Given Points in Space-Time?

Many of the considerations discussed previously are relevant in designing research to answer this question. One that has not yet been discussed is the selection of a methodology for measuring attitudes. Several methodologies have been developed for this purpose (see Edwards, 1957). The one that appears to have been used most frequently in education and psychotherapy outcome research is the *semantic differential* (Osgood, Suci, and Tannenbaum, 1957).

The semantic differential technique was developed by Professor Charles Osgood and his associates at the University of Illinois in the 1940s. With this approach, clients would be provided with a set of seven-step, bipolar adjectival scales and instructed to indicate for each scale the direction and intensity of its association to the stimulus being rated. If, for example, we wished to determine a client's attitude toward a hearing aid, one scale that might be included in the semantic differential for this purpose would be:

acceptable ___:___:___:___:___:___:___ unacceptable

If a client's attitude toward the hearing aid was *very closely related* to one or the other of these adjectives, he or she would mark the scale in the following manner:

acceptable _x_:___:___:___:___:___:___ unacceptable

or

acceptable ___:___:___:___:___:___:_x_ unacceptable

If a client's attitude toward the hearing aid was *quite closely* (but not extremely) *related* to one or the other of these adjectives, he or she would mark the scale in the following manner:

acceptable ___ : x : ___ : ___ : ___ : ___ : ___ unacceptable

or

acceptable ___ : ___ : ___ : ___ : ___ : x : ___ unacceptable

If a client's attitude toward the hearing aid was *only slightly related* to one or the other of these adjectives, he or she would mark the scale in the following manner:

acceptable ___ : ___ : x : ___ : ___ : ___ : ___ unacceptable

or

acceptable ___ : ___ : ___ : ___ : x : ___ : ___ unacceptable

Finally, a client who felt that his or her attitude toward the hearing aid was either *neutral* on the scale or was that both adjectives were *completely irrelevant* would mark in the following manner:

acceptable ___ : ___ : ___ : x : ___ : ___ : ___ unacceptable

A semantic differential developed for assessing the impact of a therapy upon stutterers (from videotape recordings) is reproduced for purposes of illustration as Figure 11.2.

Both the construction and administration of semantic differentials have been described in considerable detail (Osgood, Suci, and Tannenbaum, 1957; Snider and Osgood, 1968). This section will therefore be devoted primarily to a discussion of specific considerations in constructing and analyzing semantic differentials to measure attitudes toward therapies.

Constructing a Semantic Differential. One of the first considerations in constructing a semantic differential is generating the set of bipolar adjectival scales. The specific scales selected will be determined by the stimulus to which reactions are desired. The stimulus, incidentally, does not have to be a word or words—any observable object or event (e.g., tape recordings) could serve as the stimulus.

Three approaches, singly or in combination, are useful for generating a set of scales for a semantic differential. The first is to consult the thesaurus sample of bipolar adjectival scales that Osgood and his associates included in *The Measurement of Meaning* (pp. 53–61). The second is to conduct a brainstorming session in which the members of a group are asked to suggest scales

THE PERSON WHO IS SPEAKING

afraid	___:___:___:___:___:___:___	not afraid
mature	___:___:___:___:___:___:___	immature
unlovable	___:___:___:___:___:___:___	lovable
speech intelligible	___:___:___:___:___:___:___	speech unintelligible
intelligent	___:___:___:___:___:___:___	unintelligent
secure	___:___:___:___:___:___:___	insecure
natural	___:___:___:___:___:___:___	unnatural
no sense of humor	___:___:___:___:___:___:___	sense of humor
speaks rapidly	___:___:___:___:___:___:___	speaks slowly
unselfish	___:___:___:___:___:___:___	selfish
dishonest	___:___:___:___:___:___:___	honest
fluent	___:___:___:___:___:___:___	disfluent
cautious	___:___:___:___:___:___:___	rash
witty	___:___:___:___:___:___:___	dull
speech monotonous	___:___:___:___:___:___:___	speech not monotonous
stable	___:___:___:___:___:___:___	unstable
employable	___:___:___:___:___:___:___	unemployable
unsociable	___:___:___:___:___:___:___	sociable
loud	___:___:___:___:___:___:___	soft
old	___:___:___:___:___:___:___	young
coordinated	___:___:___:___:___:___:___	uncoordinated
dominant	___:___:___:___:___:___:___	submissive
speech dysrhythmic	___:___:___:___:___:___:___	speech rhythmic
speech unpleasant	___:___:___:___:___:___:___	speech pleasant
hesitant	___:___:___:___:___:___:___	not hesitant
boring	___:___:___:___:___:___:___	interesting
unfriendly	___:___:___:___:___:___:___	friendly
cowardly	___:___:___:___:___:___:___	brave
confused	___:___:___:___:___:___:___	orientated
superior	___:___:___:___:___:___:___	inferior
speech slow	___:___:___:___:___:___:___	speech fast
reputable	___:___:___:___:___:___:___	disreputable
optimistic	___:___:___:___:___:___:___	pessimistic
excitable	___:___:___:___:___:___:___	calm
handicapped	___:___:___:___:___:___:___	not handicapped
untrustworthy	___:___:___:___:___:___:___	trustworthy
relaxed	___:___:___:___:___:___:___	tense
contrary	___:___:___:___:___:___:___	agreeable
reliable	___:___:___:___:___:___:___	unreliable
extrovert	___:___:___:___:___:___:___	introvert
rich	___:___:___:___:___:___:___	poor
insane	___:___:___:___:___:___:___	sane
contented	___:___:___:___:___:___:___	discontented
soothing	___:___:___:___:___:___:___	aggravating
not frightened	___:___:___:___:___:___:___	frightened
not frustrating	___:___:___:___:___:___:___	frustrating
alert	___:___:___:___:___:___:___	not alert

FIGURE 11.2. *Semantic differential task for stutterers.*

FIGURE 11.2 *(Continued)*

THE PERSON WHO IS SPEAKING

speaks poorly	speaks well
discourteous	courteous
quarrelsome	congenial
lazy	industrious
deaf	not deaf
emotional	unemotional
realistic	idealistic
approachable	unapproachable
not talkative	talkative
not aggressive	aggressive
weak	strong
positive self concept	negative self concept
uneducated	educated
deliberate	impulsive
nervous	calm
sensitive	insensitive
able to carry on conversation	unable to carry on conversation
scrupulous	unscrupulous
independent	dependent
masculine	feminine
confident	not confident
frustrated	not frustrated
competent	incompetent
inhibited	uninhibited
depressed	happy
organized	unorganized
accept	reject
isolated	not isolated
comfortable	uncomfortable
insincere	sincere
enthusiastic	unenthusiastic
soothing	aggravating
kind	cruel
naive	sophisticated

relevant to their reactions to the stimulus. The third is to solicit responses from a number of persons to a statement such as this: "Please list all the adjectives you can think of that describe (the stimulus)." Bipolar scales are constructed from adjectives listed by two or more persons.

After they have been selected, the scales are ordered by means of a table of random numbers. Whether the positive or negative adjective in each pair appears on the left is also randomly determined. Ordering the scales for the response sheet (see Figure 11.2) can be facilitated by writing or typing each pair of adjectives on a separate card.

Administering a Semantic Differential. To administer a semantic differential, present a response sheet to each subject along with a set of instructions. The author has found the set included in *The Measurement of Meaning* (pp. 82–84) quite satisfactory. To maximize the probability that a subject will understand what is required, it is advisable to read the instructions aloud while the subject follows along on his copy.

Analyzing Semantic Differential Ratings. To facilitate analysis of semantic differential ratings, the seven points between pairs of adjectives are each assigned a numeral. The set usually assigned is either

$$1, 2, 3, 4, 5, 6, 7$$

or

$$-3, -2, -1, 0, +1, +2, +3$$

If the first set is used, the numeral 4 would be assigned to the center of the scale, 1 to the lower end, and 7 to the upper end. The lower end of the scale could be associated with the negative adjective and the upper end with the positive.

The numerals in the second set are more descriptive of the bipolar nature of the adjectives than those in the first. However, they are more difficult to manipulate arithmetically because some have negative values. Since both sets lead to the same result, and since the numerals in the 1 to 7 set are easier to manipulate arithmetically than those in the -3 to $+3$ set, the 1 to 7 set is usually used.

The numerals assigned to a semantic differential scale can be viewed as having either ordinal, interval, or ratio properties depending upon the assumptions made. The -3 to $+3$ set will be used to illustrate this point. If these numerals are viewed as having ordinal properties, it is only necessary to assume that the further a rating is from the center of a scale, the more intense will be the association between the polar adjective defining that end of the scale and the stimulus rated. If, on the other hand, the numerals are viewed as possessing interval properties, it is necessary to assume in addition that the differences in intensity of association between the polar adjective and the stimulus between adjacent points on the scale are subjectively equal. That is, we must be willing to assume that the difference in intensity of association between 0 and $+1$ is the same as between $+1$ and $+2$ and between $+2$ and $+3$. Finally, if the numerals are viewed as having ratio properties, it is necessary to assume, in addition to the previous two assumptions, that the 0 point at the center of a scale is an absolute, or true, zero. With these assumptions, a rating of $+3$ would signify an association three times as intense between the stimulus and the positive polar adjective than a rating of

+1 would signify. The numerals assigned to semantic differential scales are usually assumed to have interval properties.

Information on clients' attitudes toward a therapy and its effects upon them can be abstracted for individuals and groups from semantic differential ratings. Obviously, the ratings assigned by clients to individual scales can provide information about their reaction to, or attitude toward, the stimulus. Comparable information for the "typical" member of a group can be derived by computing the mean or median of the ratings assigned to each scale. The closer an individual or average rating is to the center of a scale, the less likely the adjectives defining that scale are to be relevant to reactions to the stimulus.

The emotional tone of an individual's or group's reaction to a stimulus can be at least partially evaluated from semantic differential ratings of that stimulus. Several analyses will provide this information. All require, as a preliminary step, the identification of the polar adjective in each pair that is most likely to be associated by a subject with feelings of approach, favorableness, positive feeling, and/or desirability. One approach that can be used to identify these adjectives is to have a small group of persons from the same population that will be rating the stimulus indicate the polar adjective in each pair they feel is most closely associated with the feelings mentioned. The polar adjective of each pair that is identified by the majority of the group members would be the one classified as possessing these qualities.

Three indices of the emotional tone of a person's reaction to a stimulus can be derived by assigning his or her rating of each pair of polar adjectives to one of the following categories: (1) the neutral point, or center, of the scale, i.e., 0 or 4, (2) the three points associated with the positive adjective, and (3) the three points associated with the negative adjective. We will use this notation for these indices:

X = the number (or percentage) of scales with positive ratings,
Y = the number (or percentage) of scales with negative ratings, and
Z = the number (or percentage) of scales with neutral ratings.

The first of these indices, the *Overall-Tone Index*, is defined by the following ratio:

$$\text{Overall-Tone Index} = \frac{X}{Y}$$

A quotient of less than 1.0 indicates a negative reaction to a stimulus; a quotient of greater than 1.0, a positive reaction. A quotient of approximately 1.0 indicates that there was no overall tone to a person's reaction to a stimulus. The numbers generated by this ratio should be interpreted as having ordinal properties. A quotient of 2.4, for example, would indicate a more positive reaction toward a stimulus than one of 1.2, but not necessarily a reaction that is twice as positive.

The second of these indices, the *Negativity Index*, is defined by the following ratio:

$$\text{Negativity Index} = \frac{Y}{X + Y + Z}$$

The possible values of this index range from 0.0 to 1.0. The higher the quotient, the more negative the reaction to the stimulus will be. It would be safest to interpret the numbers generated by this ratio as having ordinal properties.

The third of these indices, the *Positivity Index*, is defined by the following ratio:

$$\text{Positivity Index} = \frac{X}{X + Y + Z}$$

Both the range of values and interpretation of this index are the same as for the Negativity Index.

Specifically, how might measures derived from semantic differential ratings be used to assess clients' attitudes toward a therapy and its effects on their communicative and other behaviors? First, to assess their attitudes toward a therapy, you might ask them to complete a semantic differential with the stimulus being the therapy to which their reactions are desired. They could be asked to do the task before receiving the therapy, which would provide information about their expectations concerning its effectiveness, or after receiving the therapy. Each client's reaction to the therapy would be at least partially defined by his or her ratings of individual scales. In addition, the emotional tone of each client's reaction to the therapy could be inferred from Overall-Tone, Negativity, and Positivity Indices computed from individual ratings. This same approach also could be used for assessing clients' reaction to the effects of a therapy on their behavior. It probably would be desirable to have clients rate their reaction to their behavior both before and after receiving the therapy.

What Are the Attitudes of a Client's Clinician, Family, Friends, and Others toward the Therapy and toward Its Effects upon the Client's Communicative Behavior at Given Points in Space-Time?

The considerations in designing research to answer this question are the same as for the previous question. The semantic differential in Figure 11.2 was developed to partially answer this question for a stuttering therapy (Silverman and Trotter, 1973).

What Investment Is Required of Client and Clinician at Given Points in Space-Time?

To answer this question, both the client and the clinician will have to keep careful records of their time and financial investment in the therapy being evaluated. The client's emotional investment in a therapy can be partially inferred from comments he or she makes to the clinician during the course of therapy and from interviews conducted by the clinician (or someone else) following termination of the therapy.

What Is the Probability of Relapse following Termination of the Therapy?

An investigator should assess the long-term effects of a therapy in addition to its immediate effects. Clinicians would be naive to assume that their client's status following termination of therapy will necessarily remain unchanged over a relatively long period of time. Based upon reports by clinical psychologists, psychiatrists, educators (as well as speech pathologists) on the stability of behavior change, we would expect many clients who receive a therapy to experience some regression following termination of that therapy. The degree of regression would vary, i.e., the effects of some therapies would be expected to hold up better than those of others. Since the objective of most therapy is to produce a *permanent* behavior change in a client, and since therapies can be expected to vary with regard to the permanence of such a change, it would obviously be desirable to incorporate in the design the making of criterion measures following termination of therapy.

Investigators who wish to incorporate some type of follow-up into their design—i.e., who wish to continue to make criterion measures following termination of therapy—will have to make three decisions: (1) which measures to make, (2) the intervals at which to make these measures, and (3) the length of time to continue to make these measures.

You should decide whether your design will include follow-up before you select criterion measures. Some measures that would be sufficiently reliable and valid for your purposes would be difficult or impossible to make following termination of therapy, particularly for those clients who live some distance from where they received therapy. It may be necessary, therefore, to select criterion measures that can be made by telephone or by using a "paper and pencil" task.

How frequently should criterion measures be made following termination of therapy? This is a decision for which it is difficult to provide guidelines. However, if the design included periodic sampling during the course of therapy (e.g., a time series design), it probably would be desirable to make measures following termination of therapy at the same interval as during therapy.

The final decision—the length of time to follow up—is also a difficult one for which to provide guidelines. There is insufficient data on the long-term effects of therapies for communicative disorders to provide a sound basis for making this decision. Perhaps until adequate data are available, it would be advisable to be conservative and adopt a five-year follow-up period, as have many investigators in the fields of medicine and psychotherapy as well as in speech pathology (Van Riper, 1958).

REFERENCES

CAMPBELL, D. T., From description to experimentation: Interpreting trends as quasi-experiments. In C. W. HARRIS (Ed.), *Problems in Measuring Change*. Madison: University of Wisconsin Press (1963).

CAMPBELL, D. T., and STANLEY, J. C., *Experimental and Quasi-Experimental Designs in Research*. Chicago: Rand McNally & Company (1963).

EDWARDS, A. L., *Techniques of Attitude Scale Construction*. New York: Appleton-Century-Crofts (1957).

EDWARDS, A. L., and CRONBACH, L. J., Experimental design for research in psychotherapy. In Arnold P. Goldstein and Stanford J. Dean (Eds.), *The Investigation of Psychotherapy: Commentaries and Readings*. New York: John Wiley & Sons, Inc., 71–79 (1966).

ELBERT, M., SHELTON, R., and ARNDT, W., A task for evaluation of articulation change: I. Development of methodology. *Journal of Speech and Hearing Research*, 10, 281–288 (1967).

OSGOOD, C. E., SUCI, G. J., and TANNENBAUM, P. H., *The Measurement of Meaning*. Urbana: University of Illinois Press (1957).

ROSENTHAL, R., Interpersonal expectations: Effects of the experimenter's hypothesis. In Robert Rosenthal and Ralph Rosnow (Eds.), *Artifacts in Behavioral Research*. New York: Academic Press, Inc. (1969).

ROSENTHAL, R., and ROSNOW, R., *Artifacts in Behavioral Research*. New York: Academic Press, Inc. (1969).

SHAPIRO, A. K., Factors contributing to the placebo effect: Implications for psychotherapy. *American Journal of Psychotherapy*, 18 (Supplement 1), 73–88 (1964).

SILVERMAN, F. H., and TROTTER, W. D., Impact of pacing speech with a miniature electronic metronome upon the manner in which a stutterer is perceived. *Behavior Therapy*, 4, 414–419 (1973).

SNIDER, J. G., and OSGOOD, C. E. (Eds.), *Semantic Differential Technique: A Sourcebook*. Chicago: Aldine Publishing Company (1968).

VAN RIPER, C., Experiments in stuttering therapy. In Jon Eisenson (Ed.), *Stuttering: A Symposium*. New York: Harper & Row, Publishers, 273–390 (1958).

TWELVE

ESTABLISHING A COMMUNICATIVE DISORDERS RESEARCH PROGRAM IN A CLINICAL SETTING

This book has attempted to demonstrate what benefits speech pathologists and audiologists would derive from doing clinical research (i.e., functioning as clinician-investigators) and to provide the information that they need to do it. Suppose a speech pathologist or audiologist wished to function as a clinician-investigator. How might he or she go about achieving the necessary administrative and financial support? We will attempt to partially answer this question here. Specifically, we will indicate several strategies a speech pathologist or audiologist may find helpful when attempting to convince the administration of an institution that it would be *of benefit to them* if he or she functioned as a clinician-investigator. We will also deal here with research funding and the use of consultants, particularly research design consultants.

ACHIEVING ADMINISTRATIVE SUPPORT

It would be difficult (though certainly not impossible) for a speech pathologist or audiologist employed in a clinical setting to do clinical research without at least some administrative support. Doing such research obviously requires an investment of time. Since most master's level speech pathologists and audiologists are hired for the purpose of providing clinical services, they will have to convince their administrators that it would benefit them—the clinicians, the clients, and the institution—if they were permitted some time for clinical research. This time investment could be relatively small if the question, or questions, a speech pathologist or audiologist sought to answer could be answered by observations that could be made while providing clinical services (e.g., questions dealing with therapy outcome).

What arguments for the need to do clinical research are apt to be considered cogent by the administrators of the clinical program in which you are employed? Several can be summarized as follows:

1. Accountability is an important consideration. Research assessing the impact of your clinical program (therapy outcome research, and so on) on the communicatively handicapped could be used by your administrator or administrators to demonstrate its value to various groups, including: (a) administrators of the institution in which the program is located, (b) potential consumers of the services offered, i.e., the communicatively handicapped and their families, (c) third parties who are paying for the services, e.g., voluntary organizations, governmental agencies, and insurance companies, (d) governmental agencies and private foundations that award grants, and (e) the community.
2. Evaluating your clinical programs systematically will provide you with information you need to maximize their effectiveness. If you do not systematically evaluate the impact of your clinical programs on your clients, how can you tell if they are achieving their objectives?
3. The presence of an ongoing clinical research program is likely to bring local, state, national, and international recognition to the institution that should help in attracting grants and gifts from individuals, private foundations, and governmental sources.
4. Outcome research on your clinical programs should not be very costly either in time or in money, since you can gather the data necessary to answer your questions as a part of your clinical routine. It should therefore not interfere significantly with your ability to provide clinical services.

Of course, not every administrator of a speech and hearing program would regard these arguments as compelling. You must decide based on your previous experience with an administrator what arguments he or she is apt to be convinced by and use them. (Incidentally, at least some of the arguments presented in Chapter 2 about the benefits of functioning as a clinician-investigator are relevant here.)

PREPARING A RESEARCH PROPOSAL

We have suggested several arguments that might be useful in securing administrative support for research. How should such arguments be communicated to the administrator or administrator whose support you are seeking? In most instances, the best way would probably be as a part of a written research proposal, or prospectus, which could be drafted in the form of a *memorandum*. The kinds of information you should present in such a proposal include:

1. the question or questions you wish to answer,
2. possible practical consequences of answering the question or questions in *your clinical setting* and others,
3. why it would be of benefit for *you* to undertake answering the question or questions in *your* clinical setting,
4. your qualifications to undertake the project,
5. the time and financial investment required and the source or sources from which you would seek financial support,
6. where you would plan to report the results of the research,
7. coinvestigators and consultants who would be involved in the project and a statement of their roles and qualifications to perform them,
8. a description of the methodology that would be used to answer each question, including a statement concerning possible dangers to subjects, and
9. a description of how the data would be analyzed to answer each question.

Let us now examine briefly the contribution of each of these kinds of information to a proposal.

Your statement of the question or questions you wish to answer should communicate to an administrator the topic of your proposed research. Since he or she may not be familiar with the technical terminology used by speech pathologists or audiologists, this should not be used unless absolutely necessary; those technical terms that are used should be defined. If data have been reported that are relevant to your questions, they should be summarized; you should indicate why additional data are needed to answer each question.

Your discussion of the possible practical consequences of answering the question or questions in your clinical setting and others will be one of the most important parts of your proposal for achieving administrative support. You should attempt to demonstrate as forcefully as you can how answering the question or questions you propose will benefit your caseload and your institution. You may also wish to indicate here possible theoretical implications of the answer to each question.

After you indicate why it would be clinically (and possibly theoretically) important to answer each question, you should attempt to demonstrate why it would be advantageous for you to attempt to answer them in your clinical setting. This part of your proposal is also important for achieving administrative support. You should indicate as cogently as you can why answering them would be beneficial both to you and to your institution. Some of the arguments summarized in the previous section of this chapter and in Chapter 2 may be applicable here.

Your next task is to demonstrate that you are qualified to make the observations necessary to answer each question. It is particularly important to specify your qualifications for administering the experimental treatments (e.g., therapies) and the instruments (e.g., tests) by which you plan to assess their effects.

You must also deal with the matter of time and financial investment required to complete the proposed research and the source or sources from which the necessary financial support might be obtained. You should provide an estimate of the amount of time that would have to be set aside for the project. This could be indicated in terms of the average number of hours per week required at various stages of the project. You should present a detailed budget and indicate the reason for each item. Sources (internal, external, or both) from which the necessary funding might be obtained should be specified.

You should give some indication of how you plan to disseminate your questions, answers, and interpretations. If this information is going to be in a written report, specify the journal to which you plan to submit it (unless, of course, the report would be intended for internal use only within your institution).

Coinvestigators and consultants who would be involved with the project should be indicated in the proposal. The role of each should be specified, along with a statement concerning his or her qualifications to perform this role.

A detailed tentative description of the methodology that would be used to make the observations necessary to answer each question should be included. You should describe who you are going to observe and how you are going to observe them in as much detail as you would for the "methods" section of a research report (see Chapter 10). Any possible negative effects of the experimental procedures on the subjects should be specified, along with a statement concerning the likelihood of their occurrence. An investigator has both an ethical and legal responsibility not to expose subjects to potentially dangerous experimental procedures without their informed consent.

You must also describe how the observations, or data, will be analyzed to answer each question. It should be clear from the proposal how the observations necessary for answering each question will be abstracted from those that were made and organized (see Chapter 8).

The kinds of information mentioned here should be included in all research proposals. They are not, however, the only information necessary to include. You would be wise before beginning to prepare a proposal to inquire whether the institution in which you are employed has a format, or set of forms, they wish used for this purpose. Many institutions in which clinical speech or hearing programs are located (e.g., Veterans' Administration hospitals) have specific forms for this purpose.

RESEARCH FUNDING

All research projects require the expenditure of some funds. The amount of funding needed to answer some questions is so small that it can often be taken from the operating budget for equipment and supplies provided by the institution. This would probably be true for many questions relevant to therapy outcome.

If the funds necessary to answer your question or questions exceed those available from your operating budget, you will probably have to apply for some sort of grant. Speech pathologists and audiologists have received funds from a variety of sources to support their research activities. For purposes of discussion we will divide such sources into two groups, internal and external.

Internal grants are awarded by the institution (school system, hospital, rehabilitation center, and so on) with which a clinical program is affiliated. Their maximum size usually is relatively small (i.e., less than one thousand dollars). Internal grants are generally intended both to support research that only requires relatively low levels of funding (which would include almost all therapy outcome research in speech pathology and audiology) and to provide "seed" money for the preliminary research of investigators who plan to apply for external grant support. These grants are usually easier for beginning investigators to obtain than external ones. They also tend to require a less complex application procedure than the latter.

If the funds necessary to answer your question or questions exceed one thousand dollars, you will probably have to apply for an external grant. An external grant is one from any source other than the institution with which you are affiliated. Such a source could be an organization (e.g., the Heart Association or United Cerebral Palsy), a private foundation (e.g., the Ford Foundation), or a governmental agency (e.g., the National Institute of Health, the Office of Education, or the National Science Foundation). Funds for research in speech pathology and audiology have been secured from all three sources. The federal government, through such agencies as the National Institute of Health (NIH), the Office of Education (OE) and the National Science Foundation (NSF), has provided more funds for this purpose than any other source. These agencies support a variety of research support programs, some of which beginning investigators are eligible to apply for. Information on their current programs can be obtained by writing directly to the agency. In 1975 the American Speech and Hearing Association published a directory, *Foundations: Potential Funding Sources for Speech Pathology and*

Audiology, which indicates some possible sources of research funding in the private sector.

Almost all external research grants are highly competitive, and their application processing procedures tend to be quite complex (see Lore and Gutter, 1968, for a description of such procedures at NIH). More proposals usually are submitted than can be funded. Also, most granting agencies look for evidence of "demonstrated research potential," or previous successful research experience as evidenced by publication. This stress places a beginning investigator's proposal at a disadvantage. You would probably be wise, therefore, to select as your *first* research projects those that could be *funded internally*.

USE OF CONSULTANTS

This book has attempted to provide you with information to help you develop an intuitive understanding of how to function as a clinician-investigator —i.e., how to ask and answer questions in a manner consistent with the scientific method. Obviously, the information presented here may not be sufficient to bring you to the point where you could safely undertake a research project without having your design checked by a person or persons knowledgeable in research methodology. Such individuals would serve as consultants on your research project.

Many institutions with speech and hearing facilities (including hospitals, school systems, and rehabilitation centers) employ individuals knowledgeable in statistics and research methodology for consultation with members of their staff who wish to do research. As previously mentioned, there may also be faculty at local colleges and universities who are competent in this area and would be willing to consult with you.

It is important to contact a consultant, particularly a research design consultant, before you begin data collection. If something is wrong with the design you are using, the data you collect may be useless for your purpose. It may not possess adequate validity, reliability, and generality to answer your question or questions with a sufficient degree of accuracy. It is crucial, therefore, to have your proposal checked before you begin collecting data.

Any recommendations that are made by a consultant, of course, have to be carefully evaluated because they might be inappropriate. They may not result in a design that will yield the data necessary to answer your question or questions. Or they may not result in the most efficient or practical design for this purpose.

Why might a consultant's recommendations be inappropriate? There are several possible reasons. First, he or she may commit what Kimball (1957) has referred to as an "error of the third kind"—i.e., giving the right answer to the wrong question. Here, the consultant does not understand the question or questions the investigator is attempting to answer. Hence, his or her recommendations are appropriate not for answering these questions, but for those he thinks the investigator is trying to answer. A consultant is most likely to make this type of error when he or she is completely unfamiliar with the content area in which the research is being done.

A consultant's recommendations may also be inappropriate because they are not sufficiently practical or efficient. For assessing the impact of a particular therapy, a consultant may recommend using a typical subject design (see Chapter 5), in which forty persons who have a particular communicative disorder are randomly assigned to one of two groups: the members of one group receive the experimental therapy and the members of the other do not. Such a design may not be practical because forty persons with that communicative disorder are not available to serve as subjects and it is not ethical (or possible) to deprive half of them of therapy for the duration of the program. Even if it were practical to use such a design, it might not be efficient, because of the time needed to administer therapy to twenty clients and evaluate its impact on a group of this size. An individual subject design (see Chapter 5) using ten persons, in which each served as his own "control," could well be both more efficient and more practical for collecting the necessary data.

A third reason a consultant's recommendations may be inappropriate is that he or she has made a mistake. Consultants, like all humans, are fallible. A certain percentage of the time their recommendations will be erroneous.

What should you do if you feel a consultant's recommendations may be inappropriate? Your best strategy would probably be to seek one or more additional opinions, weigh them (considering the reasons for them), and then make the best decision you can. This, of course, is similar to the situation you sometimes find yourself in when you are forced to make clinical decisions from equivocal or incomplete data.

Our emphasis in this discussion has been on research design consultants. However, most of these comments are relevant to other types of consultants as well.

REFERENCES

KIMBALL, A. W., Errors of the third kind in statistical consulting. *Journal of the American Statistical Association*, 52, 133–142 (1957).

LORE, J. I., and GUTTER, F. J., The embryogeny of an NIH research grant. *Asha*, 10, 7–9 (1968).

Appendices

APPENDIX A

Computational Formulas, Worked Examples, and Exercises for Selected Descriptive and Inferential Statistics that are Practical to Compute with a Desk or Slide Rule Calculator

CONTENTS

		Page
I.	Data Table	281
II.	Notation	282
III.	Descriptive Statistics	
	A. Measures of Central Tendency	
	1. Mean	283
	2. Median	284
	3. Mode	285
	B. Measures of Variability	
	1. Range	286
	2. Interquartile Range	287
	3. Standard Deviation	288
	C. Measures of Association	
	1. Contingency Coefficient	289
	2. Phi Coefficient	290
	3. Spearman Rank-Order Coefficient	292
	4. Pearson Product-Moment Correlation Coefficient	293

Appendices

- IV. Inferential Statistical Tests
  - A. Nominal Data
    1. Chi Square 294
  - B. Ordinal Data
    1. Sign Test 296
    2. Mann-Whitney U Test 298
    3. Friedman Two-Way Analysis of Variance 301
    4. Kruskal-Wallis One-Way Analysis of Variance 302
  - C. Interval and Ratio Data
    1. t-Test for Related Measures 304
    2. t-Test for Independent Measures 306
    3. t-Test for the Significance of Pearson Product-Moment Correlation Coefficients 308
    4. One-Way Analysis of Variance (F-Test) for Dependent Measures 309
    5. One-Way Analysis of Variance (F-Test) for Independent Measures 312
- V. Confidence Interval Estimation
  - A. Mean 314
  - B. Median 315
  - C. Difference between Means 317
- VI. Tables for Chi Square, Binomial, Normal, t-, and F-Distributions 319

Note

A single set of data is used for all statistical analyses in this Appendix. This was done both to permit comparisons between alternative statistical analyses that could be used to answer a question and to permit the data (i.e., numbers being analyzed) to remain in the background. The statistics included are discussed in Chapter 8.

TABLE A.1. Frequencies per 100 words of interjection of sounds and syllables (I), part-word repetition (PW), word repetition (W) and revision-incomplete phrase (R-IP) produced by 56 second- through sixth-grade nonstutterers during their performance of a spontaneous speech task.

Subject Number	School Grade	I	PW	W	R-IP
1	2	0.50	1.16	0.50	2.16
2	2	2.13	1.42	0.35	5.67
3	2	1.40	0.00	0.00	5.14
4	2	0.40	1.21	0.40	1.62
5	2	0.31	0.94	0.63	2.52
6	2	0.00	0.35	0.35	1.74
7	2	0.00	0.00	1.28	3.21
8	2	0.47	2.37	0.95	1.90
9	2	0.30	1.80	1.50	4.49
10	2	0.50	1.00	1.33	6.16
11	2	8.53	0.34	2.39	2.73
12	2	1.04	1.04	1.04	1.56
13	2	1.46	0.29	0.44	4.54
14	2	0.36	0.36	0.72	1.08
15	2	1.87	0.00	0.75	2.24
16	3	0.46	1.14	1.60	3.65
17	3	3.78	1.13	2.64	3.02
18	3	2.23	1.49	2.97	4.83
19	3	0.33	0.99	0.99	1.64
20	3	0.49	0.00	0.49	0.49
21	3	1.07	1.43	1.07	6.79
22	3	0.55	4.42	3.31	6.08
23	3	0.84	0.28	0.28	1.68
24	3	0.28	0.41	0.28	3.72
25	3	3.40	1.51	1.89	1.89
26	3	1.80	0.90	0.60	2.40
27	4	0.44	1.54	0.00	3.30
28	4	0.94	1.57	0.78	2.83
29	4	0.00	2.41	2.78	3.33
30	4	0.33	0.65	0.49	3.41
31	4	0.56	1.29	0.88	5.31
32	4	0.00	0.12	0.12	0.97
33	4	0.43	0.22	0.65	4.13
34	4	0.00	1.21	2.02	4.48
35	4	3.67	0.83	0.83	3.33
36	5	0.84	0.84	0.42	3.38
37	5	0.16	0.82	0.82	8.20
38	5	1.61	0.00	0.36	1.97
39	5	1.76	1.58	3.25	4.55
40	5	0.28	0.14	1.14	1.99

TABLE A.1. (Continued)

Subject Number	School Grade	I	PW	W	R-IP
41	5	2.92	0.93	0.80	4.77
42	5	1.72	0.81	1.26	2.80
43	5	0.72	0.21	0.21	1.65
44	5	0.00	0.54	0.27	2.41
45	5	1.82	0.61	1.70	3.64
46	5	0.52	0.34	2.41	4.83
47	6	0.00	0.28	0.28	0.86
48	6	0.00	0.19	0.77	0.96
49	6	1.99	0.00	0.85	3.42
50	6	0.00	0.47	0.47	1.10
51	6	0.00	0.93	0.00	1.39
52	6	0.69	0.00	0.00	1.72
53	6	0.00	0.66	0.99	1.32
54	6	0.73	0.91	0.18	3.09
55	6	0.78	0.26	0.26	1.03
56	6	0.30	0.41	0.51	2.03

SOME NOTATION USED IN THIS APPENDIX

Symbol	Operation(s) Necessary to Compute, or Meaning
ΣX	Sum (or add) scores on variable labeled X.
ΣX^2	Square scores on variable labeled X and then sum (or add) them.
$(\Sigma X)^2$	Sum (or add) scores on variable labeled X and then square this sum.
$\bar{X}$	Sum (or add) scores on variable labeled X and then divide total by number of scores summed.
$\bar{X}^2$	Compute mean of variable labeled X (as indicated above) and square it.
ΣY	Sum (or add) scores on variable labeled Y.
ΣY^2	Square scores on variable labeled Y and then sum (or add) them.
$(\Sigma Y)^2$	Sum (or add) scores on variable labeled Y and then square this sum.

$\bar{Y}$ — Sum (or add) scores on variable labeled Y and then divide total by number of scores summed.

$\bar{Y}^2$ — Compute mean of variable labeled Y (as indicated above) and square it.

ΣXY — Multiply each individual's X-score by his Y-score and then sum (or add) the results of these multiplications.

N — The number of individuals in the sample.

$\sqrt{}$ — Compute square root.

(Other notation is defined when used.)

DESCRIPTIVE STATISTICS: MEASURES OF CENTRAL TENDENCY

1. Mean ($\bar{X}$)

QUESTION: How many instances of interjection per 100 words did the *average* child produce during his performance of the spontaneous speech task?

$$\bar{X} = \frac{\Sigma X}{N} = \frac{57.71}{56} = 1.03$$

ANSWER: The average child produced 1.03 instances of interjection per 100 words during his performance of the spontaneous speech task.

QUESTION: How many instances of part-word repetition per 100 words did the *average* child produce during his performance of the spontaneous speech task?

$$\bar{X} = \frac{\Sigma X}{N} = \frac{46.75}{56} = 0.83$$

ANSWER: The average child produced 0.83 instances of part-word repetition per 100 words during his performance of the spontaneous speech task.

EXERCISE: (Number 1) Determine the mean numbers of word repetitions and revisions-incomplete phrases per 100 words that were produced by these 56 children. (Your answers should be approximately 0.97 and 3.06 for word repetition and revision-incomplete phrase, respectively.)

2. Median (Mdn)

QUESTION: How many instances of interjection per 100 words did the *typical* child produce during his performance of the spontaneous speech task?

The first step in computing the median is to order the 56 interjection frequencies from lowest to highest.

.00	.30	.52	1.61
.00	.30	.55	1.72
.00	.31	.56	1.76
.00	.33	.69	1.80
.00	.33	.72	1.82
.00	.36	.73	1.87
.00	.40	.78	1.99
.00	.43	.84	2.13
.00	.44	.84	2.23
.00	.46	.94	2.92
.00	.47	1.04	3.40
.16	.49	1.07	3.67
.28	.50	1.40	3.78
.28	.50	1.46	8.53

Since there is an *even* number of scores, the median score would be midway between the $N/2$ score (.50) and $N/2 + 1$ score (.52). The median interjection frequency, therefore, would be 0.51. (If there had been an *odd* number of scores, the median score would have been the middle one.)

ANSWER: The typical child produced 0.51 instances of interjection per 100 words during his performance of the spontaneous speech task.

REMARK: Note that the mean interjection frequency (1.03) is approximately twice as high as the median interjection frequency (.51). This discrepancy is primarily due to five children who had relatively high interjection frequencies, i.e., frequencies greater than 2.5 per 100 words. A few persons who have relatively high (or relatively low) scores on a task can substantially influence the mean score on that task.

QUESTION: How many instances of part-word repetition per 100 words did the typical child produce during his performance of the spontaneous speech task?

The first step in computing the median is to order the 56 part-word repetition frequencies from lowest to highest.

.00	.28	.82	1.21
.00	.29	.83	1.21
.00	.34	.84	1.29
.00	.34	.90	1.42
.00	.35	.91	1.43
.00	.36	.93	1.49
.00	.41	.93	1.51
.12	.41	.94	1.54
.14	.47	.99	1.57
.19	.54	1.00	1.58
.21	.61	1.04	1.80
.22	.65	1.13	2.37
.26	.66	1.14	2.41
.28	.81	1.16	4.42

Since there is an even number of scores, the median score would be midway between the $N/2$ score (.81) and $N/2 + 1$ score (.82). The median part-word repetition frequency, therefore, would be 0.815.

ANSWER: The typical child produced 0.815 instances of part-word repetition per 100 words during his performance of the spontaneous speech task.

REMARK: Note that the mean part-word repetition frequency (.83) is approximately the same as the median part-word repetition frequency (.815). The lack of discrepancy is primarily due to the fact that only one child had a relatively high part-word repetition frequency (i.e., greater than 2.5 per 100 words).

EXERCISE: (Number 2) Determine the median numbers of word repetitions and revisions-incomplete phrases per 100 words that were produced by these 56 children. (Your answers should be approximately 0.76 and 2.82 for word repetition and revision-incomplete phrase, respectively.)

3. Mode

QUESTION: What frequency of interjection per 100 words was most typical (i.e., occurred most often) during the children's performance of the spontaneous speech task?

Since the mode is the most frequently occurring score, the modal interjection frequency per 100 words would be .00. (Note that in the frequency distribution on p. 284, .00 occurs 11 times. No other frequency occurred this often.)

ANSWER: The frequency of interjection per 100 words that was most typical during the children's performance of the spontaneous speech task was .00.

QUESTION: What frequency of part-word repetition per 100 words was most typical (i.e., occurred most often) during the children's performance of the spontaneous speech task?

Since the mode is the most frequently occurring score, the modal part-word repetition frequency per 100 words would be .00. (Note that in the frequency distribution on p. 285, .00 occurs seven times. No other frequency occurred this often.)

ANSWER: The frequency of part-word repetition per 100 words that was most typical during the children's performance of the spontaneous speech task was .00.

EXERCISE: Determine the modal numbers of word repetitions and
(Number 3) revisions-incomplete phrases per 100 words that were produced by these 56 children. (Your answers should be 0.00 and 3.33, 4.83 for word repetition and revision-incomplete phrase, respectively.)

DESCRIPTIVE STATISTICS: MEASURES OF VARIABILITY

1. Range

QUESTION: What was the range of interjection frequencies produced by these children during their performance of the spontaneous speech task?

The range is the difference between the largest score in the data and the smallest score in the data. The interjection frequencies for the 56 children range from .00 to 8.53 (see p. 284). The range of interjection frequencies would be 8.53, since $8.53 - .00 = 8.53$.

ANSWER: The interjection frequencies produced by these children during their performance of the spontaneous speech task ranged from

.00 to 8.53. The difference between the highest and lowest frequencies produced by these children was 8.53 per 100 words.

QUESTION: What was the range of part-word repetition frequencies produced by these children during their performance of the spontaneous speech task?

The part-word repetition frequencies for the 56 children range from .00 to 4.42 (see p. 285). The range of part-word repetition frequencies would be 4.42, since $4.42 - .00 = 4.42$.

ANSWER: The part-word repetition frequencies produced by these children during their performance of the spontaneous speech task ranged from .00 to 4.42. The difference between the highest and lowest frequencies produced by these children was 4.42 per 100 words.

EXERCISE: (Number 4) Determine the ranges of word repetition frequencies and revision-incomplete phrase frequencies for these 56 children. (Your answers should be 3.31 and 7.71 for word repetition and revision-incomplete phrase, respectively.)

2. Interquartile Range

QUESTION: Within what range of interjection frequencies did the middle 50 percent of children fall during their performance of the spontaneous speech task?

The interquartile range (Q) is the difference between the third quartile (Q_3)—i.e., the score below which 75 percent of the scores fall—and the first quartile (Q_1)—i.e., the score below which 25 percent of the scores fall. For the interjection frequencies

$$Q = Q_3 - Q_1 = 1.535 - .29 = 1.245$$

Q_1 and Q_3 values were determined from the frequency distribution on p. 284.

ANSWER: The interjection frequencies for the middle 50 percent of the children differed from each other by a maximum of 1.245 instances per 100 words.

QUESTION: Within what range of part-word repetition frequencies did the middle 50 percent of children fall during their performance of the spontaneous speech task?

The interquartile range for the part-word repetition frequencies (based on Q_1 and Q_3 values derived from the frequency distribution on p. 285) would be:

$$Q = Q_3 - Q_1 = 1.185 - .28 = .905$$

ANSWER: The part-word repetition frequencies for the middle 50 percent of the children differed from each other by a maximum of .905 instances per 100 words.

EXERCISE: Determine the interquartile ranges of word repetition frequencies and revision-incomplete phrase frequencies for these 56 children. (Your answers should be approximately 0.92 and 2.61 for word repetition and revision-incomplete phrase, respectively.)
(Number 5)

3. Standard Deviation (S)

QUESTION: How different were the children's interjection frequencies from each other during their performance of the spontaneous speech task?

The standard deviation is a measure of how different various scores are from each other. The larger the standard deviation, the more different they would be. The standard deviation of the children's interjection frequencies is:

$$S = \sqrt{\frac{\Sigma X^2}{N} - \bar{X}^2} = \sqrt{\frac{166.92}{56} - (1.03)^2} = \sqrt{1.92} = 1.39$$

ANSWER: The children's interjection frequencies were quite different from each other judging by the fact that the standard deviation (1.39) was larger than the mean (1.03).

QUESTION: How different were the children's part-word repetition frequencies from each other during their performance of the spontaneous speech task?

The standard deviation of the children's part-word repetition frequencies is:

$$S = \sqrt{\frac{\Sigma X^2}{N} - \bar{X}^2} = \sqrt{\frac{71.68}{56} - (.83)^2} = \sqrt{.59} = .77$$

ANSWER: The children's part-word repetition frequencies differed from each other to a considerable extent, judging by the fact that the standard deviation (.77) was almost as large as the mean (.83). However, they did not differ as much from each other as their interjection frequencies, since their standard deviation was smaller.

EXERCISE: Determine the standard deviations of the children's word
(Number 6) repetition frequencies and revision-incomplete phrase frequencies. (Your answers should be approximately 0.85 and 1.66 for word repetition and revision-incomplete phrase, respectively.)

DESCRIPTIVE STATISTICS: MEASURES OF ASSOCIATION

1. Contingency Coefficient (C)

QUESTION: Were the children who produced the highest frequencies of interjection per 100 words on the spontaneous speech task the same ones who produced the highest frequencies of part-word repetition per 100 words on this task, and vice versa?

The first step in computing the contingency coefficient is to assign each of the 56 children to one of the four cells of a 2 × 2 table:

	INTERJECTION Below Median	INTERJECTION Above Median
PART-WORD REPETITION Above Median	13 (a)	15 (b)
PART-WORD REPETITION Below Median	15 (c)	13 (d)

If a child's interjection frequency was below the median (i.e., less than .51) and his part-word repetition frequency was above the median (i.e., greater than .815), he was assigned to cell a. If his interjection frequency was above the median (i.e., greater than .51) and his part-word repetition frequency also was above the median (i.e., greater than .815), he was assigned to cell b. If both his interjection and part-word repetition frequencies were below their respective medians, he was assigned to cell c. And if his interjection frequency was above the median and his part-word repetition frequency was below the median, he was assigned to cell d.

The next step is to compute the value of chi square (χ^2) for the frequencies in the table. The value of chi square that was computed for this table (see p. 295) is .07. The contingency coefficient for this table would be:

$$C = \sqrt{\frac{\chi^2}{N + \chi^2}} = \sqrt{\frac{.07}{56 + .07}} = \sqrt{.0012} = .035$$

Since the possible values of the contingency coefficient vary between .00 and a number somewhat less than 1.00, and the closer the value is to .00 the weaker the association between the two variables, the degree of association for these children between level of interjection production and level of part-word repetition production would appear to be quite weak.

ANSWER: There was little, if any, tendency for the children who produced the highest frequencies of interjection on the spontaneous speech task to be the same children who produced the highest frequencies of part-word repetition on this task, and vice versa.

EXERCISE: (Number 7) Determine whether the children who produced the highest frequencies of word repetition per 100 words on the spontaneous speech task were the same ones who produced the highest frequencies of revision-incomplete phrase per 100 words on this task, and vice versa, through the use of a contingency coefficient. (The value of the contingency coefficient you compute should be approximately 0.31.)

2. Phi Coefficient (ϕ)

QUESTION: Were the children who produced the highest frequencies of interjection per 100 words on the spontaneous speech task the same ones who produced the highest frequencies of part-word repetition per 100 words on this task, and vice versa?

The first step in computing the phi coefficient is to assign each of the 56 children to one of the four cells of a 2 × 2 table in the same manner as for the contingency coefficient (see p. 289). The next step is to compute the value of phi (ϕ) for the frequencies in the table (see p. 289) through the use of the following formula:

$$\phi = \frac{(bc - ad)}{\sqrt{(a+b)(c+d)(a+c)(b+d)}}$$

$$= \frac{(15)(15) - (13)(13)}{\sqrt{(13+15)(15+13)(13+15)(15+13)}} = \frac{56}{\sqrt{614656}}$$

$$= \frac{56}{784} = .071$$

Since the possible values of the phi coefficient range from −1.00 to +1.00, and the closer the value is to .00 the weaker the association between the two variables, the degree of association for these children between level of interjection production and level of part-word repetition production would appear to be quite weak.

ANSWER: There was little, if any, tendency for the children who produced the highest frequencies of interjection on the spontaneous speech task to be the same children who produced the highest frequencies of part-word repetition on this task and vice versa.

REMARKS: The values of the contingency coefficient and phi coefficient computed for this table are slightly different due to differences in the computational procedures involved. The phi coefficient only can be used for 2 × 2 tables. The contingency coefficient can be used as a measure of association for larger tables as well. The magnitude of the phi coefficient is simpler to interpret than that of the contingency coefficient because the highest possible value is always the same, i.e., 1.00.

EXERCISE: Determine whether the children who produced the highest
(Number 8) frequencies of word repetition per 100 words on the spontaneous speech task were the same ones who produced the highest frequencies of revision-incomplete phrase per 100 words on this task, and vice versa, through the use of a phi coefficient. (The value of the phi coefficient you compute should be approximately 0.36.)

3. Spearman Rank-Order Coefficient (r_s)

QUESTION: How similar was the ordering of the second graders with regard to their interjection frequencies and part-word repetition frequencies during their performance of the spontaneous speech task?

The first step in computing a Spearman rank-order correlation coefficient between the interjection frequencies and part-word repetition frequencies of the 15 second graders (see p. 281) is to determine each child's rank for interjection frequency and each child's rank for part-word repetition frequency. The child who had the lowest frequency of part-word repetition would be assigned the rank 1; the one who had the second lowest, the rank 2; the one who had the third lowest, the rank 3; and so on. If more than one child had the same frequency, each would be assigned the mean of the tied ranks. The ranks assigned to the 15 children for their interjection frequencies and part-word repetition frequencies are indicated in the table that follows. Also included in the table is the difference between each child's two ranks (d_i) and this difference squared (d_i^2). The sum of the squared differences between ranks for the 15 children is used for computing the Spearman rank-order coefficient (r_s).

Subject Number	Rank I	Rank PW	d_i	d_i^2
1	8.5	11.0	−2.5	6.25
2	14.0	13.0	1.0	1.00
3	11.0	2.0	9.0	81.00
4	6.0	12.0	−6.0	36.00
5	4.0	8.0	−4.0	16.00
6	1.5	6.0	−4.5	20.25
7	1.5	2.0	−0.5	0.25
8	7.0	15.0	−8.0	64.00
9	3.0	14.0	−11.0	121.00
10	8.5	9.0	−0.5	0.25
11	15.0	5.0	10.0	100.00
12	10.0	10.0	0.0	0.00
13	12.0	4.0	8.0	64.00
14	5.0	7.0	−2.0	4.00
15	13.0	2.0	11.0	121.00
			$\Sigma d_i^2 =$	635.00

Computational Formulas, Worked Examples, and Exercises 293

The value of r_s for these data would be:

$$r_s = 1 - \frac{6\Sigma d_i^2}{N^3 - N} = 1 - \frac{(6)(635)}{(15)^3 - 15}$$

$$= 1 - \frac{3810}{3375 - 15} = 1 - 1.13 = -0.13$$

Since the possible values range from -1.00 to $+1.00$, and the closer the value is to .00 the weaker the association between the two variables, the degree of association for these children between level of interjection production and level of part-word repetition production would appear to be quite weak.

ANSWER: There was little, if any, similarity in the ordering of the second graders with regard to their interjection frequencies and part-word repetition frequencies during their performance of the spontaneous speech task.

EXERCISE: Determine the degree of similarity of the ordering of the third
(Number 9) graders with regard to their interjection frequencies and part-word repetition frequencies during their performance of the spontaneous speech task through the use of r_s. (The value of r_s you compute should be approximately 0.40.)

4. Pearson Product-Moment Correlation Coefficient (r)

QUESTION: Were the levels of the children's interjection frequencies related to those of their part-word repetition frequencies during their performances of the spontaneous speech task?

The first step in computing a Pearson product-moment correlation coefficient between the interjection frequencies and part-word repetition frequencies of the 56 children (see Table A.1) is to compute the following sums:

$\Sigma X =$ sum of the 56 interjection frequencies $= 57.71$
$\Sigma Y =$ sum of the 56 part-word repetition frequencies
$= 46.75$
$\Sigma X^2 =$ sum of the squares of the 56 interjection frequencies $= 166.92$
$\Sigma Y^2 =$ sum of the squares of the 56 part-word repetition frequencies $= 71.68$
$\Sigma XY =$ sum of the products of the 56 pairs of frequencies $= 47.00$

The Pearson product-moment correlation coefficient for these data would be:

$$r = \frac{N \Sigma XY - (\Sigma X)(\Sigma Y)}{\sqrt{[N \Sigma X^2 - (\Sigma X)^2][N \Sigma Y^2 - (\Sigma Y)^2]}}$$

$$= \frac{(56)(47.00) - (57.71)(46.75)}{\sqrt{[(56)(166.92) - (57.71)^2][(56)(71.68) - (46.75)^2]}}$$

$$= \frac{2632.00 - 2697.94}{\sqrt{[9347.52 - 3330.44][4014.08 - 2185.56]}}$$

$$= \frac{-65.94}{\sqrt{11002351}} = \frac{-65.94}{3316.98}$$

$$= -0.02$$

Since the possible values of r range from -1.00 to $+1.00$, and the closer the value is to .00 the weaker the association between the two variables, there would appear to be little, if any, association between these children's interjection and part-word repetition frequencies.

ANSWER: There was little or no relationship between the children's interjection frequency levels and part-word repetition frequency levels during their performance of the spontaneous speech task.

EXERCISE: Determine the degree of relationship between the children's (Number 10) word repetition frequencies and revision-incomplete phrase frequencies through the use of r. (The value of r you compute should be approximately 0.37.)

INFERENTIAL STATISTICAL TESTS: NOMINAL DATA

1. Chi Square Test (χ^2)

QUESTION: Was there a tendency for the children who had interjection frequencies above the median for the group also to have part-word repetition frequencies above the median for the group, or vice versa?

The first step in performing a chi square test is selecting an *alpha* level, or a maximum acceptable probability for a *Type I* error (i.e., concluding that the children who had interjection frequencies that were above the median for the group also tended to have part-word repetition frequencies that were above the median for the group, or vice versa, when there was no such tendency). A 0.05 alpha level will be used for this test. Since to answer the question it would be necessary to detect both positive and negative relationships between interjection level and part-word repetition level, the region of rejection for the test will be *two-tailed*.

The next step is to compute the value of chi square. Each of the 56 children is assigned to one of the four cells in a 2 × 2 table in the same manner as for the contingency coefficient (see p. 289). The value of chi square would be computed from this table (see p. 289) as follows:

$$\chi^2 = \frac{N\left(|ad - bc| - \frac{N}{2}\right)^2}{(a+b)(c+d)(a+c)(b+d)}$$

$$= \frac{56\left(|(13)(13) - (15)(15)| - \frac{56}{2}\right)^2}{(13+15)(15+13)(13+15)(15+13)}$$

$$= \frac{56(|169 - 225| - 28)^2}{(28)(28)(28)(28)} = \frac{56(28)^2}{614656}$$

$$= \frac{43904}{614656} = 0.07$$

To determine whether the value of chi square computed is large enough for the null hypothesis to be rejected, the value of chi square required for rejection is located in Table A.2 (see p. 319). The degrees of freedom (df) here would be 1 (i.e., the number of rows minus one times the number of columns minus one). The value of chi square required for rejection at the 0.05 alpha level when $df = 1$ is 3.84. Since the value computed is smaller than this, i.e., 0.07, the null hypothesis would not be rejected.

ANSWER: There was no tendency for the children who had interjection frequencies above the median for the group also to have part-word repetition frequencies above the median for the group or vice versa (chi square test; alpha = 0.05).

REMARKS: This application of the chi square test illustrates that it is not limited to nominal data: it can be used with ordinal, interval, and ratio data as well. The chi square formula that was used is a special one for 2 × 2 tables when N is larger than 40. The chi square formulas for other tables can be found in most educational and psychological statistics texts.

EXERCISE: Determine whether there was a tendency for the children who
(Number 11) had word repetition frequencies above the median for the group also to have revision-incomplete phrase frequencies above the median for the group, or vice versa, through the use of the chi square test. (The value of chi square you compute should be approximately 5.78.).

INFERENTIAL STATISTICAL TESTS: ORDINAL DATA

1. Sign Test

QUESTION: Did the second graders tend to produce higher frequencies of interjection than of part-word repetition?

The first step in performing a sign test is selecting an *alpha* level, or a maximum acceptable probability for a *Type I* error (i.e., concluding there was a tendency for the second graders to produce higher frequencies of interjection than of part-word repetition when there was no such tendency). A 0.05 alpha level will be used for this test. Since to answer the question it only would be necessary to detect a difference between interjection frequency and part-word repetition frequency in one direction, the region of rejection for the test will be *one-tailed*.

The next step is to compute the value for the sign test. Each of the 15 second graders is assigned a + or a −, depending on whether his interjection frequency or part-word repetition frequency is higher. If his interjection frequency is higher than his part-word repetition frequency, he is assigned a +; if his part-word repetition frequency is higher than his interjection frequency, he is assigned a −. If his interjection and part-word repetition frequencies are the same, he is assigned a 0. The sign assignments for the 15 children are as follows:

Subject	Sign	Subject	Sign
1	−	9	−
2	+	10	−
3	+	11	+
4	−	12	0
5	−	13	+
6	−	14	0
7	0	15	+
8	−		

The number of subjects for whom the two frequencies are not the same (N), and the number of times the sign occurs which occurs *least* often (x), are determined for this distribution. The values of N and x are 12 and 5, respectively. Based on the binomial distribution (see p. 320) when $N = 12$, the probability of five pluses (x) occurring by chance is .387. Since this value is larger than .05, the null hypothesis would not be rejected.

ANSWER: The second graders did not exhibit a tendency to produce higher frequencies of interjection than of part-word repetition (sign test; alpha $= 0.05$).

REMARK: This procedure can be used to compute the probability value for the sign test when the number of subjects for whom the two frequencies are not the same (N) is 25 or fewer. When the value of N exceeds 25, the procedure used to answer the next question is appropriate.

QUESTION: Did the second, third, and fourth graders tend to produce higher frequencies of interjection than of part-word repetition?

The alpha level that will be used for this sign test is 0.05. The region of rejection will be *one-tailed* for the same reason as indicated for the previous question.

Next, each of the 35 second, third, and fourth graders is assigned a sign in the same manner as for the previous question. The sign assignments for these children are as follows:

Subject	Sign	Subject	Sign
1	−	19	−
2	+	20	+
3	+	21	−
4	−	22	−
5	−	23	+
6	−	24	−
7	0	25	+
8	−	26	+
9	−	27	−
10	−	28	−
11	+	29	−
12	0	30	−
13	+	31	−
14	0	32	−
15	+	33	+
16	−	34	−
17	+	35	+
18	+		

The values of N and x for this distribution (which were determined in the same manner as for the previous question) are 32 and 13, respectively. The probability of 13 pluses (x) occurring by chance when $N = 32$ can be estimated by means of the following formula (which is based on the "normal curve"):

$$Z = \frac{(x \pm .5) - \frac{1}{2}N}{\frac{1}{2}\sqrt{N}} \quad \text{where } x + .5 \text{ is used when } x < \frac{1}{2}N,$$
$$\text{and } x - .5 \text{ is used when } x > \frac{1}{2}N.$$

$$= \frac{(13 + .5) - \frac{1}{2}(32)}{\frac{1}{2}\sqrt{32}}$$

$$= \frac{13.5 - 16.0}{\frac{1}{2}(5.66)} = \frac{-2.5}{2.83} = -.88$$

Based on the normal distribution (see p. 321) the probability of this outcome occurring by chance is .189. Since this value is larger than 0.05, the null hypothesis would not be rejected.

ANSWER: The second, third, and fourth graders did not exhibit a tendency to produce higher frequencies of interjection than of part-word repetition (sign test; alpha = 0.05).

EXERCISE: Determine whether the second and third graders exhibited a tendency to produce higher frequencies of revision-incomplete phrase than of word repetition through the use of *both* sign test computational procedures. (The probability values you compute by the "small" sample and the "large" sample computational procedures should be approximately 0.001 and 0.00003, respectively.)

2. Mann-Whitney U Test

QUESTION: Did the typical (i.e., median) second or third grader have a higher frequency of interjection than did the typical fourth, fifth, or sixth grader?

The first step in performing a Mann-Whitney U Test is selecting an *alpha* level, or a maximum acceptable probability for a *Type I* error (i.e., concluding the median second or third grader had a higher frequency of interjection than did the median fourth, fifth, or sixth grader when there was no such difference). A 0.05 alpha level will be used for this test. Since to answer the question it only would be necessary to detect a difference between the two groups in one direction, the region of rejection for the test will be *one-tailed*.

The next step is to compute the value for the Mann-Whitney U Test. The 56 children are ordered on the basis of their interjection frequencies, and the rank is assigned to each child that designates his place in the ordering. The child who had the lowest interjection frequency would be assigned the rank 1; the one who had the second lowest, the rank 2; the one who had the third lowest, the rank 3; and so on. If more than one child had the same frequency, each would be assigned the mean of the tied ranks. The ranks assigned to the children are indicated as follows:

2nd and 3rd Graders		4th, 5th, and 6th Graders	
Frequency	Rank	Frequency	Rank
0.00	6.0	0.00	6.0
0.00	6.0	0.00	6.0
0.28	13.5	0.00	6.0
0.30	15.5	0.00	6.0
0.31	17.0	0.00	6.0
0.33	18.5	0.00	6.0
0.36	20.0	0.00	6.0
0.40	21.0	0.00	6.0
0.46	24.0	0.00	6.0
0.47	25.0	0.16	12.0
0.49	26.0	0.28	13.5
0.50	27.5	0.30	15.5
0.50	27.5	0.33	18.5
0.55	30.0	0.43	22.0
0.84	36.5	0.44	23.0
1.04	39.0	0.52	29.0
1.07	40.0	0.56	31.0
1.40	41.0	0.69	32.0
1.46	42.0	0.72	33.0
1.80	46.0	0.73	34.0
1.87	48.0	0.78	35.0
2.13	50.0	0.84	36.5
2.23	51.0	0.94	38.0
3.40	53.0	1.61	43.0
3.78	55.0	1.72	44.0
8.53	56.0	1.76	45.0
		1.82	47.0
		1.99	49.0
		2.92	52.0
		3.67	54.0
$R_1 = 835.0$		$R_2 = 761.0$	
$n_1 = 26$		$n_2 = 30$	

Next, two estimates of U are computed from the sums of the ranks of the second and third graders (R_1) and of the fourth, fifth, and sixth graders (R_2). In these formulas, n_1 refers to the number of second and third graders and n_2 to the number of fourth, fifth, and sixth graders.

$$U = n_1 n_2 + \frac{n_1(n_1 + 1)}{2} - R_1$$

$$= (26)(30) + \frac{26(26 + 1)}{2} - 835.0$$

$$= 780.0 + 351.0 - 835.0 = 296.0$$

$$U = n_1 n_2 + \frac{n_2(n_2 + 1)}{2} - R_2$$

$$= (26)(30) + \frac{30(30 + 1)}{2} - 761.0$$

$$= 780.0 + 465.0 - 761.0 = 484.0$$

The *lowest* estimate of U then is used to compute the value of Z, the test statistic.

$$Z = \frac{U - \frac{n_1 n_2}{2}}{\sqrt{\frac{(n_1)(n_2)(n_1 + n_2 + 1)}{12}}}$$

$$= \frac{296 - \frac{(26)(30)}{2}}{\sqrt{\frac{(26)(30)(26 + 30 + 1)}{12}}}$$

$$= \frac{296 - 390}{\sqrt{3705}} = \frac{-94}{60.87} = -1.54$$

Based on the normal distribution (see p. 321), the probability of this outcome occurring by chance is 0.062. Since this value is larger than 0.05, the null hypothesis would not be rejected.

ANSWER: The typical second or third grader did not have a higher frequency of interjection than the typical fourth, fifth, or sixth grader (Mann-Whitney U Test; alpha = 0.05).

REMARK: This computational procedure is appropriate when the number of subjects in the larger of the groups is more than 20. Appropriate computational procedures when this number is 20 or smaller can be found in several educational and psychological statistical texts, including that of Siegel (1956).

EXERCISE: Determine whether the typical (i.e., median) second or third
(Number 13) grader had a higher frequency of part-word repetition than did the typical fourth, fifth, or sixth grader through the use of the

Mann-Whitney U Test. (The value you compute for Z should be approximately −1.40.)

3. Friedman Two-Way Analysis of Variance (χ_r^2)

QUESTION: Did the second graders tend to produce higher frequencies of some of the four disfluency types (i.e., interjection, part-word repetition, word repetition, and revision-incomplete phrase) than of others?

The first step in performing a Friedman Two-Way Analysis of Variance is selecting an *alpha* level, or a maximum acceptable probability for a *Type I* error (i.e., concluding there was a tendency for the second graders to produce higher frequencies of some of the disfluency types than of others when there was no such tendency). A 0.05 alpha level will be used for this test.

The next step is to compute the value of χ_r^2. Each second grader's disfluency frequencies for interjection, part-word repetition, word repetition, and revision-incomplete phrase are ordered from lowest to highest. The rank is then assigned to each that designates its position in the ordering (1 is assigned to the lowest frequency, 2 to the second lowest frequency, and so on). If more than one disfluency type has the same frequency, each is assigned the mean of the tied ranks. The ranks assigned to the 15 second graders which were based on the frequencies of the four disfluency types they produced (see page 281) are as follows:

Subject Number	I	PW	W	R-IP
1	1.5	3.0	1.5	4.0
2	3.0	2.0	1.0	4.0
3	3.0	1.5	1.5	4.0
4	1.5	3.0	1.5	4.0
5	1.0	3.0	2.0	4.0
6	1.0	2.5	2.5	4.0
7	1.5	1.5	3.0	4.0
8	1.0	4.0	2.0	3.0
9	1.0	3.0	2.0	4.0
10	1.0	2.0	3.0	4.0
11	4.0	1.0	2.0	3.0
12	2.0	2.0	2.0	4.0
13	3.0	1.0	2.0	4.0
14	1.5	1.5	3.0	4.0
15	3.0	1.0	2.0	4.0
$R_j =$	29.0	32.0	31.0	58.0

Appendices

The formula for computing the value of χ_r^2 is:

$$\chi_r^2 = \frac{12}{Nk(k+1)} \sum_{j=1}^{k} (R_j)^2 - 3N(k+1)$$

where R_j = a column sum (i.e., total)
N = number of rows
k = number of columns

The value of χ_r^2 for these data is:

$$\chi_r^2 = \frac{12}{(15)(4)(4+1)}[(29)^2 + (32)^2 + (31)^2 + (58)^2] - (3)(15)(4+1)$$

$$= \frac{12}{300}(6190) - 225$$

$$= 247.6 - 225.0 = 22.6$$

To determine whether this value of χ_r^2 is large enough for the null hypothesis to be rejected, the value of chi square required for rejection is located in Table A.2 (see p. 319). The degrees of freedom (df) here would be 3 (i.e., the number of columns minus one). The value of chi square required for rejection at the 0.05 alpha level when $df = 3$ is 7.82. Since the value computed is larger than this, i.e., 22.6, the null hypothesis would be rejected.

ANSWER: The second graders tended to produce higher frequencies of some of the disfluency types than of others (Friedman Two-Way Analysis of Variance; alpha = 0.05).

EXERCISE: Determine whether the third graders tended to produce higher
(Number 14) frequencies of some of the four disfluency types than of others through the use of the Friedman Two-Way Analysis of Variance. (The value of χ_r^2 you compute should be approximately 12.74.)

4. Kruskal-Wallis One-Way Analysis of Variance (H)

QUESTION: Was there a tendency for the amount of part-word repetition produced by the children to vary as a function of grade level?

The first step in performing a Kruskal-Wallis One-Way Analysis of Variance is selecting an *alpha* level, or a maximum acceptable probability for a *Type I* error (i.e., concluding there was a tendency for the amount of part-word repetition produced by the children to vary as a function of grade level when there was no such tendency). A 0.05 alpha level will be used for this test.

The next step is to compute the value of H. First, the 56 children are ordered on the basis of their part-word repetition frequency. The rank is then assigned to each that designated his position in the ordering (1 is assigned to the child with the lowest frequency, 2 to the one with the second lowest frequency, and so on). If more than one child has the same frequency, each is assigned the mean of the tied ranks. The ranks assigned to the children in each grade are as follows:

2nd Grade	3rd Grade	4th Grade	5th Grade	6th Grade
4.0	4.0	8.0	4.0	4.0
4.0	14.5	12.0	9.0	4.0
4.0	21.5	26.0	11.0	10.0
16.0	32.0	30.0	17.5	13.0
17.5	37.0	43.5	24.0	14.5
19.0	40.0	45.0	25.0	21.5
20.0	41.0	50.0	28.0	23.0
36.0	47.0	51.0	29.0	27.0
38.0	48.0	55.0	31.0	33.0
39.0	49.0		34.5	34.5
42.0	56.0		52.0	
43.5				
46.0				
53.0				
54.0				
R_j = 436.0	390.0	320.5	265.0	184.5

The formula for computing the value of H is:

$$H = \frac{12}{N(N+1)} \sum_{j=1}^{k} \frac{R_j^2}{n_j} - 3(N+1)$$

where R_j = a column sum (i.e., total)
N = the number of subjects
n_j = the number of subjects in a column

The value of H for these data is:

$$H = \frac{12}{56(56+1)} \left[\frac{(436)^2}{15} + \frac{(390)^2}{11} + \frac{(320.5)^2}{9} + \frac{(265)^2}{11} + \frac{(184.5)^2}{10} \right]$$
$$- 3(56+1)$$
$$= \frac{12}{3192} [12673.07 + 13827.27 + 11413.36 + 6384.09 + 3404.02]$$
$$- 171$$
$$= .004 [47701.81] - 171$$
$$= 190.81 - 171 = 19.81$$

To determine whether this value of H is large enough for the null hypothesis to be rejected, the value of H required for rejection is located in Table A.2 (see p. 319). (H is distributed as chi square, provided that the number of groups is greater than 3 and that there are more than 5 subjects in each of the groups.) The degrees of freedom (df) here would be 4 (i.e., the number of columns minus one). The value of chi square required for rejection at the 0.05 alpha level when $df = 4$ is 9.49. Since the value of H computed is larger than this, i.e., 19.81, the null hypothesis would be rejected.

ANSWER: There was a tendency for the amount of part-word repetition produced by the children to vary as a function of grade level (Kruskal-Wallis One-Way Analysis of Variance; alpha = 0.05).

REMARK: See Siegel, 1956, for probabilities associated with various values of H when the number of groups is 3 and the number of subjects in each group is 5 or fewer.

EXERCISE: (Number 15) Determine whether there was a tendency for the amount of word repetition produced by the children to vary as a function of grade level through the use of the Kruskal-Wallis One-Way Analysis of Variance. (The value of H you compute should be approximately 19.14.)

INFERENTIAL STATISTICAL TESTS: INTERVAL AND RATIO DATA

1. t-Test for Related Measures (t)

QUESTION: Did the children on the average tend to produce higher frequencies of interjection than of part-word repetition?

The first step in performing a *t*-test for related measures is selecting an *alpha* level, or a maximum acceptable probability for a *Type I* error (i.e., concluding that the children on the average tended to produce higher frequencies of interjection than of part-word repetition when there was no such tendency). A 0.05 alpha level will be used for this test. Since to answer the question it only would be necessary to detect a difference between interjection frequency and part-word repetition frequency in one direction, the region of rejection for the test will be *one-tailed*.

The next step is to compute the value for t. Each child's part-word repetition frequency is subtracted from his interjection frequency (see Table A.1). If his part-word repetition frequency is smaller than his interjection frequency, this difference is assigned a + sign. If his part-word repetition frequency is larger than his interjection frequency, this difference is assigned a − sign. The difference frequencies for the 56 children are as follows:

Subject	Difference (D)	Subject	Difference (D)
1	−0.66	29	−2.41
2	+0.71	30	−0.32
3	+1.40	31	−0.73
4	−0.81	32	−0.12
5	−0.63	33	+0.21
6	−0.35	34	−1.21
7	0.00	35	+2.84
8	−1.90	36	0.00
9	−1.50	37	−0.66
10	−0.50	38	+1.61
11	+8.19	39	+0.18
12	0.00	40	+0.14
13	+1.17	41	+1.99
14	0.00	42	+0.91
15	+1.87	43	+0.51
16	−0.68	44	−0.54
17	+2.65	45	+1.21
18	+0.74	46	+0.18
19	−0.66	47	−0.28
20	+0.49	48	−0.19
21	−0.36	49	+1.99
22	−3.87	50	−0.47
23	+0.56	51	−0.93
24	−0.13	52	+0.69
25	+1.89	53	−0.66
26	+0.90	54	−0.18
27	−1.10	55	+0.52
28	−0.63	56	−0.11

The following are computed from these difference frequencies:

ΣD = the algebraic difference between the sum of the differences which have plus signs and the sum of the differences which have minus signs = 33.55 (i.e., plus sum) − 22.59 (i.e., minus sum) = 10.96

$\bar{D}$ = the mean of the algebraic sum of the differences = 10.96/56 = 0.196

ΣD^2 = the sum of the squared difference frequencies = 144.596

The value of t here is:

$$t = \frac{\bar{D}\sqrt{N-1}}{\sqrt{\frac{\Sigma D^2}{N} - \bar{D}^2}} = \frac{.196\sqrt{56-1}}{\sqrt{\frac{144.596}{56} - (.196)^2}}$$

$$= \frac{.196(7.416)}{\sqrt{2.582 - .038}} = \frac{1.454}{1.579}$$

$$= 0.92$$

To determine whether this value of t is large enough for the null hypothesis to be rejected, the value of t required for rejection is located in Table A.5 (see p. 322). The degrees of freedom (df) here would be 55 (i.e., the number of subjects minus one). The value of t required for rejection at the 0.05 alpha level when $df = 55$ is 1.67. Since the value computed—i.e., 0.92—is smaller than this, the null hypothesis would not be rejected.

ANSWER: The children on the average did not tend to produce higher frequencies of interjection than of part-word repetition (t-test for related measures; alpha $= 0.05$).

EXERCISE: Determine whether the children on the average exhibited a
(Number 16) tendency to produce higher frequencies of revision-incomplete phrase than of word repetition through the use of the t-test for related measures. (The value of t you compute should be approximately 9.88.)

2. t-Test for Independent Measures (t)

QUESTION: Did the second and third graders tend to produce higher frequencies of interjection on the average than the fourth, fifth, and sixth graders?

The first step in performing a t-test for independent measures is selecting an *alpha* level, or a maximum acceptable probability for a *Type I* error (i.e., concluding that the second and third graders tend to produce higher frequencies of interjection on the average than the fourth, fifth, and sixth graders when there was no such tendency). A 0.05 alpha level will be used for this test. Since to answer the question it only would be necessary to detect a difference between second and third graders and fourth, fifth, and sixth graders in one direction, the region of rejection for the test will be *one-tailed*.

The next step is to compute the value for t. The following values are computed from the interjection frequencies in Table A.1 for each group of children:

2nd and 3rd Grade

$n_1 = 26$
$\Sigma X_1 = 34.50$
$\bar{X}_1 = 1.33$
$\Sigma X_1^2 = 124.02$
$S_1^2 = \dfrac{\Sigma X_1^2}{N_1} - \bar{X}_1^2$
$= \dfrac{124.02}{26} - (1.33)^2$
$= 4.77 - 1.77 = 3.00$

4th, 5th, and 6th Grade

$n_2 = 30$
$\Sigma X_2 = 23.21$
$\bar{X}_2 = 0.77$
$\Sigma X_2^2 = 42.91$
$S_2^2 = \dfrac{\Sigma X_2^2}{N_2} - \bar{X}_2^2$
$= \dfrac{42.91}{30} - (.77)^2$
$= 1.43 - .59 = .84$

The value of t here would be:

$$t = \dfrac{\bar{X}_1 - \bar{X}_2}{\sqrt{\dfrac{n_1 S_1^2 + n_2 S_2^2}{n_1 + n_2 - 2}\left(\dfrac{1}{n_1} + \dfrac{1}{n_2}\right)}}$$

$$= \dfrac{1.33 - .77}{\sqrt{\dfrac{(26)(3.00) + (30)(.84)}{26 + 30 - 2}\left(\dfrac{1}{26} + \dfrac{1}{30}\right)}}$$

$$= \dfrac{.56}{\sqrt{\dfrac{103.2}{54}(.07)}}$$

$$= \dfrac{.56}{\sqrt{.1337777}} = \dfrac{.56}{.37}$$

$$= 1.51$$

To determine whether this value of t is large enough for the null hypothesis to be rejected, the value of t required for rejection is located in Table A.5 (see p. 322). The degrees of freedom (df) here would be 54 (i.e., the number of subjects minus two). The value of t required for rejection at the 0.05 alpha level when $df = 54$ is 1.67. Since the value computed—i.e., 1.51—is smaller than this, the null hypothesis would not be rejected.

ANSWER: The second and third graders did not tend to produce higher frequencies of interjection on the average than the fourth, fifth, and sixth graders (*t*-test for independent measures; alpha = 0.05).

EXERCISE: Determine whether the second and third graders tended to
(Number 17) produce higher frequencies of part-word repetition on the average than the fourth, fifth, and sixth graders through the use of the *t*-test for independent measures. (The value of *t* you compute should be approximately 1.52.)

3. t-Test for the Significance of Pearson Product-Moment Correlation Coefficients

QUESTION: Was there any relationship between the children's interjection frequencies and part-word repetition frequencies during their performances of the spontaneous speech task?

The first step in performing a *t*-test for the significance of the Pearson product-moment correlation coefficient (r) is selecting an *alpha* level, or a maximum acceptable probability for a *Type I* error (i.e., concluding there was a relationship between the children's interjection frequencies and part-word repetition frequencies when there was no such relationship). A 0.05 alpha level will be used for this test. Since to answer this question it would be necessary to detect both positive and negative relationships between interjection frequency and part-word repetition frequency, the region of rejection for the test will be *two-tailed*.

The next step is to compute the value of *t*. The Pearson product-moment correlation coefficient for the relationship between interjection frequency and part-word repetition frequency for the 56 children is −0.02 (see p. 294). The value of *t* here would be:

$$t = \frac{r}{\sqrt{1-r^2}} \sqrt{N-2}$$

$$= \frac{-.02}{\sqrt{1-(-.02)^2}} \sqrt{56-2}$$

$$= \frac{-.02}{\sqrt{1-.0004}} \sqrt{54}$$

$$= \frac{-.02}{.9998} 7.3485 = (-.0200)(7.3485)$$

$$= -.1470$$

To determine whether this value of t is large enough for the null hypothesis to be rejected, the value of t required for rejection is located in Table A.5 (see p. 322). The degrees of freedom (df) here would be 54 (i.e., the number of subjects minus two). The value of t required for rejection at the 0.05 alpha level, when $df = 54$ and the region of rejection is two-tailed, is 2.00. Since the value computed, i.e., -0.147, is smaller than this, the null hypothesis would not be rejected.

ANSWER: There was no relationship between the children's interjection frequencies and part-word repetition frequencies during their performances of the spontaneous speech task (t-test for the significance of a Pearson product-moment correlation coefficient; alpha = 0.05).

EXERCISE: (Number 18) Determine whether there was any relationship between the children's word repetition frequencies and revision-incomplete phrase frequencies during their performances of the spontaneous speech task through the use of the t-test for the significance of Pearson product-moment correlation coefficients. (The value of t you compute should be approximately 3.02.)

4. One-Way Analysis of Variance (F-Test) for Dependent Measures

QUESTION: Did the second graders on the average tend to produce higher frequencies of some of the four disfluency types (i.e., interjection, part-word repetition, word repetition, and revision-incomplete phrase) than of others?

The first step in performing a one-way analysis of variance for dependent measures (F) is selecting an *alpha* level, or a maximum acceptable probability for a *Type I* error (i.e., concluding there was a tendency for the second graders on the average to produce higher frequencies of some of the four disfluency types than of others when there was no such tendency). A 0.05 alpha level will be used for this test.

The next step is to compute the value of F. The sum of each second grader's four disfluency frequencies (T) and the square of the sum of his four disfluency frequencies divided by the number of disfluency frequencies summed ($T^2/4$) based on Table A.1 are as follows:

Subject	T_r	$T_r^2/4$
1	4.32	4.666
2	9.57	22.896
3	6.54	10.693
4	3.63	3.294
5	4.40	4.84
6	2.44	1.488
7	4.49	5.040
8	5.69	8.094
9	8.09	16.362
10	8.99	20.205
11	13.99	48.930
12	4.68	5.476
13	6.73	11.323
14	2.52	1.588
15	4.86	5.905
	$T = 90.94$	$170.800 = \Sigma T_r^2/4$

The following computations are then made from the frequencies in each column—i.e., the disfluency frequencies of each of the four types produced by the 15 second graders.

Measure	I	PW	W	R-IP	
T_c	19.27	12.28	12.63	46.76	$T = 90.34$
$\bar{X}_c$	1.285	0.819	0.842	3.117	
$T_c^2/15$	24.756	10.053	10.634	145.766	$\Sigma T_c^2/15 = 191.209$
ΣX^2	87.164	17.100	15.680	183.938	$\Sigma\Sigma X^2 = 303.782$

Next, *four* sum of square (SS) values are computed from these row and column data analyses. The first is the sum of squares (SS) for columns (c), or disfluency types.

$$SS_c = \frac{\Sigma T_c^2}{r} - \frac{T^2}{cr}$$

$$= 191.209 - \frac{(90.94)^2}{(4)(15)}$$

$$= 191.209 - 137.835 = 53.374$$

The second is the sum of squares (SS) for rows (r), or subjects.

$$SS_r = \frac{\Sigma T_r^2}{c} - \frac{T^2}{cr}$$

$$= 170.800 - \frac{(90.94)^2}{(4)(15)}$$

$$= 170.800 - 137.835 = 32.965$$

The third is the total (T) sum of squares.

$$SS_T = \Sigma\Sigma X^2 - \frac{T^2}{cr} = 303.782 - \frac{(90.94)^2}{(4)(15)}$$

$$= 303.782 - 137.835 = 165.947$$

The fourth is the residual sum of squares, labeled SS_{cr}, which is assumed to represent random measurement error.

$$SS_{cr} = SS_T - SS_c - SS_r = 165.947 - 53.374 - 32.965$$
$$= 79.608$$

The value of F can be computed by means of the following formula:

$$F = \frac{SS_c/c - 1}{SS_{cr}/(c-1)(r-1)}$$

where $c - 1$ is the degrees of freedom for SS_c and $(c-1)(r-1)$ is the degrees of freedom for SS_{cr}. The first is df_1 and the second df_2 (see Table A.6).

The value of F here is:

$$F = \frac{53.374/3}{79.608/42} = \frac{17.791}{1.895} = 9.39$$

To determine whether this value of F is large enough for the null hypothesis to be rejected, the value of F required for rejection is located in Table A.6 (see p. 323). There are two degrees of freedom: df_1 would be 3 (i.e., the number of columns minus one) and df_2 would be 42 (i.e., the number of columns minus one times the number of rows minus one). The value of F required for rejection at the 0.05 alpha level when $df_1 = 3$ and $df_2 = 42$ is 2.84. Since the value computed—i.e., 9.39—exceeds this value, the null hypothesis would be rejected.

ANSWER: The second graders on the average tended to produce higher frequencies of some of the disfluency types than of others (F-test; alpha $= 0.05$).

REMARK: This example and the one that follows illustrate the simplest possible applications of analysis of variance. Other applications are described in a number of psychological and educational statistical texts, including those of Lindquist (1956) and Winer (1962).

EXERCISE: Determine whether the third graders tended to produce higher
(Number 19) frequencies of some of the four disfluency types than of others through the use of analysis of variance. (The value of F you compute should be approximately 7.77.)

5. One-Way Analysis of Variance (F-Test) for Independent Measures

QUESTION: Was there a tendency for the amount of part-word repetition produced by the children to vary as a function of grade level?

The first step in performing a one-way analysis of variance for independent measures (F) is selecting an *alpha* level, or maximum acceptable probability for a *Type I* error (i.e., concluding there was a tendency for the amount of part-word repetition produced by the children to vary as a function of grade level when there was no such tendency). A 0.05 alpha level will be used for this test.

The next step is to compute the value of F. The following computations are made from the part-word repetition frequencies of the children at each grade level (see Table A.1).

Measure	2nd Grade	3rd Grade	4th Grade	5th Grade	6th Grade	
n_c	15	11	9	11	10	$N = 56$
T_c	12.28	13.70	9.84	6.82	4.11	$T = 46.75$
$\bar{X}_c$	0.819	1.245	1.093	0.620	0.411	
T_c^2/n_c	10.053	17.063	10.758	4.228	1.689	$\Sigma T_c^2/n_c = 43.791$
ΣX_c^2	17.100	30.695	14.947	6.238	2.700	$\Sigma\Sigma X^2 = 71.680$

Next, three sum of square (SS) values are computed from these column data analyses. The first is the sum of squares (SS) for columns (c) or grade levels.

$$SS_c = \frac{\Sigma T_c^2}{n_c} - \frac{T^2}{N}$$

$$= 43.791 - \frac{(46.75)^2}{56}$$

$$= 43.791 - 39.028$$

$$= 4.763$$

The second is the total (T) sum of squares.

$$SS_T = \Sigma\Sigma X^2 - \frac{T^2}{N}$$

$$= 71.680 - \frac{(46.75)^2}{56}$$

$$= 71.680 - 39.028$$

$$= 32.652$$

The third is the within group (w), or residual, sum of squares, which is assumed to represent random measurement error.

$$SS_w = SS_T - SS_c = 32.652 - 4.763 = 27.889$$

The value of F can be computed by means of the following formula:

$$F = \frac{SS_c/c - 1}{SS_w/N - c}$$

where $c - 1$ is the degrees of freedom for SS_c and $N - c$ is the degrees of freedom for SS_w. The first is df_1 and the second df_2 (see p. 212). The value of F here is:

$$F = \frac{4.763/5 - 1}{27.889/56 - 5}$$

$$= \frac{1.191}{.547}$$

$$= 2.18$$

To determine whether this value of F is large enough for the null hypothesis to be rejected, the value of F required for rejection is located in Table A.6 (see p. 323). There are two degrees of freedom: df_1 would be 4 (i.e., the number of columns minus one), and df_2 would be 51 (i.e., the number of subjects minus the number of columns). The value of F required for rejection at the 0.05 alpha level, when $df_1 = 4$ and $df_2 = 51$, is 2.56. Since the value computed—i.e., 2.18—is smaller than this value, the null hypothesis would not be rejected.

ANSWER: There did not appear to be a tendency for the amount of part-word repetition produced by the children to vary as a function of grade level (F-test; alpha = 0.05).

EXERCISE: (Number 20) Determine whether there was a tendency for the amount of word repetition produced by the children to vary as a function of grade level through the use of analysis of variance. (The value of F you compute should be approximately 2.32.)

CONFIDENCE INTERVAL ESTIMATION

A. Mean

QUESTION: Within what range is the mean interjection frequency of the *population* from which the children were selected (i.e., second- through sixth-grade nonstutterers) most likely to fall?

To answer this question, a *95 percent confidence interval* will be computed. Theoretically, the limits of this interval define a range within which we can be 95 percent certain to find the mean interjection frequency for the *population* from which the sample was drawn. This 95 percent figure, however, should be regarded as only approximate, since certain assumptions underlying the computational procedure may not have been met (see Chapter 8).

The upper ($\bar{\mu}$) and lower ($\underline{\mu}$) limits of the confidence interval can be computed by means of the following formulas:

$$\bar{\mu} = \bar{X} + \frac{SD}{\sqrt{N-1}}(1.96)$$

$$\underline{\mu} = \bar{X} - \frac{SD}{\sqrt{N-1}}(1.96)$$

where

$\bar{X}$ = the mean frequency for the sample = 1.03 (see p. 283)

SD = the standard deviation for the sample = 1.39 (see p. 288)

N = the number of subjects = 56
1.96 = a constant for 95 percent confidence intervals

The *mean* value that would represent the *upper limit* of the confidence interval would be:

$$\bar{\mu} = 1.03 + \frac{1.39}{\sqrt{56-1}}(1.96)$$
$$= 1.03 + (.187)(1.96)$$
$$= 1.40$$

The *mean* value that would represent the *lower limit* of the confidence interval would be:

$$\underline{\mu} = 1.03 - \frac{1.39}{\sqrt{56-1}}(1.96)$$
$$= 1.03 - (.187)(1.96)$$
$$= 0.66$$

ANSWER: The mean interjection frequency of the population from which the children were selected is *approximately* 95 percent certain to fall between 0.66 and 1.40.

REMARK: The width of the confidence interval can be changed by substituting a different constant for 1.96. For a 99 percent confidence interval, for example, 2.58 would be used as the constant.

EXERCISE: Compute a 95 percent confidence interval for the mean part-word repetition frequency of the population from which the children were selected (see p. 283 and p. 288 for the sample mean and standard deviation). (The upper limit of the confidence interval you compute should be approximately 1.03, and the lower limit should be approximately 0.63.)
(Number 21)

B. Median

QUESTION: Within what range is the median interjection frequency of the *population* from which the children were selected (i.e., second-through sixth-grade nonstutterers) most likely to fall?

To answer this question, a *95 percent confidence interval* will be computed. Theoretically, the limits of this interval define a range within which we can be 95 percent certain of finding the median interjection frequency for the population from which the sample was drawn. This 95 percent figure, however, should be regarded as only approximate since certain assumptions underlying the computational procedure may not have been met (see Chapter 8).

The upper ($\bar{\xi}$) and lower ($\underline{\xi}$) limits of the confidence interval can be computed by means of the following formulas:

$$\bar{\xi} = \text{mdn} + \frac{1.25\ SD}{\sqrt{N-1}}(1.96)$$

$$\underline{\xi} = \text{mdn} - \frac{1.25\ SD}{\sqrt{N-1}}(1.96)$$

where

mdn = the median frequency for the sample = 0.51 (see p. 284)

SD = the standard deviation for the sample = 1.39 (see p. 288)

N = the number of subjects = 56

1.96 = a constant for 95 percent confidence intervals

1.25 = a constant

The median value that would represent the *upper boundary* of the confidence interval would be:

$$\bar{\xi} = .51 + \frac{(1.25)(1.39)}{\sqrt{56-1}}(1.96)$$

$$= .51 + (.234)(1.96)$$

$$= 0.97$$

The median value that would represent the *lower boundary* of the confidence interval would be:

$$\underline{\xi} = .51 - \frac{(1.25)(1.39)}{\sqrt{56-1}}(1.96)$$

$$= .51 - (.234)(1.96)$$

$$= 0.05$$

ANSWER: The median interjection frequency of the population from which the children were selected is *approximately* 95 percent certain to fall between 0.05 and 0.97.

REMARK: The width of the confidence interval can be changed by substituting a different constant for 1.96. For a 99 percent confidence interval, for example, 2.58 would be used as the constant.

EXERCISE: Compute a 95 percent confidence interval for the median part-
(Number 22) word repetition frequency of the population from which the children were selected (see p. 285 and p. 288 for the sample median and standard deviation). (The upper boundary of the confidence interval you compute should be approximately 1.07, and the lower boundary should be approximately 0.56.)

C. Difference between Means

QUESTION: Within what range is the *difference between mean* part-word repetition frequencies for third graders and sixth graders in the *populations* from which the children were selected (i.e., third-grade nonstutterers and sixth-grade nonstutterers) most likely to fall?

To answer this question, a *95 percent confidence interval* will be computed. Theoretically, the limits of this interval define a range within which we can be 95 percent certain of finding the difference between mean part-word repetition frequencies for third graders and sixth graders in the populations from which the samples were drawn. This 95 percent figure, however, should only be regarded as approximate, since certain assumptions underlying the computational procedure may not have been met (see Chapter 8).

The upper ($\bar{\Delta}$) and lower ($\underline{\Delta}$) limits of the confidence interval can be computed by means of the following formulas:

$$\bar{\Delta} = \bar{D}_1 + (1.96)\sqrt{\frac{S_1^2}{n_1 - 1} + \frac{S_2^2}{n_2 - 1}}$$

$$\underline{\Delta} = \bar{D}_1 - (1.96)\sqrt{\frac{S_1^2}{n_1 - 1} + \frac{S_2^2}{n_2 - 1}}$$

where

$\bar{D}_1 = \bar{X}_1 - \bar{X}_2 = 1.245 - 0.411 = 0.834$ (*see p. 281*)
$n_1 = $ the number of third graders $= 11$
$n_2 = $ the number of sixth graders $= 10$

S_1^2 = the variance of the third graders' part-word repetition frequencies =

$$\frac{\Sigma X_1^2}{n_1} - \bar{X}_1^2 = \frac{30.695}{11} - (1.245)^2 = 2.790 - 1.550 = 1.240$$

S_2^2 = the variance of the sixth graders' part-word repetition frequencies =

$$\frac{\Sigma X_2^2}{n_2} - \bar{X}_2^2 = \frac{2.700}{10} - (.411)^2 = .270 - .169 = .101$$

The mean difference that would represent the *upper boundary* of the confidence interval would be:

$$\bar{\Delta} = .834 + (1.96)\sqrt{\frac{1.240}{11-1} + \frac{.101}{10-1}}$$
$$= .834 + (1.96)(.368) = 1.56$$

The mean difference that would represent the *lower boundary* of the confidence interval would be:

$$\underline{\Delta} = .834 - (1.96)\sqrt{\frac{1.240}{11-1} + \frac{.101}{10-1}}$$
$$= .834 - (1.96)(.368) = .11$$

ANSWER: The difference between the means of the populations from which the children were selected is *approximately* 95 percent certain to fall between 0.11 and 1.56.

REMARK: The width of the confidence interval can be changed by substituting a different constant for 1.96. For a 99 percent confidence interval, for example, 2.58 would be used as the constant.

EXERCISE: (Number 23) Compute a 95 percent confidence interval for the difference between mean part-word repetition frequencies for fourth graders and fifth graders in the populations from which the children were selected (see p. 281 for the values you will need). (The upper boundary of the confidence interval you compute should be approximately 1.01 and the lower boundary should be approximately −0.07.)

TABLE A.2. Table of critical values of chi square[a]

df	.99	.98	.95	.90	.80	.70	.50	.30	.20	.10	.05	.02	.01	.001
					Probability under H_0 that $\chi^2 \geq$ chi square									
1	.00016	.00063	.0039	.016	.064	.15	.46	1.07	1.64	2.71	3.84	5.41	6.64	10.83
2	.02	.04	.10	.21	.45	.71	1.39	2.41	3.22	4.60	5.99	7.82	9.21	13.82
3	.12	.18	.35	.58	1.00	1.42	2.37	3.66	4.64	6.25	7.82	9.84	11.34	16.27
4	.30	.43	.71	1.06	1.65	2.20	3.36	4.88	5.99	7.78	9.49	11.67	13.28	18.46
5	.55	.75	1.14	1.61	2.34	3.00	4.35	6.06	7.29	9.24	11.07	13.39	15.09	20.52
6	.87	1.13	1.64	2.20	3.07	3.83	5.35	7.23	8.56	10.64	12.59	15.03	16.81	22.46
7	1.24	1.56	2.17	2.83	3.82	4.67	6.35	8.38	9.80	12.02	14.07	16.62	18.48	24.32
8	1.65	2.03	2.73	3.49	4.59	5.53	7.34	9.52	11.03	13.36	15.51	18.17	20.09	26.12
9	2.09	2.53	3.32	4.17	5.38	6.39	8.34	10.66	12.24	14.68	16.92	19.68	21.67	27.88
10	2.56	3.06	3.94	4.86	6.18	7.27	9.34	11.78	13.44	15.99	18.31	21.16	23.21	29.59
11	3.05	3.61	4.58	5.58	6.99	8.15	10.34	12.90	14.63	17.28	19.68	22.62	24.72	31.26
12	3.57	4.18	5.23	6.30	7.81	9.03	11.34	14.01	15.81	18.55	21.03	24.05	26.22	32.91
13	4.11	4.76	5.89	7.04	8.63	9.93	12.34	15.12	16.98	19.81	22.36	25.47	27.69	34.53
14	4.66	5.37	6.57	7.79	9.47	10.82	13.34	16.22	18.15	21.06	23.68	26.87	29.14	36.12
15	5.23	5.98	7.26	8.55	10.31	11.72	14.34	17.32	19.31	22.31	25.00	28.26	30.58	37.70
16	5.81	6.61	7.96	9.31	11.15	12.62	15.34	18.42	20.46	23.54	26.30	29.63	32.00	39.29
17	6.41	7.26	8.67	10.08	12.00	13.53	16.34	19.51	21.62	24.77	27.59	31.00	33.41	40.75
18	7.02	7.91	9.39	10.86	12.86	14.44	17.34	20.60	22.76	25.99	28.87	32.35	34.80	42.31
19	7.63	8.57	10.12	11.65	13.72	15.35	18.34	21.69	23.90	27.20	30.14	33.69	36.19	43.82
20	8.26	9.24	10.85	12.44	14.58	16.27	19.34	22.78	25.04	28.41	31.41	35.02	37.57	45.32
21	8.90	9.92	11.59	13.24	15.44	17.18	20.34	23.86	26.17	29.62	32.67	36.34	38.93	46.80
22	9.54	10.60	12.34	14.04	16.31	18.10	21.24	24.94	27.30	30.81	33.92	37.66	40.29	48.27
23	10.20	11.29	13.09	14.85	17.19	19.02	22.34	26.02	28.43	32.01	35.17	38.97	41.64	49.73
24	10.86	11.99	13.85	15.66	18.06	19.94	23.34	27.10	29.55	33.20	36.42	40.27	42.98	51.18
25	11.52	12.70	14.61	16.47	18.94	20.87	24.34	28.17	30.68	34.38	37.65	41.57	44.31	52.62
26	12.20	13.41	15.38	17.29	19.82	21.79	25.34	29.25	31.80	35.56	38.88	42.86	45.64	54.05
27	12.88	14.12	16.15	18.11	20.70	22.72	26.34	30.32	32.91	36.74	40.11	44.14	46.96	55.48
28	13.56	14.85	16.93	18.94	21.59	23.65	27.34	31.39	34.03	37.92	41.34	45.42	48.28	56.89
29	14.26	15.57	17.71	19.77	22.48	24.58	28.34	32.46	35.14	39.09	42.56	46.69	49.59	58.30
30	14.95	16.31	18.49	20.60	23.36	25.51	29.34	33.53	36.25	40.26	43.77	47.96	50.89	59.70

[a] Adapted from Table IV of Fisher and Yates: *Statistical Tables for Biological, Agricultural, and Medical Research* (6th edition), Copyright 1974 by Longman Group, Ltd. With permission of Longman Group, Ltd.

TABLE A.3. Table of probabilities associated with values as small as observed values of x in the sign test.[a]

Given in the body of this table are one-tailed probabilities under H_0 for the binomial test when $P = Q = \frac{1}{2}$. To save space, decimal points are omitted in the p's.

N \ x	0	1	2	3	4	5	6	7	8	9	10	11	12	13	14	15
5	031	188	500	812	969	†										
6	016	109	344	656	891	984	†									
7	008	062	227	500	773	938	992	†								
8	004	035	145	363	637	855	965	996	†							
9	002	020	090	254	500	746	910	980	998	†						
10	001	011	055	172	377	623	828	945	989	999	†					
11		006	033	113	274	500	726	887	967	994	†	†				
12		003	019	073	194	387	613	806	927	981	997	†	†			
13		002	011	046	133	291	500	709	867	954	989	998	†	†		
14		001	006	029	090	212	395	605	788	910	971	994	999	†	†	
15			004	018	059	151	304	500	696	849	941	982	996	†	†	†
16			002	011	038	105	227	402	598	773	895	962	989	998	†	†
17			001	006	025	072	166	315	500	685	834	928	975	994	999	†
18			001	004	015	048	119	240	407	593	760	881	952	985	996	999
19				002	010	032	084	180	324	500	676	820	916	968	990	998
20				001	006	021	058	132	252	412	588	748	868	942	979	994
21				001	004	013	039	095	192	332	500	668	808	905	961	987
22					002	008	026	067	143	262	416	584	738	857	933	974
23					001	005	017	047	105	202	339	500	661	798	895	953
24					001	003	011	032	076	154	.271	419	581	729	846	924
25						002	007	022	054	115	212	345	500	655	788	885

†1.0 or approximately 1.0
[a] Adapted from Table IV, B, of Walker, Helen, and Lev, J. 1953. *Statistical Inference.* New York: Holt, p. 458, with permission of the authors and publisher.

TABLE A.4. Table of probabilities associated with values as extreme as observed values of z in the normal distribution.[a]

z	.00	.01	.02	.03	.04	.05	.06	.07	.08	.09
.0	.5000	.4960	.4920	.4880	.4840	.4801	.4761	.4721	.4681	.4641
.1	.4602	.4562	.4522	.4483	.4443	.4404	.4364	.4325	.4286	.4247
.2	.4207	.4168	.4129	.4090	.4052	.4013	.3974	.3936	.3897	.3859
.3	.3821	.3783	.3745	.3707	.3669	.3632	.3594	.3557	.3520	.3483
.4	.3446	.3409	.3372	.3336	.3300	.3264	.3228	.3192	.3156	.3121
.5	.3085	.3050	.3015	.2981	.2946	.2912	.2877	.2843	.2810	.2776
.6	.2743	.2709	.2676	.2643	.2611	.2578	.2546	.2514	.2483	.2451
.7	.2420	.2389	.2358	.2327	.2296	.2266	.2236	.2206	.2177	.2148
.8	.2119	.2090	.2061	.2033	.2005	.1977	.1949	.1922	.1894	.1867
.9	.1841	.1814	.1788	.1762	.1736	.1711	.1685	.1660	.1635	.1611
1.0	.1587	.1562	.1539	.1515	.1492	.1469	.1446	.1423	.1401	.1379
1.1	.1357	.1335	.1314	.1292	.1271	.1251	.1230	.1210	.1190	.1170
1.2	.1151	.1131	.1112	.1093	.1075	.1056	.1038	.1020	.1003	.0985
1.3	.0968	.0951	.0934	.0918	.0901	.0885	.0869	.0853	.0838	.0823
1.4	.0808	.0793	.0778	.0764	.0749	.0735	.0721	.0708	.0694	.0681
1.5	.0668	.0655	.0643	.0630	.0618	.0606	.0594	.0582	.0571	.0559
1.6	.0548	.0537	.0526	.0516	.0505	.0495	.0485	.0475	.0465	.0455
1.7	.0446	.0436	.0427	.0418	.0409	.0401	.0392	.0384	.0375	.0367
1.8	.0359	.0351	.0344	.0336	.0329	.0322	.0314	.0307	.0301	.0294
1.9	.0287	.0281	.0274	.0268	.0262	.0256	.0250	.0244	.0239	.0233
2.0	.0228	.0222	.0217	.0212	.0207	.0202	.0197	.0192	.0188	.0183
2.1	.0179	.0174	.0170	.0166	.0162	.0158	.0154	.0150	.0146	.0143
2.2	.0139	.0136	.0132	.0129	.0125	.0122	.0119	.0116	.0113	.0110
2.3	.0107	.0104	.0102	.0099	.0096	.0094	.0091	.0089	.0087	.0084
2.4	.0082	.0080	.0078	.0075	.0073	.0071	.0069	.0068	.0066	.0064
2.5	.0062	.0060	.0059	.0057	.0055	.0054	.0052	.0051	.0049	.0048
2.6	.0047	.0045	.0044	.0043	.0041	.0040	.0039	.0038	.0037	.0036
2.7	.0035	.0034	.0033	.0032	.0031	.0030	.0029	.0028	.0027	.0026
2.8	.0026	.0025	.0024	.0023	.0023	.0022	.0021	.0021	.0020	.0019
2.9	.0019	.0018	.0018	.0017	.0016	.0016	.0015	.0015	.0014	.0014
3.0	.0013	.0013	.0013	.0012	.0012	.0011	.0011	.0011	.0010	.0010
3.1	.0010	.0009	.0009	.0009	.0008	.0008	.0008	.0008	.0007	.0007
3.2	.0007									
3.3	.0005									
3.4	.0003									
3.5	.00023									
3.6	.00016									
3.7	.00011									
3.8	.00007									
3.9	.00005									
4.0	.00003									

[a] Adapted from Table A of Siegel: Nonparametric Statistics for the Behavioral Sciences. Copyright 1956 by McGraw-Hill Inc. With permission of McGraw-Hill Book Company.

TABLE A.5. Table of critical values of t[a]

df	Level of significance for one-tailed test					
	.10	.05	.025	.01	.005	.0005
	Level of significance for two-tailed test					
	.20	.10	.05	.02	.01	.001
1	3.078	6.314	12.706	31.821	63.657	636.619
2	1.886	2.920	4.303	6.965	9.925	31.598
3	1.638	2.353	3.182	4.541	5.841	12.941
4	1.533	2.132	2.776	3.747	4.604	8.610
5	1.476	2.015	2.571	3.365	4.032	6.859
6	1.440	1.943	2.447	3.143	3.707	5.959
7	1.415	1.895	2.365	2.998	3.499	5.405
8	1.397	1.860	2.306	2.896	3.355	5.041
9	1.383	1.833	2.262	2.821	3.250	4.781
10	1.372	1.812	2.228	2.764	3.169	4.587
11	1.363	1.796	2.201	2.718	3.106	4.437
12	1.356	1.782	2.179	2.681	3.055	4.318
13	1.350	1.771	2.160	2.650	3.012	4.221
14	1.345	1.761	2.145	2.624	2.977	4.140
15	1.341	1.753	2.131	2.602	2.947	4.073
16	1.337	1.746	2.120	2.583	2.921	4.015
17	1.333	1.740	2.110	2.567	2.898	3.965
18	1.330	1.734	2.101	2.552	2.878	3.922
19	1.328	1.729	2.093	2.539	2.861	3.883
20	1.325	1.725	2.086	2.528	2.845	3.850
21	1.323	1.721	2.080	2.518	2.831	3.819
22	1.321	1.717	2.074	2.508	2.819	3.792
23	1.319	1.714	2.069	2.500	2.807	3.767
24	1.318	1.711	2.064	2.492	2.797	3.745
25	1.316	1.708	2.060	2.485	2.787	3.725
26	1.315	1.706	2.056	2.479	2.779	3.707
27	1.314	1.703	2.052	2.473	2.771	3.690
28	1.313	1.701	2.048	2.467	2.763	3.674
29	1.311	1.699	2.045	2.462	2.756	3.659
30	1.310	1.697	2.042	2.457	2.750	3.646
40	1.303	1.684	2.021	2.423	2.704	3.551
60	1.296	1.671	2.000	2.390	2.660	3.460
120	1.289	1.658	1.980	2.358	2.617	3.373
∞	1.282	1.645	1.960	2.326	2.576	3.291

[a] *Adapted from Table III of Fisher and Yates:* Statistical Tables for Biological, Agricultural, and Medical Research (*6th edition*). Copyright 1974 by Longman Group, Ltd. With permission of Longman Group, Ltd.

TABLE A.6. Percent points in the distribution of F [a]

df_2		df_1 1	2	3	4	5	6	8	12	24	∞
1	0.1%	405284	500000	540379	562500	576405	585937	598144	610667	623497	636619
	0.5%	16211	20000	21615	22500	23056	23437	23925	24426	24940	25465
	1%	4052	4999	5403	5625	5764	5859	5981	6106	6234	6366
	2.5%	647.79	799.50	864.16	899.58	921.85	937.11	956.66	976.71	997.25	1018.30
	5%	161.45	199.50	215.71	224.58	230.16	233.99	238.88	243.91	249.05	254.32
	10%	39.86	49.50	53.59	55.83	57.24	58.20	59.44	60.70	62.00	63.33
	20%	9.47	12.00	13.06	13.73	14.01	14.26	14.59	14.90	15.24	15.58
2	0.1	998.5	999.0	999.2	999.2	999.3	999.3	999.4	999.4	999.5	999.5
	0.5	198.50	199.00	199.17	199.25	199.30	199.33	199.37	199.42	199.46	199.51
	1	98.49	99.00	99.17	99.25	99.30	99.33	99.36	99.42	99.46	99.50
	2.5	38.51	39.00	39.17	39.25	39.30	39.33	39.37	39.42	39.46	39.50
	5	18.51	19.00	19.16	19.25	19.30	19.33	19.37	19.41	19.45	19.50
	10	8.53	9.00	9.16	9.24	9.29	9.33	9.37	9.41	9.45	9.49
	20	3.56	4.00	4.16	4.24	4.28	4.32	4.36	4.40	4.44	4.48
3	0.1	167.5	148.5	141.1	137.1	134.6	132.8	130.6	128.3	125.9	123.5
	0.5	55.55	49.80	47.47	46.20	45.39	44.84	44.13	43.39	42.62	41.83
	1	34.12	30.81	29.46	28.71	28.24	27.91	27.49	27.05	26.60	26.12
	2.5	17.44	16.04	15.44	15.10	14.89	14.74	14.54	14.34	14.12	13.90
	5	10.13	9.55	9.28	9.12	9.01	8.94	8.84	8.74	8.64	8.53
	10	5.54	5.46	5.39	5.34	5.31	5.28	5.25	5.22	5.18	5.13
	20	2.68	2.89	2.94	2.96	2.97	2.97	2.98	2.98	2.98	2.98
4	0.1	74.14	61.25	56.18	53.44	51.71	50.53	49.00	47.41	45.77	44.05
	0.5	31.33	26.28	24.26	23.16	22.46	21.98	21.35	20.71	20.03	19.33
	1	21.20	18.00	16.69	15.98	15.52	15.21	14.80	14.37	13.93	13.46
	2.5	12.22	10.65	9.98	9.60	9.36	9.20	8.98	8.75	8.51	8.26
	5	7.71	6.94	6.59	6.39	6.26	6.16	6.04	5.91	5.77	5.63
	10	4.54	4.32	4.19	4.11	4.05	4.01	3.95	3.90	3.83	3.76
	20	2.35	2.47	2.48	2.48	2.48	2.47	2.47	2.46	2.44	2.43
5	0.1	47.04	36.61	33.20	31.09	29.75	28.84	27.64	26.42	25.14	23.78
	0.5	22.79	18.31	16.53	15.56	14.94	14.51	13.96	13.38	12.78	12.14
	1	16.26	13.27	12.06	11.39	10.97	10.67	10.29	9.89	9.47	9.02
	2.5	10.01	8.43	7.76	7.39	7.15	6.98	6.76	6.52	6.28	6.02
	5	6.61	5.79	5.41	5.19	5.05	4.95	4.82	4.68	4.53	4.36
	10	4.06	3.78	3.62	3.52	3.45	3.40	3.34	3.27	3.19	3.10
	20	2.18	2.26	2.25	2.24	2.23	2.22	2.20	2.18	2.16	2.13
6	0.1	35.51	27.00	23.70	21.90	20.81	20.03	19.03	17.99	16.89	15.75
	0.5	18.64	14.54	12.92	12.03	11.46	11.07	10.57	10.03	9.47	8.88
	1	13.74	10.92	9.78	9.15	8.75	8.47	8.10	7.72	7.31	6.88
	2.5	8.81	7.26	6.60	6.23	5.99	5.82	5.60	5.37	5.12	4.85
	5	5.99	5.14	4.76	4.53	4.39	4.28	4.15	4.00	3.84	3.67
	10	3.78	3.46	3.29	3.18	3.11	3.05	2.98	2.90	2.82	2.72
	20	2.07	2.13	2.11	2.09	2.08	2.06	2.04	2.02	1.99	1.95
7	0.1	29.22	21.69	18.77	17.19	16.21	15.52	14.63	13.71	12.73	11.69
	0.5	16.24	12.40	10.88	10.05	9.52	9.16	8.68	8.18	7.65	7.08
	1	12.25	9.55	8.45	7.85	7.46	7.19	6.84	6.47	6.07	5.65
	2.5	8.07	6.54	5.89	5.52	5.29	5.12	4.90	4.67	4.42	4.14
	5	5.59	4.74	4.35	4.12	3.97	3.87	3.73	3.57	3.41	3.23
	10	3.59	3.26	3.07	2.96	2.88	2.83	2.75	2.67	2.58	2.47
	20	2.00	2.04	2.02	1.99	1.97	1.96	1.93	1.91	1.87	1.83
8	0.1	25.42	18.49	15.83	14.39	13.49	12.86	12.04	11.19	10.30	9.34
	0.5	14.69	11.04	9.60	8.81	8.30	7.95	7.50	7.01	6.50	5.95
	1	11.26	8.65	7.59	7.01	6.63	6.37	6.03	5.67	5.28	4.86
	2.5	7.57	6.06	5.42	5.05	4.82	4.65	4.43	4.20	3.95	3.67
	5	5.32	4.46	4.07	3.84	3.69	3.58	3.44	3.28	3.12	2.93
	10	3.46	3.11	2.92	2.81	2.73	2.67	2.59	2.50	2.40	2.29
	20	1.95	1.98	1.95	1.92	1.90	1.88	1.86	1.83	1.79	1.74
9	0.1	22.86	16.39	13.90	12.56	11.71	11.13	10.37	9.57	8.72	7.81
	0.5	13.61	10.11	8.72	7.96	7.47	7.13	6.69	6.23	5.73	5.19
	1	10.56	8.02	6.99	6.42	6.03	5.80	5.47	5.11	4.73	4.31
	2.5	7.21	5.71	5.08	4.72	4.48	4.32	4.10	3.87	3.61	3.33
	5	5.12	4.26	3.86	3.63	3.48	3.37	3.23	3.07	2.90	2.71
	10	3.36	3.01	2.81	2.69	2.61	2.55	2.47	2.38	2.28	2.16
	20	1.91	1.94	1.90	1.87	1.85	1.83	1.80	1.76	1.72	1.67

[a] *Adapted from Table V of Fisher and Yates:* Statistical Tables for Biological, Agricultural, and Medical Research *(6th edition). Copyright 1974 by Longman Group, Ltd. With permission of Longman Group, Ltd. The 0.5% and 2.5% points are reprinted by permission of the Biometrika Trustees from* Biometrika, volume 33 *(April, 1943), pp. 73–78.*

TABLE A.6. Continued

df_2	df_1	1	2	3	4	5	6	8	12	24	∞
10	0.1%	21.04	14.91	12.55	11.28	10.48	9.92	9.20	8.45	7.64	6.76
	0.5%	12.83	9.43	8.08	7.34	6.87	6.54	6.12	5.66	5.17	4.64
	1%	10.04	7.56	6.55	5.99	5.64	5.39	5.06	4.71	4.33	3.91
	2.5%	6.94	5.46	4.83	4.47	4.24	4.07	3.85	3.62	3.37	3.08
	5%	4.96	4.10	3.71	3.48	3.33	3.22	3.07	2.91	2.74	2.54
	10%	3.28	2.92	2.73	2.61	2.52	2.46	2.38	2.28	2.18	2.06
	20%	1.88	1.90	1.86	1.83	1.80	1.78	1.75	1.72	1.67	1.62
11	0.1	19.69	13.81	11.56	10.35	9.58	9.05	8.35	7.63	6.85	6.00
	0.5	12.23	8.91	7.60	6.88	6.42	6.10	5.68	5.24	4.76	4.23
	1	9.65	7.20	6.22	5.67	5.32	5.07	4.74	4.40	4.02	3.60
	2.5	6.72	5.26	4.63	4.28	4.04	3.88	3.66	3.43	3.17	2.88
	5	4.84	3.98	3.59	3.36	3.20	3.09	2.95	2.79	2.61	2.40
	10	3.23	2.86	2.66	2.54	2.45	2.39	2.30	2.21	2.10	1.97
	20	1.86	1.87	1.83	1.80	1.77	1.75	1.72	1.68	1.63	1.57
12	0.1	18.64	12.97	10.80	9.63	8.89	8.38	7.71	7.00	6.25	5.42
	0.5	11.75	8.51	7.23	6.52	6.07	5.76	5.35	4.91	4.43	3.90
	1	9.33	6.93	5.95	5.41	5.06	4.82	4.50	4.16	3.78	3.36
	2.5	6.55	5.10	4.47	4.12	3.89	3.73	3.51	3.28	3.02	2.72
	5	4.75	3.88	3.49	3.26	3.11	3.00	2.85	2.69	2.50	2.30
	10	3.18	2.81	2.61	2.48	2.39	2.33	2.24	2.15	2.04	1.90
	20	1.84	1.85	1.80	1.77	1.74	1.72	1.69	1.65	1.60	1.54
13	0.1	17.81	12.31	10.21	9.07	8.35	7.86	7.21	6.52	5.78	4.97
	0.5	11.37	8.19	6.93	6.23	5.79	5.48	5.08	4.64	4.17	3.65
	1	9.07	6.70	5.74	5.20	4.86	4.62	4.30	3.96	3.59	3.16
	2.5	6.41	4.97	4.35	4.00	3.77	3.60	3.39	3.15	2.89	2.60
	5	4.67	3.80	3.41	3.18	3.02	2.92	2.77	2.60	2.42	2.21
	10	3.14	2.76	2.56	2.43	2.35	2.28	2.20	2.10	1.98	1.85
	20	1.82	1.83	1.78	1.75	1.72	1.69	1.66	1.62	1.57	1.51
14	0.1	17.14	11.78	9.73	8.62	7.92	7.43	6.80	6.13	5.41	4.60
	0.5	11.06	7.92	6.68	6.00	5.56	5.26	4.86	4.43	3.96	3.44
	1	8.86	6.51	5.56	5.03	4.69	4.46	4.14	3.80	3.43	3.00
	2.5	6.30	4.86	4.24	3.89	3.66	3.50	3.29	3.05	2.79	2.49
	5	4.60	3.74	3.34	3.11	2.96	2.85	2.70	2.53	2.35	2.13
	10	3.10	2.73	2.52	2.39	2.31	2.24	2.15	2.05	1.94	1.80
	20	1.81	1.81	1.76	1.73	1.70	1.67	1.64	1.60	1.55	1.48
15	0.1	16.59	11.34	9.34	8.25	7.57	7.09	6.47	5.81	5.10	4.31
	0.5	10.80	7.70	6.48	5.80	5.37	5.07	4.67	4.25	3.79	3.26
	1	8.68	6.36	5.42	4.89	4.56	4.32	4.00	3.67	3.29	2.87
	2.5	6.20	4.77	4.15	3.80	3.58	3.41	3.20	2.96	2.70	2.40
	5	4.54	3.68	3.29	3.06	2.90	2.79	2.64	2.48	2.29	2.07
	10	3.07	2.70	2.49	2.36	2.27	2.21	2.12	2.02	1.90	1.76
	20	1.80	1.79	1.75	1.71	1.68	1.66	1.62	1.58	1.53	1.46
16	0.1	16.12	10.97	9.00	7.94	7.27	6.81	6.19	5.55	4.85	4.06
	0.5	10.58	7.51	6.30	5.64	5.21	4.91	4.52	4.10	3.64	3.11
	1	8.53	6.23	5.29	4.77	4.44	4.20	3.89	3.55	3.18	2.75
	2.5	6.12	4.69	4.08	3.73	3.50	3.34	3.12	2.89	2.63	2.32
	5	4.49	3.63	3.24	3.01	2.85	2.74	2.59	2.42	2.24	2.01
	10	3.05	2.67	2.46	2.33	2.24	2.18	2.09	1.99	1.87	1.72
	20	1.79	1.78	1.74	1.70	1.67	1.64	1.61	1.56	1.51	1.43
17	0.1	15.72	10.66	8.73	7.68	7.02	6.56	5.96	5.32	4.63	3.85
	0.5	10.38	7.35	6.16	5.50	5.07	4.78	4.39	3.97	3.51	2.98
	1	8.40	6.11	5.18	4.67	4.34	4.10	3.79	3.45	3.08	2.65
	2.5	6.04	4.62	4.01	3.66	3.44	3.28	3.06	2.82	2.56	2.25
	5	4.45	3.59	3.20	2.96	2.81	2.70	2.55	2.38	2.19	1.96
	10	3.03	2.64	2.44	2.31	2.22	2.15	2.06	1.96	1.84	1.69
	20	1.78	1.77	1.72	1.68	1.65	1.63	1.59	1.55	1.49	1.42
18	0.1	15.38	10.39	8.49	7.46	6.81	6.35	5.76	5.13	4.45	3.67
	0.5	10.22	7.21	6.03	5.37	4.96	4.66	4.28	3.86	3.40	2.87
	1	8.28	6.01	5.09	4.58	4.25	4.01	3.71	3.37	3.00	2.57
	2.5	5.98	4.56	3.95	3.61	3.38	3.22	3.01	2.77	2.50	2.19
	5	4.41	3.55	3.16	2.93	2.77	2.66	2.51	2.34	2.15	1.92
	10	3.01	2.62	2.42	2.29	2.20	2.13	2.04	1.93	1.81	1.66
	20	1.77	1.76	1.71	1.67	1.64	1.62	1.58	1.53	1.48	1.40
19	0.1	15.08	10.16	8.28	7.26	6.61	6.18	5.59	4.97	4.29	3.52
	0.5	10.07	7.09	5.92	5.27	4.85	4.56	4.18	3.76	3.31	2.78
	1	8.18	5.93	5.01	4.50	4.17	3.94	3.63	3.30	2.92	2.49
	2.5	5.92	4.51	3.90	3.56	3.33	3.17	2.96	2.72	2.45	2.13
	5	4.38	3.52	3.13	2.90	2.74	2.63	2.48	2.31	2.11	1.88
	10	2.99	2.61	2.40	2.27	2.18	2.11	2.02	1.91	1.79	1.63
	20	1.76	1.75	1.70	1.66	1.63	1.61	1.57	1.52	1.46	1.39

TABLE A.6. Continued

df_2	df_1	1	2	3	4	5	6	8	12	24	∞
20	0.1%	14.82	9.95	8.10	7.10	6.46	6.02	5.44	4.82	4.15	3.38
	0.5%	9.94	6.99	5.82	5.17	4.76	4.47	4.09	3.68	3.22	2.69
	1 %	8.10	5.85	4.94	4.43	4.10	3.87	3.56	3.23	2.86	2.42
	2.5%	5.87	4.46	3.86	3.51	3.29	3.13	2.91	2.68	2.41	2.09
	5 %	4.35	3.49	3.10	2.87	2.71	2.60	2.45	2.28	2.08	1.84
	10 %	2.97	2.59	2.38	2.25	2.16	2.09	2.00	1.89	1.77	1.61
	20 %	1.76	1.75	1.70	1.65	1.62	1.60	1.56	1.51	1.45	1.37
21	0.1	14.59	9.77	7.94	6.95	6.32	5.88	5.31	4.70	4.03	3.26
	0.5	9.83	6.89	5.73	5.09	4.68	4.39	4.01	3.60	3.15	2.61
	1	8.02	5.78	4.87	4.37	4.04	3.81	3.51	3.17	2.80	2.36
	2.5	5.83	4.42	3.82	3.48	3.25	3.09	2.87	2.64	2.37	2.04
	5	4.32	3.47	3.07	2.84	2.68	2.57	2.42	2.25	2.05	1.81
	10	2.96	2.57	2.36	2.23	2.14	2.08	1.98	1.88	1.75	1.59
	20	1.75	1.74	1.69	1.65	1.61	1.59	1.55	1.50	1.44	1.36
22	0.1	14.38	9.61	7.80	6.81	6.19	5.76	5.19	4.58	3.92	3.15
	0.5	9.73	6.81	5.65	5.02	4.61	4.32	3.94	3.54	3.08	2.55
	1	7.94	5.72	4.82	4.31	3.99	3.76	3.45	3.12	2.75	2.31
	2.5	5.79	4.38	3.78	3.44	3.22	3.05	2.84	2.60	2.33	2.00
	5	4.30	3.44	3.05	2.82	2.66	2.55	2.40	2.23	2.03	1.78
	10	2.95	2.56	2.35	2.22	2.13	2.06	1.97	1.86	1.73	1.57
	20	1.75	1.73	1.68	1.64	1.61	1.58	1.54	1.49	1.43	1.35
23	0.1	14.19	9.47	7.67	6.69	6.08	5.65	5.09	4.48	3.82	3.05
	0.5	9.63	6.73	5.58	4.95	4.54	4.26	3.88	3.47	3.02	2.48
	1	7.88	5.66	4.76	4.26	3.94	3.71	3.41	3.07	2.70	2.26
	2.5	5.75	4.35	3.75	3.41	3.18	3.02	2.81	2.57	2.30	1.97
	5	4.28	3.42	3.03	2.80	2.64	2.53	2.38	2.20	2.00	1.76
	10	2.94	2.55	2.34	2.21	2.11	2.05	1.95	1.84	1.72	1.55
	20	1.74	1.73	1.68	1.63	1.60	1.57	1.53	1.49	1.42	1.34
24	0.1	14.03	9.34	7.55	6.59	5.98	5.55	4.99	4.39	3.74	2.97
	0.5	9.55	6.66	5.52	4.89	4.49	4.20	3.83	3.42	2.97	2.43
	1	7.82	5.61	4.72	4.22	3.90	3.67	3.36	3.03	2.66	2.21
	2.5	5.72	4.32	3.72	3.38	3.15	2.99	2.78	2.54	2.27	1.94
	5	4.26	3.40	3.01	2.78	2.62	2.51	2.36	2.18	1.98	1.73
	10	2.93	2.54	2.33	2.19	2.10	2.04	1.94	1.83	1.70	1.53
	20	1.74	1.72	1.67	1.63	1.59	1.57	1.53	1.48	1.42	1.33
25	0.1	13.88	9.22	7.45	6.49	5.88	5.46	4.91	4.31	3.66	2.89
	0.5	9.48	6.60	5.46	4.84	4.43	4.15	3.78	3.37	2.92	2.38
	1	7.77	5.57	4.68	4.18	3.86	3.63	3.32	2.99	2.62	2.17
	2.5	5.69	4.29	3.69	3.35	3.13	2.97	2.75	2.51	2.24	1.91
	5	4.24	3.38	2.99	2.76	2.60	2.49	2.34	2.16	1.96	1.71
	10	2.92	2.53	2.32	2.18	2.09	2.02	1.93	1.82	1.69	1.52
	20	1.73	1.72	1.66	1.62	1.59	1.56	1.52	1.47	1.41	1.32
26	0.1	13.74	9.12	7.36	6.41	5.80	5.38	4.83	4.24	3.59	2.82
	0.5	9.41	6.54	5.41	4.79	4.38	4.10	3.73	3.33	2.87	2.33
	1	7.72	5.53	4.64	4.14	3.82	3.59	3.29	2.96	2.58	2.13
	2.5	5.66	4.27	3.67	3.33	3.10	2.94	2.73	2.49	2.22	1.88
	5	4.22	3.37	2.98	2.74	2.59	2.47	2.32	2.15	1.95	1.69
	10	2.91	2.52	2.31	2.17	2.08	2.01	1.92	1.81	1.68	1.50
	20	1.73	1.71	1.66	1.62	1.58	1.56	1.52	1.47	1.40	1.31
27	0.1	13.61	9.02	7.27	6.33	5.73	5.31	4.76	4.17	3.52	2.75
	0.5	9.34	6.49	5.36	4.74	4.34	4.06	3.69	3.28	2.83	2.29
	1	7.68	5.49	4.60	4.11	3.78	3.56	3.26	2.93	2.55	2.10
	2.5	5.63	4.24	3.65	3.31	3.08	2.92	2.71	2.47	2.19	1.85
	5	4.21	3.35	2.96	2.73	2.57	2.46	2.30	2.13	1.93	1.67
	10	2.90	2.51	2.30	2.17	2.07	2.00	1.91	1.80	1.67	1.49
	20	1.73	1.71	1.66	1.61	1.58	1.55	1.51	1.46	1.40	1.30
28	0.1	13.50	8.93	7.19	6.25	5.66	5.24	4.69	4.11	3.46	2.70
	0.5	9.28	6.44	5.32	4.70	4.30	4.02	3.65	3.25	2.79	2.25
	1	7.64	5.45	4.57	4.07	3.75	3.53	3.23	2.90	2.52	2.06
	2.5	5.61	4.22	3.63	3.29	3.06	2.90	2.69	2.45	2.17	1.83
	5	4.20	3.34	2.95	2.71	2.56	2.44	2.29	2.12	1.91	1.65
	10	2.89	2.50	2.29	2.16	2.06	2.00	1.90	1.79	1.66	1.48
	20	1.72	1.71	1.65	1.61	1.57	1.55	1.51	1.46	1.39	1.30
29	0.1	13.39	8.85	7.12	6.19	5.59	5.18	4.64	4.05	3.41	2.64
	0.5	9.23	6.40	5.28	4.66	4.26	3.98	3.61	3.21	2.76	2.21
	1	7.60	5.42	4.54	4.04	3.73	3.50	3.20	2.87	2.49	2.03
	2.5	5.59	4.20	3.61	3.27	3.04	2.88	2.67	2.43	2.15	1.81
	5	4.18	3.33	2.93	2.70	2.54	2.43	2.28	2.10	1.90	1.64
	10	2.89	2.50	2.28	2.15	2.06	1.99	1.89	1.78	1.65	1.47
	20	1.72	1.70	1.65	1.60	1.57	1.54	1.50	1.45	1.39	1.29

TABLE A.6. Continued

df₂	df₁	1	2	3	4	5	6	8	12	24	∞
30	0.1%	13.29	8.77	7.05	6.12	5.53	5.12	4.58	4.00	3.36	2.59
	0.5%	9.18	6.35	5.24	4.62	4.23	3.95	3.58	3.18	2.73	2.18
	1 %	7.56	5.39	4.51	4.02	3.70	3.47	3.17	2.84	2.47	2.01
	2.5%	5.57	4.18	3.59	3.25	3.03	2.87	2.65	2.41	2.14	1.79
	5 %	4.17	3.32	2.92	2.69	2.53	2.42	2.27	2.09	1.89	1.62
	10 %	2.88	2.49	2.28	2.14	2.05	1.98	1.88	1.77	1.64	1.46
	20 %	1.72	1.70	1.64	1.60	1.57	1.54	1.50	1.45	1.38	1.28
40	0.1	12.61	8.25	6.60	5.70	5.13	4.73	4.21	3.64	3.01	2.23
	0.5	8.83	6.07	4.98	4.37	3.99	3.71	3.35	2.95	2.50	1.93
	1	7.31	5.18	4.31	3.83	3.51	3.29	2.99	2.66	2.29	1.80
	2.5	5.42	4.05	3.46	3.13	2.90	2.74	2.53	2.29	2.01	1.64
	5	4.08	3.23	2.84	2.61	2.45	2.34	2.18	2.00	1.79	1.51
	10	2.84	2.44	2.23	2.09	2.00	1.93	1.83	1.71	1.57	1.38
	20	1.70	1.68	1.62	1.57	1.54	1.51	1.47	1.41	1.34	1.24
60	0.1	11.97	7.76	6.17	5.31	4.76	4.37	3.87	3.31	2.69	1.90
	0.5	8.49	5.80	4.73	4.14	3.76	3.49	3.13	2.74	2.29	1.69
	1	7.08	4.98	4.13	3.65	3.34	3.12	2.82	2.50	2.12	1.60
	2.5	5.29	3.93	3.34	3.01	2.79	2.63	2.41	2.17	1.88	1.48
	5	4.00	3.15	2.76	2.52	2.37	2.25	2.10	1.92	1.70	1.39
	10	2.79	2.39	2.18	2.04	1.95	1.87	1.77	1.66	1.51	1.29
	20	1.68	1.65	1.59	1.55	1.51	1.48	1.44	1.38	1.31	1.18
120	0.1	11.38	7.31	5.79	4.95	4.42	4.04	3.55	3.02	2.40	1.56
	0.5	8.18	5.54	4.50	3.92	3.55	3.28	2.93	2.54	2.09	1.43
	1	6.85	4.79	3.95	3.48	3.17	2.96	2.66	2.34	1.95	1.38
	2.5	5.15	3.80	3.23	2.89	2.67	2.52	2.30	2.05	1.76	1.31
	5	3.92	3.07	2.68	2.45	2.29	2.17	2.02	1.83	1.61	1.25
	10	2.75	2.35	2.13	1.99	1.90	1.82	1.72	1.60	1.45	1.19
	20	1.66	1.63	1.57	1.52	1.48	1.45	1.41	1.35	1.27	1.12
∞	0.1	10.83	6.91	5.42	4.62	4.10	3.74	3.27	2.74	2.13	1.00
	0.5	7.88	5.30	4.28	3.72	3.35	3.09	2.74	2.36	1.90	1.00
	1	6.64	4.60	3.78	3.32	3.02	2.80	2.51	2.18	1.79	1.00
	2.5	5.02	3.69	3.12	2.79	2.57	2.41	2.19	1.94	1.64	1.00
	5	3.84	2.99	2.60	2.37	2.21	2.09	1.94	1.75	1.52	1.00
	10	2.71	2.30	2.08	1.94	1.85	1.77	1.67	1.55	1.38	1.00
	20	1.64	1.61	1.55	1.50	1.46	1.43	1.38	1.32	1.23	1.00

REFERENCES

LINDQUIST, E. F., *Design and Analysis of Experiments in Psychology and Education.* Boston: Houghton Mifflin Company (1956).

SIEGEL, S., *Nonparametric Statistics for the Behavioral Sciences.* New York: McGraw-Hill Book Company (1956).

WINER, B. J., *Statistical Principles in Experimental Design.* New York: McGraw-Hill Book Company (1962).

APPENDIX B

18,000 COMPUTER-GENERATED RANDOM DIGITS

NOTE

The computer program used to generate this table did not print some zeros. Missing digits therefore should be interpreted as zeros. The table can be entered at any point in any row or column; any consecutive series of digits is random.

Appendices

```
169 413 585 482 750  94 222 716 722 835 776 401 336 986 858
288 208 464 387 354 416 136 196 469 685 436 230 388  54 194
205 524 517 986 377 653 818 728 320 588 629 773 298 449 439
638 274 921 431  72 173 682 607 693 363 845 564 294 208 879
980 925 878 708  35 156 728  85 276 884 405 428  85 205 325
132  75 975 370 561 375 222  42 419  40 829 490 857 358  37
975 129 942 843  45 844 782 488  29 281 325  85 380 302 296
656  94 875 727 221 689 689 549 405 323 487 102 562 585 441
160 401 772 769 921 532  92 895 164 407 990 841 952 793 980
 53 558 756  74 536 994 352 433 340 537 558 125 652 488 916
879 736 583 520 925 173 283 539 560 556 436 180 345 786 669
797 388 695 449 727  86 527 332 300 497 589 954 197 325 768
866 708 922  18  34 962 609 139 759 980 611 102  77 872 591
 22 750 272  60 663 992 908 840 848 402 365  23 690 307 629
336 126 338 200 669 294 967 793 259 589 685 220 444 996 451
812   3 576 652  43 830 629 195 917 914 829 112 455 212  43
851 881 411 111 235 337  74  25 174 185 801 687 729 300 199
796 260 277 799  21 544 778 396 788 882 347 113 277 896 803
112 628 963 791  10 232   1 149 158 624 869 492  99 672  23
507 420 285 556 868 495   4 329 856 808  88 934  97 964 905
 30 870  39 216 119 878  12 632 712 228 707 171 688 730 223
619 434 668 292 898 814  35 833 563  94 446 616 253 708 193
443 776 655 805 315 981 102 306 970 514 308 160 324 670 146
 85 747 912 198 805 561 299 338 750 233 832 411 669 652 140
517 492 578 941 995 534 867 271 771 771 221  26  93 875 525
338 230 260 863 719 146 513 583 873 527 836 455 535 380 834
366 946 353 708 358  74 274  57 291 222  27 489 377 409 581
155 606 779 475 675 128  23  97 893 581 638 842 443  31 530
635 117 495 479 826  94 668  67 732 488 578 650 262 499 947
414 251 954 592 874 410 796 524 354 698 727 315 580 712 908
768 449 266 238 810 618 766 541 535 797 156  42 123 781 921
883 434   6 103 989  15 425 523  20 501 390 413 515 277 353
383 558 647 473 643 523 655 267 302 830 929  99 980 630 822
352 438 821 909 955   2 108 895 632 466  68 872 239 285 757
664 606 103 193 945 301 749 966  73 322  39 339 618  32 142
811 690 229 974  71 788 521 742 749 737 620 184 553 630  38
888 688 442 104 924  16 384 756 836 524 373  52 751 486 942
 30 912 587 854 898   2 612 852 272 506 655 660 530 248 309
183 278 544 186  72 867 217 308 105 318 569 487 413 112 378
826 463 978 428 349 178 791 178 178 356 515 979 707 439 485
312 275 971 888 446 266 790 300 125 273 966 488 529 618 503
431 476  25 477 532 992 619 195 144 432 157 113 806 760 657
778 380 406 870 179 558 599 466 739 131 247 285  72 995 408
788 992 210 922 285 413  21  33 133 896  69 691 175 122 532
731 535 608 701 101 457 730   8 148 192 192 578 404 781 523
289 277 754 907  35  23 194 745 689  86 529 248 842 582 345
153 847  48 131 299  27 592 398 797 781 444 286 418 461 366
312 588 501 616 479 953 802 682 579 913 902 479 921 527  84
492 901 576 520 185 471 483 502 301 448 412 305 769  12 212
141 116 945 571 794 244 678 873 592 469 352 514 318 328 514
```

```
860 318  47 356 961 580  83 659 443 740 476 724  87 505 438
425 431 866  97 209 792 392  18  10 719 866  98 173 338 918
807 721 771 375 599 525 603 174  69 654 904  76 249 486 566
 13 443 836 380 716  24  92 882 325 454 632 569 940 866 129
819 168  69 903 899 416 125 724 324 833 655 726 391 823 681
793  18 892 995 949 273 914 406  18 911 234 237 887 142 919
382 593 727 839 605 893 359 919 189 967 512 885 800 444 381
150 394 332  75  81 898 929 857 972 602 963 172 817 389  18
467  22 451 895  44 350 341 871 127 905 165  69 698 330 678
443 584 716 695 531  19 677 509  10   7 317 866 829 483 900
460 309 233 113 789 960 995 215 918 899 418 570 690 923 297
766 594 950 418 953 589 872 703 415 324 653 625 680 191 678
455 781 603 489 616 896 281 287 223 853 158 617 867 833 393
836 336  69 170 112  68 833 388 602 201  68  78  77 279 255
921 987 980 617 129 345 463 743 601 527 985 911 656 173 990
999 900 260 170 759 455 283 966 187 356 299 764 239 525 637
705 512 740 466 395 618 532 107 713 388 927 382 530 587 912
234 973  94 264 533 616 637 947 592 124 864 408  25 798 739
 53 230 900 386 643 132  34 718 137 252 846  14 376 496 224
213 619 558 938  57 242 470 788 488 395 293 406  31 795 689
802 641 245 145 555 264 515 263 696 102 144 309 798 304 118
890 273 444 432 816 405 859 484 781  55 226 196 506 673 502
118 866 453 281 900  45 516 535 425 408  56 393 853 295 953
696 734 723 798  53 629 360 853 515 947 305 595 562 714 195
110 614 258 260 218 364 515 304 262   9 323  35 690 626 589
397  72  34 375 826 521 848 146 939 530 189 849  79 331 782
391 904 883 911 994 850 452 132 275  99 231 776 262 351 387
772 778 987  85 528 408  80 479 197 822 679  16 857 121 283
105 527 972 312 223 796 412 683 701  42 993 111 781 569 216
686 160 949  99 583 105 748 788 433 856 846 522 966 321 745
167 218 942 787 485 464 780 578 290 751 141 125 769 807 529
822 865 107 828 665 835 944 369 839 799 229  55 915 951 465
432 228 161 886 621 829 647  11 428  39  99 198 564 434  31
186 581   6 860 734 460 381 745  10  40 529 694 149  49 994
231 436 584 182 816 295 463 371 211 884 285 378 818 384 683
708 385 446 346 286 630 345 521 172 939 947  21 566 859 153
169 383 416 442 377 123 897 781 132 678 113 725  36 692 766
638 836 479 532 679  67 278 999 239 617 157 155 119 422 220
307 561 129 215 685 290 593 965 243 601 921 404 386 302 427
 98 845 461 501 996 137  51 792 305  50 111  26 247   7 577
825  18 604  64 804 208 971  66 642 890 373 523   2 327 620
 65 494 472 872 857  13 366 267 102 886 240 899 789 896 523
966 804 390 660 907 209 452   5 835 300  78 684 712 428 556
207 375  93 105 728 135 416 620  88 825 306  14 168 503 626
545  15  49 690 206 922 427 677   7 246 131 924 595 160 752
402 712 453 195 679 320 817 481 252  52  35 422  56 432 877
510 132 275 957 220 615  56 788 441  97  26 208 984 147 495
438 382 567 986 204 812 985 398 379 112 844 451 395 993  73
 37  99 926 305 246 332 403 295 304 798 826 831 513 633 987
275 157 448 951 632 678 548 183 413 777 360 928 521 856 261
```

Appendices

```
921 334  51 779 471 642 518 946 719 448 303 950 696 344 479
693 805 887 991 416 647 799 347 110 857 539  90 865 214 331
867 822 855 931 256 104 128 565 188 113 508 985 923 188 668
958 692 148 664 795 797 572 265 134 962 192  98 757 198  29
947 746 189 603 461 847 280 504 106 754 580 725 232 496 158
 56 252 806 639 610 910 526 635 434 860 753 467 572 191 684
817 792 131 409 514 832 640 274 645 374 291 275 346 683 681
393 481 528 699 589 800  98 929 963 500 971 445 922 377 933
  4 757 988 506 908 311 826 107 973 634 201 191 414 114 466
484 212 178 745 145 665  79 278 165 302 464 137 188 288 395
869 455 170 914 700 193  33 706 232 109 973 100 396 694 177
851 820 418 781 887 171 486 732 901 930 661 362 687 571 504
285 824 975 458  22 286 620  34 320 599 209 272 557 181 431
 54 558  80 718 150 176 340 614 805 221 306 369 153 946  47
750 933 708 179 699 479 459 372 950 928 956 766 904  44 400
 18 573 520 615 843 284 693 704 453 581 976 273  44 754 976
351  37 751  70 767 392  23 872 163 131 250 739 128 124 255
945  62 822 886  15 797 898 898 903 557 718 980 371 954 745
504  42 169 687 188 248 181 539 950 158  51 227  77 603 167
518 685 614 143 990 316   5 147 568 932 844 537 116  31 300
573 735 160 672 243 662 398  33 855 169 608 175   3 752 290
772 240 430 745 542 127 342 871  15 630  46 215 973 233  42
473 827 135 420  68 803 469 927 396 254 804 713 806 629 639
884 797 938 818 524 674 733 723 238 851 408 344  75 676 456
 46 338 414 121 534 816 178 998 868 821 208 646 194 393 979
321 853  39 364 485 830 470 476  60 262 572 774 489 271 770
512  73 512  91 102 632 215 871 548 184 555 829 184  90 810
180 760 718 274 241 324  57 936 747 741 183  11 699  97 927
469 902 693 821 530 253 403 777 553 789  96 602 538 766 270
190 566 696 454  10 601 900 241 592  63 928 507 931 725 275
918 276 938 332 288 323 771 449 568 275 704 626 747 453 217
793 562 361 909 634 529 528 522  80  82 869 187  98 189 825
496 887 719 462 210 259 223  84 366  18 877 491 860  62 998
839 262  60 587 555 797 583 807 472 367 433 259 280 666 559
569 586 890 358 440 443 496  87 540  33 704 133 934 434 367
863 155 799 868 644 487 724 253 986 893 328 465  86 610 174
 52 652 785 981 899 933 875 733  54  62 630 593 108 748 732
545 515 514  72 598 215 735 120 450 332 824 369 873 994 830
799 222  19 598 492 887 531 120 209 429 270 870 263 232 387
886 693 490 938 571 386 568 640 201 588 204 901 719 446 846
123 159 767 239 995 335 629 757 326 663 790 573 948 585 596
764 713 185 991 829 536 659 775 146 688 903 329 210 497 958
473 849 208 795  17 197 288 837 940 157 306 816 729 712 381
962 675 579 845 636 354 798  45 324 745 709 933 482 797 664
509 404 597 915 660 352 194 737 477  60 494 251 333 375 553
397 344 369 885 235 920 985  19 950 649 583 103 653  75 333
797 433 838  71 469 352 159 478 400 355  53 357 918  73  25
204 493 708 461 700 825  90 695 849 284  63 219 635 762 148
 51  62 704 126 980 780 104 861 493 505 902  93 543 913 662
466 936 854 601 578 257 814 911 314 475 845 590 539 616 637
```

```
 25  495  202  571  873  355  432  122  329  807  642  743  366  872  911
955  919  588  669  920  512  632  773  578  756  495  960  858  711  404
510   62  705  876  657  875  904  536  511  267  183   69  853  419  229
456   98  939  233  661  642  736  256  859  797  648  772  397  109  735
150   25  288  510   49  974  277  707  553  381  234   11  701  882  344
790  266  273  960  342   63   32  939  587  108  571  112  636  309  445
389  370   45  174  613  608  700  271  538  215  321  574  503  918  572
226  825  808  398  595   81  910  170  947  319  786  434  289  721  424
853  613  442  819   58   12  158  577  836  979  822  435  209   65  398
 77  256  383  333  984  338  761  932  487    2  856  704  649  896  565
785   13  312  621  385  921  138  390  399  198  742  306   11  789  809
 14  775  429  728  451  478  980  954    2  164  741  495  228  669  768
 15  529  761  780  234  579  638  211  424  203  768  215  260  911  320
961  196  705  128  348  170    1  682  523  742  936  832  512  439    9
625  413  376  743  978  809  269  192  318  621  700   49  729  435  174
100  715  908  303  734  321  597    5  204   50  777  808  762  658  963
978  571   59  131  603  640  160  306  361  706  362  405    5   35  204
964  984  181   62    7  954  591  784  325  789  176  157  175  288  558
981  764  554  187  615  959  103  953  695  374  798  293    1  406  510
207  726  698  564  620  166  293  654  248  142  202  344  426  844   38
409  481  198  700  183  365  828  346  229  484   29  422  548  409  636
591  345  900  117  520  696  336  193  138  628  355  431  450  852  469
863  739  621  401  467  891  557   41  761  410  868  790  766  428   88
860  330  623  352  119   77  318  502  326  804   12  455  540  900  309
386  324  145  501  510  444  890  643  105  128  259   18  345  546   58
574  972  265  840  989  971  480  340  693  535  443  415  206  176  570
971  921  281  525  343  827  865  249  210   54  322  320  127  136  895
656  771  296  589  160  221  873  431   21  506  942  185  911  232  235
199  336  244  803  872  879  449  338  239  551  754  229  318  170  356
285   79  802  548  784  282  833  150  243  747   43  708  708  928   16
917  445  613   11  856  776  959  851  299  519  468  186  387   36  890
937  959  453  131   81  121  254  756  608  392  417  743  946  862  194
373  747  201  687  775  736  891  878  954  680  291  779  190  843  157
797  850  133  940  921  326   56  461  251  545  986  989  628  295  190
424  369  980  455  550  332  318  866  919  151  299  922   54  186  727
370  564  687  267   11   61  400   42  254  996  916  628  670  456  650
407   64  298  504  116  370  533  458  254  618  805  468  538   63  355
108  305  600  614  591  672  598  363  236  742  583  155  194  276  275
984  252  916  152  501  700  788   57  127  883  248  719  316   84  452
931  765   94  377  682  154  347   76  636  622  239  914  152   16  237
733  326  317  898  582  621  986  935  667  778  198   17   64  340  350
 16   66   54  991  354  337  790  925  277   71   34  871   11  892  968
491  460  468  861  825  433  868  136  658  419  415   72  488  293  660
803  163  317  247  122  563   92  489  452  875  181  590  830  726  241
397  834  690  728  763  474  739  708  790  478  354  890  583  722  506
152  533  289  144  481  777  604  843  667  987  490   26   29  794  864
340  690  518  306   17  394  966  689  893  624  754  148  918  267  629
668  341  504  539  774  373  359  545  350  854  111  652  251  453  999
948  838  363  482  487  689  465   66   65  510  880  577  238  310  329
672  958  639   35  957  773  551  488  232  373  277  593  169  784  981
```

```
955 405 213 516 563 201 406 983 757 590 229 492 501 657 739
  3 526 549 426 339 767  79 619 307 665 371 814 802 470 600
423 503 374 909 966 794 812 867  29 678 161 456 300 912 945
509 288 304 618 744 860 160 631 412  85 625 409 582 236 272
242 193 458 529 764   6 655 979 210 405 304 349 786 206 125
872 565   7 613 886 299 487 192 547 663 194 406 474 110 294
 46 655 924 909 438 736  22 339 393 332 429 297 772 801 639
430 842 477 938 648 723 750 302 431  22 828 125 360 814 189
164 155 541 445 947 707 300 760  49 140 101  74 216 676 376
112 347 951 225 846 735  52 837 415 639 155 324  54 728 553
192 691 836 341 554  45 611 181  46 573  17 270 371 281 935
140  18 453  20 705 655 196 552 537 688 705 707 744 135 627
108 889 190  50 246 521 671 682 806 969  78 808 120 283 350
387 165  62 125 124 229 266 126   5 616 124 483  19 477 449
347 988 653 292 531 685 552 613 770 977  35 626  34 313 545
595 447 362 631  64  50 916 541 576 311  96 405  35 581 231
445 787 294 153 604 129 523 730 519  73 252 793 902 670 474
308 693 502 234  48 324 888 508 931 639 651 117  90 783 766
346  77 366  29 852 786 623 479 909 170 634 561 423 670 326
301 219 680  66 673 795 743 302  75 272 943 310 722 972  63
189 621 780 131 371 696 847 499 270  98 954 808 526 797 442
423 747 562 191 167  17 400 276 938 142 231  57 656  31  82
833 896 346 964 664 835 769 160 198 963 797  71 199   9 512
188 652  14  65 475 856  16 476 746 500 706 908 291 774 331
634 842 572 709 872 613 168 413 689 332  55 808 953 562 374
108 183 706 664 957 977 868 196 421 490 979 674  99 411 257
937 519 483 605 894 341 692 453 322 947 371 767  15 401 180
647 464 542 648 748 255 337 954 139 272 418 534 199 708 761
448 107 901 442 444 453 792 645 934 102 162 296  56 632 945
867 468 528 824 930 423 713 288 348 164 209 972 538 424 821
170 845  59 961 581 463 149 921 683  66 800 164 724 847 420
213 854 605 346 112 970 479 926 963 913 912 230 502 271 129
743 514  93 431 444 649 532 268 627 888 273 903 498 996 991
538 399 112 469 655 159 878 270  90 108 424 343 464 535 777
544 764 829 929 931 112 475 212 894 648  86 935 303 245 741
419 990 965 352 683 234 947 838 553 915 699 517 635 657 457
612  65 331 746 722 395 407 116 272 661 416 688  86 734  70
901 478 300 310 180 262 915 148 655 728 202 473 796 491 302
901 283 819 142 586  16 824 848 482 417 469 637   3 335 178
291 398 208  59 889 734 702 751 995 947 995 568 853 588 352
636 839 873  74  61 255 798 872 632 930 743 669  85 515 505
199 448 369 909 362 927 468 472 836  55 501 905 830 791 863
466 133 356 785 617 262 625 976 323 964 321 405 217 112 630
 10 765 809 526 443 227 535 610 415 283 415 283 826 551  10
858 395 648  85  98   2 581 871 582  17 600  53   7 296 387
 58 481 606 775 603 969 666 740 754 558 861 765 604 812 232
625 329 802 885 732 797 766 597 284 193 761 112 555 208 911
225 640 357 330 964  57 604 915 914 131 820 785 894 939 375
725 882 918  14 195 166 726 118 925  49  66 700 369 757  48
323 525 296 115 493 484 919 470 319 111  15 134 163  92 910
```

18,000 Computer-Generated Random Digits

```
 65 229 808  37  54 528 773 170 718 235 210 512 149 979 733
833 550 879 965 155 898  69 251 377 343 548  37 775 772 158
408 237   2 452 442 628 452 970 801 936 392 614 311 821 352
955 473 102  30 256 687  87 564 406 531 419 351 887 977 688
 55 699 591 107 556 470 457 649 227 755 988 576 519 472 954
730 935 624 368  27 634 954 818 709 752 153 299 127  40 532
885 316 428 242 153 572 607  63 203 712  22 605  88 987 601
735 479 949 138 677 729  60  21 838 505 755 940 378 559 815
443  31 836 651 679 223 893 555 196 618 324 190 477 469 477
 41 873 476 661 978 773 815 136 637 160 152 676 458 787 527
257 960 328 108 760 634 850 818  51 391 989 349 457 496 868
170 902 686 696 752 842 763 682 575 906 568   6 616 888 466
703 772 161 203 672 345 925 726 988 916 499 890 583 867 978
685 509 784 948 261 490 683 217 752 339 885 283 955 205 678
786 106 254 862 516 834 768 767 616 789 816 687 481 422 261
542  48 470 637 746 587 461 644 933 683 929 573 289 690 463
180 336 529  59 828  21 849 959  50   0 226 249 403 337 427
202 581 941 615 249 835 946 952 896 849 995 335 812 807 388
587 464 885 161  45 824  28  82 926  86 928 767 241 810 488
702 551 838 429  27 424 651 923 493 879 614 584 137 594 432
929 129  56 123 749 127 655 796 622 494 331 598 649 268 194
251 811 793 877 254 942  72 471 290  55 456 325 666 262 273
141 703 253 152 781 507 532 657 142 879 751 565 149 161 895
589 913 385  16 396 556 546 700 241 780 401 468 899 605 908
262 154  27 730 343 774 484 286 165 762 647 719  48 179 389
270 705 696 236 495 639 986 414 817 552 267  99 197 626 162
263 839 936 840 881 864 557 911 413 452 780 125 743 145 470
149 689 344 915 826 431 471 734 121 737 275 855 685 234 358
522 576 641 930  28 808 807 201   8 356 628   8 423  99 914
792 258 748 341 726 964 602 604 960 495 295 349 374 487 258
 50 359 718 673 107 514 347 810 688 765 116  17 435  27 321
171 833 572 967 104 403 658 422 484 135  39 961 235 777 604
576 760 968 744 660 786 823 238 710 924 188 609 499 419 731
913  65 656 756  19  93  16 625 900 331 778   0 872 515 949
290 548 225 841 175 480 683 608  11 665 973 519 741 316 116
521 702 441 244 877  41 954  25 958  14 834 114 599 258 150
519 277 625 888 683 923 572 672 648  97 249   6 920 706 856
420 339 774 133 203 165 845 809 267 448 982  11 126 914 784
844 545  18 801  73 683 923 803 769 816 651   9 475 125 996
284 214 140 614 609 607 930 538 206 863  63 947 712 520 923
105 378 676 470 991 498 268 996 317 831 514 601 995 996 567
 74 336 792 292 461 522 237 131  47 221 519  81 561 287  94
497 614 668 515 850 647   6 819 422 839 481  79 405 762 459
311 661 876 465 944 177 901 731 108  48 216 743 384 983 911
393 438 244 149  13 241 356  15 854 734 959 741 653  42 330
551 680 581 709 581 851  21 506 147 965 812 758 461 401 779
774 134 286 910 367 931 924 398 194 185 236 877 891  26 705
680 679 488  76 971 926 349 833 837 418 111 437 190 547 215
109 870 348 265 517 178 779 915 275 844 538 733 121  47 947
536 107 695 907 363 730 530 992 119 301 226 457  11 360 747
```

Appendices

```
679 954 223  51 638  72  68 958 882 122 227  52  50 128  88
727 880 693 799 240 213 302 439 484 218 728 514 375 967 135
248 686 146 337 697 628 196  11 962 210 321 615 796 646  17
940 200 639 830  19 848 458 114 418 295 377  61 400 177 883
406  19 520 942 835 438 981 580 850 875 368 830 236 243 139
976 314 371 182 838 988 765 452 330 592 813 433 814 866 886
198 710 543 612 507 986 760 488 333 676 562 123 756   2  68
406 434 914  34 501  22 672 864  20 730  59 842 207 218 432
649 206 597 697 439 256 189 784 126 293 291 940 440 291 977
242 335 357 874 124 340  81 930 571 180 212  66 775 779 970
609 150 768 974 790 731 788 520 290 442 652 930 689  56  25
472 884 392 970 621 325 996 746 602  32   6 986 154 325 416
349 950 440  53 615 371 883 793 998 215 165 548 721 441 275
847 743 111 589  93 299 325  39 567   0 935 412 935 720 902
942 908 704  58  28 455   7  99 422  61 122 532 124 350 933
 25 758 223  42 325  33 111 237 424 363 312 488 326 619 475
667 373 999 724 697 108 603 533 748 632 772 134 831 559 452
777 408 980 968 252 343 619  63 667 521 825 407  53 782 439
655  92 892 288 239  90 279 578 269 440 995 240 838 663 562
935 877 526  18 168 445 106 899 613 944 546 774 549 938 415
712 433 127 515 854 859 121 193 253 704 321 477 755 660 430
855 705  26 925 604 149 770  65   0 728   6 897 580 515 846
719 329  16 911 939 165 533 649 726  32 152  86 687 145 206
618 626 856 143 196 645 263 306 348 632 850 441 900 233 619
231 792 995 657 718 385 783 992 553 505 735 872 213  93 857
824 114 262 653 547 500 326 203 189 341 755 259 181 458 570
862 559 617   6 816 531 906 283 151 497 914 706 165 914 706
756 320 338 152 971 686 500 870 209 909 689 901 354 360 110
773 893 473 859 485 338 837 671 889 980 911  50 641 928 302
831 470 797 782 166 850 525 197 451 693 258 191 656 331 819
 27 784 520 957 627  52 614 143 707 335 347 692 169 629 191
678 471 943 700 272 662 957  82 178 774 762 426 108 791 774
820 769 979 582 981 501 213 199 706 621 442 331 124  83 920
822 370 381 189 442  47 658 461 626 763 793 147 770 378 553
548 299 478 898 818 770  31 966 406 984 783 906 496 521  35
886 459 433 685 928 196 261 651 798  37 560 106  48 722 231
386  62 294  23 203 245 281 207 130 367 309 482 820 646  76
337 240 865 972 864 707 338 379 594 865 806 935 489 369 370
549 880 540 623 352  33 494 412 389 887  59 272 546 403 534
254 114 453 990 332 834 922  56 986 533  97 209 874  95 876
584 764 856 332 822 710  78 626 413 216  45 809 332 936 449
220 555  57  76 943 748 172 253 605 496 398 968 124 762 809
 57 449 633 468 263  97 325 880 908  32 977 527 751 145 807
364 703 285 124  88 846 404 997   3 726 277 449 388  13 562
667 174  10 533 156 200 497  62 841  61 868 952 562 772 103
725 712 493  77 140 582 341 392  19 836 716 670 881 511 556
340 706 866 660 433 694 570 799 543 458 480 449 226 114 408
516 822 755 270 336 924 347 260  84 228 433 660 427  82 449
 30 578 735 676 119 296 953 369 617 244 275 914 526 463  15
538  72 611 621 691 456 590 867 946 404 755 547 311  43  50
```

```
160 327 143 429 732 629 936 602 529 793 682 724 311 763 646
505 467 616 856 765 510 477 949 575  13  70 766 212 810 193
593 857 412 277   0 396 435 279 684 942 281  76 475 991 343
  8 939 923 954 115 786 316 129 928 530  54 563 939 659 313
706 920 830 233 689 153 981 261 412 700 792 691 354  28 794
166  65 668 806  94 837  40 403 121 429 266  80 678 237 938
640 105 539 739 365 647 408  65  12 268 466 254 673 166 485
341  49 215 175 340 341  87 759 982 747 396 806 139 861 464
286 346 442 398 756 226 842 967 779  72 178 548 972 669 419
647 629 713 806 473 281 268 962 835 705 509  32 584 259 335
302 659 299 256  33 651  32  71   0 584 445 254 751 529 240
991 294 376 280 946 376 774 768 483 154  88 233 247 846 424
223 832 567 370 372 394 360 962 895 670 522 113 721 313 379
415 344  16 697 718 980 188 862  19 632 343 576 100 258 458
433 573 992 852 960 327 887 507  53 758 357 434 113 732 329
163 339 806 837 295 145 628 285 149 853  48 419 776  70 852
630 876 906 354 126 922 783 140 408 301  78 610 639 828 149
315 202 179 595  95 226  40 276 110 124  33 885 846 342 224
218 319 920 375 435  53 196 392 986  33 491 816 322 596   5
468  99 908 898 756 280 810 866 919  77 644 930 316 497  12
845 718 166  10 618 204  95 667 645 161 445 239 993 614  23
856 420 824 973 905 702 279 206 592 271 872  59 117 204  25
531  55 452 747 867 372 821 230 745 178 228 201 761 699 942
475 547 291 722  59 915 411 526 140 626 518 671 514 357 422
 70 734 678 608 547 144  72  86 136 155  53 214 231 850  52
147 779 445 147 745 620 733 780 555 290 655 238 757 886 507
247 617 565 412 547 426 746 908 105 348 455 505 465 671 578
161 693 386 147 573 973 878 426 634 470 828 885 974  44 897
740 598 230 165 512   6 553 384 855 687 877 764 661 226 181
992 352 903 668 913 275 415 461 422 892 807 614 195 960  11
284 728 347 523 865 596 513 313 832 171 942 808 218 723 435
777 204 958 126 971 101 340 724 194 992 391 314 553 690 507
108 664 618  42  35 234 427 529 678 413 864 615 352 636 122
646 151  90 119 471 497 498 655 319 545 662 861 132 602 169
905 925 974 332 509 874 139 161 808 551 198 627 626 883 910
614 191  32 918 813 768 350  72 973 405 226  11 563 881 938
542 817 422 515 297 738 849 979 562 466 574 427 743 335 434
721 176 242 824 466 513 939 228 616 147 408 459 389  79 155
444 706 652 309 122 440 996 554 637 690 282 907 648 458  26
175 649 726 432 534  18 520 274 279 810  15 313 386  33 760
 55 535 491 807 103 147 158 650 938 650 553 709 481  74 323
749 369 409 957 811 715 264 434 109 613 179 436 407 146  94
  1 395  27 473 939 969 158 752 212 823  95 232 109 208 658
257  46 484 226 335 377 577 605 290 418 962 466 992 928  99
538 734 656  99 554 538  33 864 830 103 911 700 973 699 670
907 973 579 557 312 833   4 740 370 853 806   8 904 840 127
600 225 572 448 882 152 725 656 748 184 637 748 667 744 728
438 590 217 672 481 417 313 279 154 431 560 408 360 903 220
222 520 153   2 949 128 352 763 189 925 629 717 157 719 768
388 804 968 958 362  15 295  66 749 669 731 628 196 187 630
```

GLOSSARY

Many of the terms relevant to statistics and research design that were used in this book are briefly defined here. For definitions of other terms or for more complete definitions of those defined, consult the index. For a glossary of symbols used in Appendix A, see p. 282. Words set in SMALL CAPITAL LETTERS are defined elsewhere in the Glossary.

ALPHA LEVEL. See LEVEL OF CONFIDENCE.

ANSWERABLE QUESTION. A question that can be answered by observations which can be made and that implicitly or explicitly (preferably the latter) specifies the observation or observations necessary to answer it.

APPLIED RESEARCH. RESEARCH that implicitly or explicitly is intended to increase our understanding of how to prevent the development of, or modify behaviors contributing to, communicative disorders.

ATTRIBUTES OF EVENTS. Measurable or verbally describable properties of EVENTS.

"BEFORE AND AFTER" DESIGN. Research design in which measures are made before and after the administration of a TREATMENT (e.g., a therapy program).

BIVARIATE DISTRIBUTION. A DISTRIBUTION in which observations are assigned to categories on the basis of two of their ATTRIBUTES.

CAUSALITY. Assumption of the scientific method that every event has a cause.

CHANCE. See RANDOM FLUCTUATION.

CLINICIAN-INVESTIGATOR. A speech pathologist or audiologist who functions as both a clinician and a clinical investigator.

CONFIDENCE INTERVAL. An INFERENTIAL STATISTIC for estimating POPULATION values of DESCRIPTIVE STATISTICS and differences between such statistics.

CONSTANT SUMS. A PSYCHOLOGICAL SCALING METHOD.

CORRELATION COEFFICIENT. An INDEX OF ASSOCIATION.

CRITERION MEASURE. A measure of an ATTRIBUTE of an EVENT.

CUBIC RELATIONSHIP. A NONLINEAR RELATIONSHIP between VARIABLES (see Figure 5.5).

CURVILINEAR RELATIONSHIP. A NONLINEAR RELATIONSHIP between VARIABLES (see Figure 5.4).

DATA. Symbolic representations (numerical or verbal descriptive) of ATTRIBUTES of EVENTS. See QUALITATIVE and QUANTITATIVE DATA.

DEGREES OF FREEDOM. This value for a set of DATA designates the DISTRIBUTION in a table that contains the critical value of the statistic for testing the NULL HYPOTHESIS.

DEPENDENT MEASURES. Sets of measures made on the same subjects or on matched groups of subjects.

DEPENDENT VARIABLE. A VARIABLE whose value one seeks to determine.

DESCRIPTIVE STATISTICS. Indices that describe an ATTRIBUTE of a set of measures. See MEASURES OF ASSOCIATION, CENTRAL TENDENCY, and VARIABILITY.

df. Abbreviation for DEGREES OF FREEDOM.

DIRECT MAGNITUDE-ESTIMATION. A PSYCHOLOGICAL SCALING METHOD.

DISTRIBUTION. A set of categories to which measures are assigned. See BIVARIATE, MULTIVARIATE, and UNIVARIATE DISTRIBUTIONS.

END EFFECT. A piling up of ratings in one or both of the extreme intervals when the method of EQUAL-APPEARING INTERVALS is used.

EQUAL-APPEARING INTERVALS. A PSYCHOLOGICAL SCALING METHOD.

EVENT. A phenomenon that occurs in a certain place during a particular interval of time.

EXPERIMENTAL CONDITION. A set of circumstances under which observations are made.

EXPERIMENTER BIAS. The impact of an experimenter's expectations and beliefs on his observations.

EXTENSIONAL DEFINITION. Pointing to or exhibiting in some way the actual objects, phenomena, and so on which the term you wish to define refers to.

FACE VALIDITY. Refers to a test or observational procedure intuitively appearing to be valid for the purpose intended.

GENERALITY. The extent to which the persons or events observed are representative of those in the POPULATION to which a question refers.

HYPOTHESIS. A tentative theory adopted to explain certain observations.

INDEPENDENT MEASURES. Sets of measures made on different groups of persons.

INDEPENDENT VARIABLE. A VARIABLE whose values are known.

INDEX OF ASSOCIATION. See MEASURE OF ASSOCIATION.

INDEX OF CENTRAL TENDENCY. See MEASURE OF CENTRAL TENDENCY.

INDEX OF VARIABILITY. See MEASURE OF VARIABILITY.

INDIVIDUAL SUBJECT DESIGN. A research design that permits the performance of individual subjects under the experimental condition or conditions to be RELIABLY determined.

INFERENTIAL STATISTICS. Indices that allow one to answer several kinds of questions about a set of data that go beyond analyses that were made of it. See SIGNIFICANCE TESTS and CONFIDENCE INTERVALS.

INTERVAL SCALE. A measurement SCALE in which NUMERALS designate points on a continuum which have equal amounts of the ATTRIBUTE being MEASURED between them.

LABORATORY SETTING. An artificial controlled environment in which observations are made.

LEVEL OF CONFIDENCE. States how small the PROBABILITY of a NULL HYPOTHESIS being true has to be before it is rejected. See SIGNIFICANCE TESTS.

LINEAR RELATIONSHIP. When two VARIABLES are linearly related, an increase (or decrease) in the magnitude of one is associated with a proportional increase (or decrease) in the magnitude of the other. The points in a SCATTERGRAM for two VARIABLES that are linearly related lie on a straight line.

LOGARITHMIC SCALE. A measurement SCALE in which NUMERALS designate points on a continuum which have unequal, but known, mathematically defined amounts of the ATTRIBUTE being MEASURED between them.

MEAN. An INDEX OF CENTRAL TENDENCY which is the arithmetic average of a set of measures.

MEASUREMENT. The assignment of NUMERALS to ATTRIBUTES of EVENTS according to rules.

MEASUREMENT ERROR. Various forms of RANDOM and SYSTEMATIC ERROR which influence the RELIABILITY of observations.

MEASURES OF ASSOCIATION. Indices used to describe the strength and direction of the relationships between sets of measures.

MEASURES OF CENTRAL TENDENCY. Indices that designate the "average," "typical," or most frequently occurring NUMERAL in a set of numerals. See MEAN, MEDIAN, and MODE.

MEASURES OF VARIABILITY. Indices that designate the spread, dispersion, homogeneity, or variability of a set of NUMERALS.

MEDIAN. An INDEX OF CENTRAL TENDENCY; it is that measure which occurs at the midpoint of a set of measures when they are ordered from lowest to highest (or from highest to lowest).

MODE. An INDEX OF CENTRAL TENDENCY; it is the most frequently occurring measure in a set of measures.

MULTIVARIATE DISTRIBUTION. A DISTRIBUTION in which observations are assigned to categories on the basis of two or more of their attributes.

N. Abbreviation for number of subjects.

NEGATIVE RELATIONSHIP. A relationship between two VARIABLES in which individuals who tend to score highly on one tend to have relatively low scores on the other, and vice versa (see Figure 5.3).

NOMINAL SCALE. A measurement SCALE in which NUMERALS merely designate, or label, categories.

NONLINEAR RELATIONSHIP. When two VARIABLES are not linearly related, an increase (or decrease) in the magnitude of one is not associated with a proportional increase (or decrease) in the magnitude of the other. The points in a SCATTERGRAM for the two VARIABLES would not lie on a straight line.

NONRANDOM SAMPLE. A SAMPLE that was not generated by a RANDOM SAMPLING METHOD.

NORMAL DISTRIBUTION. A symmetrical, bell-shaped curve in which certain relationships hold regarding its height at specified distances from its center (see Figure 8.1).

NULL HYPOTHESIS. The hypothesis tested by a SIGNIFICANCE TEST; it states that observed differences or relationships are due to CHANCE, or RANDOM FLUCTUATION.

NUMERALS. Number symbols; their meanings are determined by the rules used to assign them.

ONE-TAILED TEST. A SIGNIFICANCE TEST intended to detect a difference between measures (e.g., means) in one direction only.

ORDER EFFECT. A phenomenon that systematically improves or impairs a subject's performance on a series of tasks (e.g., fatigue).

ORDINAL SCALE. A measurement SCALE in which NUMERALS designate locations in a rank order.

ORGANISMIC VARIABLES. Properties, or ATTRIBUTES, of the individual. Examples are sex, chronological age, and educational level.

PAIRED COMPARISONS. A PSYCHOLOGICAL SCALING METHOD.

PLACEBO EFFECT. Changes produced by placebos, i.e., therapeutic procedures that are objectively without specific activity for the condition being treated.

POPULATION. The group of persons to whom a question refers.

POSITIVE RELATIONSHIP. A relationship between two VARIABLES in which individuals who tend to score highly on one also tend to score highly on the other, and vice versa.

PROBABILITY. The likelihood of the occurrence of an event.

PSYCHOLOGICAL SCALING METHODS. Techniques for MEASURING, or quantifying, ATTRIBUTES of EVENTS through the use of observer judgments.

PURE RESEARCH. Research that implicitly or explicitly is intended to increase our understanding of the etiology of communicative disorders.

QUALITATIVE DATA (or CONCEPTS). Verbal descriptions of ATTRIBUTES of EVENTS.

QUANTITATIVE DATA (or CONCEPTS). Numerical descriptions of ATTRIBUTES of EVENTS.

RANDOM ERROR. A form of error present to some degree in all MEASUREMENT processes that does not bias the data resulting from such processes.

RANDOM FLUCTUATION. Unpredictable variation in measures of ATTRIBUTES of EVENTS.

RANDOM SAMPLE. A SAMPLE selected by a random sampling process, e.g., a table of random numbers.

RATIO SCALE. A measurement SCALE in which NUMERALS designate points on a continuum which both have equal amounts of an ATTRIBUTE between them and are related to an absolute 0.

RELIABILITY. This refers to the repeatibility of the observations used to answer a question.

REPLICATION. Repetition of a study or observational procedure used to answer a question or questions.

REPRESENTATIVENESS. Refers to the extent to which the ATTRIBUTES of the persons or EVENTS in a SAMPLE are similar to those in the POPULATION from which the sample was selected.

RESEARCH. This refers to the processes underlying the asking and answering of questions. See APPLIED RESEARCH and PURE RESEARCH.

RESEARCH HYPOTHESIS. The hypothesis an investigator seeks to test.

SAMPLE. Part of a POPULATION.

SCALE. A succession or progression of steps or degrees, or a graduated series of categories.

SCALE VALUE. The point, or value, on a SCALE to which an event (e.g., speech segment) is assigned. Scale values are computed for ratings generated by PSYCHOLOGICAL SCALING METHODS.

SCALING METHODS. See PSYCHOLOGICAL SCALING METHODS.

SCATTERGRAM. A two-dimensional graphical display used for assessing the relationship between two variables (see Figures 5.1 through 5.6).

SCIENTIFIC METHOD. A set of rules for asking and answering questions.

SEQUENCE EFFECT. Occurs when a subject's performance on a task is enhanced or impaired by his having performed a particular task prior to it.

SIGNIFICANCE TESTS. INFERENTIAL STATISTICS used to estimate the PROBABILITY that observed differences and relationships between DESCRIPTIVE STATISTICS resulted from RANDOM FLUCTUATION.

STATISTICAL INFERENCE. Statistical techniques that provide information needed to generalize beyond a set of DATA or SAMPLE of subjects. See CONFIDENCE INTERVALS and SIGNIFICANCE TESTS.

STATISTICALLY SIGNIFICANT RESULT. A finding is regarded as statistically significant if the NULL HYPOTHESIS is rejected.

STATISTICS. Numerical procedures for analyzing, organizing, and summarizing QUANTITATIVE DATA. See DESCRIPTIVE STATISTICS and INFERENTIAL STATISTICS.

SUBJECT BIAS. Results from subjects responding to experimental conditions in the manner in which they feel the experimenter either would like them to respond or expects them to respond.

SUCCESSIVE INTERVALS. A PSYCHOLOGICAL SCALING METHOD.

SYSTEMATIC ERROR. A form of error that can be present in a MEASUREMENT process which can bias the DATA resulting from that process.

SYSTEMATIC OBSERVATION. A process that permits individual ATTRIBUTES of EVENTS to be described with adequate levels of RELIABILITY and VALIDITY.

TREATMENT. An experimental condition under which subjects are observed.

TWO-TAILED TEST. A SIGNIFICANCE TEST intended to detect a difference between measures (e.g., means) in either direction.

TYPE I ERROR. Rejection of the NULL HYPOTHESIS when it should not have been rejected, i.e., when the observed difference or relationship really was the result of RANDOM FLUCTUATION.

TYPE II ERROR. Failure to reject the NULL HYPOTHESIS when it should have been rejected.

TYPICAL SUBJECT DESIGN. A research design that permits the average (i.e., mean, median, or mode) performance of the subjects in a group under the experimental condition or conditions to be RELIABLY determined.

UNIVARIATE DISTRIBUTION. A DISTRIBUTION in which observations are assigned to categories on the basis of one of their ATTRIBUTES.

VALIDITY. The appropriateness of observations for answering a question they are used to answer.

VARIABLE. A quantity that can assume more than one value. See DEPENDENT VARIABLE and INDEPENDENT VARIABLE.

AUTHOR INDEX

Abbs, J. H., 114, 161
Abelson, R. P., 163
Adams, J., 22, 25
Anderson, D., 22, 25
Angle, E., 99, 107
Arndt, W. B., 77, 87, 254, 269
Aronson, A. E., 7, 11, 16, 25, 51, 64, 230, 243

Barlett, C. J., 140, 162
Barnhart, E. N., 140, 161
Barrett, M., 140, 162
Baynes, R. A., 16, 22, 25
Beasley, D. S., 224, 227
Berry, R. C., 103, 107
Berry, W. R., 51, 64
Bloodstein, O., 39, 44, 102, 107
Bloom, C. M., 10, 12, 68, 87
Bosma, J. F., 162
Bradfield, S. S., 168, 169, 215
Bridgman, P. W., 33, 44
Brown, J. R., 7, 11, 16, 25
Buckley, W., 42, 44
Burkland, M., 22, 25
Bush, S. G., 28, 42-44

Campbell, D. T., 75, 78, 87, 94, 108, 140, 163, 254-257, 269
Campbell, S. K., 179, 215
Carmone, F. J., 199, 215
Carney, P. J., 11, 12
Carrol, J., 114, 162
Cody, R. C., 22, 25
Compton, A. J., 11, 12
Crawford, P. L., 140, 162
Cronbach, L. J., 32, 44
Cullinan, W. L., 140, 162
Curlee, R. F., 31, 45

Darley, F. L., 9, 11, 16, 25, 51, 58, 64, 159, 163
Daniloff, R. G., 10, 12
Davis, M. D., 215
Dempsey, M. E., 114, 162
Draugert, G. L., 162

Dukes, W. F., 78, 87
Dunn, L. M., 7, 11, 128, 162
Dutt, P. K., 140, 163

Ebel, R., 158, 159, 162, 195, 215
Edwards, A. L., 32, 44, 134, 152, 162, 261, 269
Egan, J. P., 6, 11
Einstein, A., 38, 45, 250
Eisler, H., 140, 162
Ekman, G., 140, 162
Elbert, M., 77, 87, 254, 269
Engen, T., 140, 162

Feigl, H., 33-39, 45
Fisher, C. G., 11, 12
Fletcher, S. G., 114, 162
Forscher, B. K., 239, 243
Freeman, G. G., 16, 25
Fruchter, B., 197, 215

Galanter, E. H., 140, 162, 164
Gall, F. J., 57
Gay, T., 114, 162
Gilbert, B. N., 114, 161
Goldstein, N. P., 51, 64
Goldstein, R., 19, 25
Golenpaul, D., 176, 215
Gottman, J. M., 15, 25, 78, 88
Green, P. E., 199, 215
Guilford, J. P., 78, 88, 134, 158, 162
Gutter, F. J., 275, 276

Halbach, M., 24, 25
Hamre, C. E., 19, 25
Hanley, T. D., 114, 162
Harris, C. W., 256, 269
Harris, K. S., 114, 162
Hays, W. L., 78, 88, 176, 215
Head, H., 42, 43, 45, 93, 107, 218, 227
Heerman, E., 140, 162
Hempel, C. G., 101, 107
Hevner, K., 140, 163
Hicks, J. M., 140, 163
Hixon, T. J., 163

Holloway, G., 114, 163
Holloway, M. S., 9, 12
Holtzman, W. H., 78, 88
Hoshiko, M., 114, 163
Hotchkiss, J. C., 224, 227
House, A. S., 224, 227
Hovland, C. I., 163

Infeld, L., 38, 45

Jenkins, J. J., 16, 26, 99, 108
Jerger, J., 11, 19, 25, 78, 88, 99, 107, 239, 243
Jiménez-Pabón, E., 16, 26, 99, 108
Johnson, W., 7, 11, 15, 20, 24, 26, 36, 45, 63, 64, 90, 93, 98, 107, 126, 159, 163
Johnston, R. G., 141, 164
Jordon, E. P., 160, 163

Kavanaugh, J. F., 58, 64
Kelley, H. H., 140, 163
Kelsey, C. A., 114, 163
Keppel, G., 78, 88
Kimball, A. W., 275, 276
King, D. J., 140, 163
King, L. S., 239, 243
King, P. S., 10, 12
Kools, J. A., 225, 227
Korzybski, A., 42, 45
Kramer, J. C., 22, 26
Kuhn, T. S., 28, 42, 43, 45
Kunnapas, T., 140, 162, 163

La Croix, Z., 22, 26
Ladefoged, P., 114, 163
Lau, A. W., 140, 163
Lauder, E., 22, 26
Lewis, D., 103, 107
Lilly, D. J., 11, 12
Lindquist, E. F., 78, 81, 88, 312, 326
Lore, J. I., 275, 276

McBurney, D. H., 140, 162
McCall, G. J., 170, 215
McClelland, K. D., 168, 169, 215
Manley, M. B., 140, 164
Manning, J. I., 224, 227
Marshall, R. C., 10, 12
Meitus, I. J., 224, 227
Messick, S., 140, 162
Minifie, F. D., 163
Misra, R. K., 140, 163
Moll, K. L., 114, 163
Moodie, C. E., 140, 164 (see also Prather, E. M.)
Moore, M. V., 239, 243
Moore, P. G., 114, 163
Morley, D. E., 11, 12, 58, 64
Mower, D., 107, 108

Orne, M. T., 112, 163
Osgood, C. E., 261, 262, 269

Paesani, A., 168, 169, 215
Palmer, B., 24, 25
Pap, A., 40, 41, 45

Perkins, W. H., 31, 45
Perloe, S. I., 140, 163
Peters, R., 114, 162
Pfeiffer, M. G., 140, 163
Polanyi, M., 60, 64
Porch, B., 92, 108
Powers, M. H., 19, 26
Prather, E. M., 134, 140, 162, 162 (see also Moodie, C. E.)

Rapoport, A., 215
Rettig, S., 140, 162
Ringel, R. L., 19, 26, 224, 227
Roberts, W. H., 19, 26
Roland, C. G., 239, 243
Rorschach, H., 128, 163
Rosenthal, R., 57, 64, 111, 163, 224, 227, 249, 258, 269
Rosnow, R., 258, 269

Saffir, M. A., 140, 164
Sanders, L. J., 114, 164
Schatzman, L., 170, 215
Schrest, L., 94, 108
Schuell, H., 16, 26, 99-108
Schultz, M. C., 19, 26
Schwartz, M., 163
Schwartz, R. D., 94, 108
Senn, D. J., 140, 164
Shapiro, A. K., 260, 269
Sheehan, J. G., 58, 64
Shelton, R. L., 77, 87, 162, 168, 169, 215, 254, 269
Sherman, D., 11, 12, 103, 107, 132, 140, 148, 160, 164, 223, 227
Shore, I., 22, 26
Shriner, T. H., 9, 12, 160, 164
Sidman, M., 49, 50, 64, 78, 88
Siegel, S., 140, 163, 195, 208, 215, 300, 326
Silverman, E.-M., 153, 164
Silverman, F. H., 10, 12, 24, 25, 68, 87, 88, 103, 107, 140, 141, 148, 152-154, 156, 158, 159, 164, 182, 215, 235, 243, 267, 269
Simmons, J. L., 170, 215
Siskind, R. P., 162
Slipakoff, E., 22, 26
Smith, C. C., 162
Snider, J. G., 262, 269
Sommers, R. F., 58-64
Soron, H. I., 114, 164
Speaks, C., 11
Spriestersbach, D. C., 159, 163, 223, 227
Stanley, J. C., 75, 78, 87, 254, 257, 269
Steer, M. D., 162
Stevens, S. S., 97, 98, 108, 140, 164
Stewart, K. C., 114, 164
Stone, G., 140, 164
Stout, M. B., 125, 164
Strauss, A. L., 170, 215
Strunk, W., 239, 243
Suci, G. J., 261, 262, 269
Summers, J., 22, 26

Author Index

Talbott, R. E., 8, 12
Tannenbaum, P. H., 261, 262, 269
Templin, M. C., 7, 11, 12, 58, 64
Torgerson, W. S., 199, 215
Trelease, S. F., 239, 243
Tretsven, V. E., 22, 26
Trotter, W. D., 225, 227, 267, 269

Van Riper, C., 269
Von Leden, H., 163

Webb, E. J., 94, 108
Wertz, R. T., 239, 243

Wessell, M., 22, 26
White, F. D., 163
Wilkstroem, I., 140, 163
Williams, D. E., 5, 12, 15, 26, 140, 162, 235, 243
Wilson, F. B., 16, 26
Winer, B. J., 78, 88, 158, 164, 312, 326
Wolfe, D., 197, 215
Woodford, F. P., 239, 243

Yairi, E., 19, 26, 169, 215
Young, M. A., 195, 215

SUBJECT INDEX

Abstracts journals:
   use of in formulating research, 58, 59
Academy of Aphasia, 241
Academy of Cerebral Palsy, 241
Acoustical Society of America, 241
Alexander Graham Bell Association, 241
Alpha level (*see* Statistics)
American Cleft Palate Association, 241
American Psychological Association, 239, 241
American Speech and Hearing Association, 14, 21, 71, 94, 153, 229, 230, 240, 274
American Statistical Association:
   listing of statisticians, 21
Analogue to digital converter, 121
Analysis of variance (*see* Statistics)
"Answerable" questions, 62-64
Answers to questions, tentative nature of, 15, 16
Aphasia (*see* Examples)
Applied research, 3
Articulation disorders (*see* Examples)
Articulation test response forms, 37
Asha, 240
ASHA Monographs, 240
ASHA Reports, 240
Asking and answering questions, 1-341
Attributes:
   of events, 5
   quantified by means of scaling methods, 132, 133
   relation to data, 89-91
   "target," 134-139
Audiogram form, 37, 38
"Authority," 61

Beliefs, need to modify, 39, 40
Bias, experimenter (*see* Experimenter bias)
Binomial distribution (*see* Statistics)
"Brainstorming," 61

Canadian Speech and Hearing Association, 241
Causality, 31, 32, 40

Chance fluctuation (*see* Random fluctuation)
Chi square distribution (*see* Statistics)
Chi square test (*see* Statistics)
Cinefluorographic techniques, 114
Cleft palate (*see* Examples)
Clinical decision making, 4, 5, 8, 14-16
Clinician-investigator:
   benefits from functioning as, 14-20
   definition, 13
   essential competencies, 25
   functions, 13
   impact of scientific method on, 27
   need for clinicians to function as, 17-20
   qualifications, 20-25
   why clinicians may be in an advantageous position to function as, 18-20
Clinician-researcher dichotomy, 19, 20
Closed watch illustration, 38
Coherence or systematic structure, 44
College of Speech Therapists, 241
Communicating research findings (*see* Reporting research findings)
Computer services, 51
Computational appendix, description of organization, 170-172
Confidence intervals (*see* Statistics)
Constant sums (*see* Scaling methods)
Consultants, use of, 19, 21, 51
Contingency coefficient (*see* Statistics)
Convention papers (*see* Reporting research findings)
Correction factors, 126, 127
Correlation coefficients (*see* Statistics)
Council of Exceptional Children, 241
Criterion measures, 69, 75, 80

Data, 89-107
   from clients' folders, 23
   clinical, 16
   definition, 5, 89-92
   examples of types of used by speech pathologists and audiologists, 91, 92

Subject Index 347

Data (*cont.*)
  measurement-related properties of quantitative data, 97-107
  normative, 7
  observational error and reliability, 66, 67
  organizing, 165-215
    approaches for, 166
    in narrative form, 168, 169
    need for, 165, 166
    qualitative, 166-170
    quantitative, 170-215
    strategies for qualitative data, 166-170
    use of tables for, 168
  qualitative, definition of, 5
  quantitative, definition of, 5
  types of, 92-97
    qualitative, 92-94
    qualitative vs. quantitative, 94
    quantitative, 94-97, 109-161
Definiteness and precision, 44
Degrees of freedom (*see* Statistics)
Describing events, 29, 30
Differential diagnosis, 5, 28
Direct magnitude-estimation (*see* Scaling methods)
Discriminant function analysis (*see* Statistics)
Dissertation Abstracts, 58, 59
dsh Abstracts, 58, 59, 229, 235, 241, 243
Dysarthria (*see* Examples)

Electrodes, 115
Electromyography, 114
Equal-appearing intervals (*see* Scaling methods)
Errors:
  gross, 125, 126, 129
  random, 125, 128-130
  systematic, 125-130
    environmental, 126, 127, 129
    instrumental, 126, 127, 129
    observational, 126-130
Events:
  definition, 29
  measurement of, 97, 98
  need for precision in defining, 35
  prediction of, 32, 40
  relation to data, 89-91
Examples:
  aphasia, 10, 28, 35, 42, 43, 53, 59, 63, 68, 69, 72, 91-93, 95, 99, 112, 166, 170, 190, 191, 195-197, 213, 218
  articulation disorders, 4, 6, 7, 9, 33, 35, 36, 63, 74, 77-80, 89-91, 95, 96, 99, 100, 104-107, 112, 128-130, 139, 140, 147, 153, 166-168, 170, 174, 185, 192, 194, 200, 201, 211, 223, 225, 253, 254
  attributes of events of interest to speech pathologists and audiologists, 133
  cleft palate, 63, 68, 159, 160, 175, 181, 223
  clinical programs, 74

Examples (*cont.*)
  dysarthria, 9, 81, 157, 168, 170, 175, 179, 207, 234
  hearing loss, 7, 8, 35, 37-39, 56, 57, 59, 60, 63, 66, 78-80, 91, 95, 99-101, 106, 112, 126, 127, 168, 169, 183, 184, 197, 198, 200, 222, 251, 261, 262
  hypernasality, 95, 131, 134-139, 145-147, 158, 159, 168, 195
  language and language disorders, 7, 9, 71, 112, 148-150, 168-170, 176-178, 181, 191, 208, 219
  laryngectomy, 160, 188, 250, 251
  scheduling therapy, 61
  stuttering, 4, 5, 7, 10, 11, 30, 34, 39, 50, 55, 56, 60, 62, 63, 66-68, 70, 73, 75-77, 79-83, 95, 101, 102, 104, 106, 122, 145-147, 152, 153, 156, 160, 172-174, 179, 180, 186-188, 194, 195, 197-199, 203, 204, 206, 210, 211, 218, 225, 226, 249-251, 262-264
  therapy outcome assessment, 75
  velopharyngeal closure, 168, 169, 197, 198
  verbal output, 9
  voice disorders, 7, 35, 51, 78, 80, 169
Experimenter bias, 57, 58, 111, 146, 165, 223-226, 249, 258, 259
Explanation as hypothetico-deductive procedure, 37, 38
Explaining events, 30-32
Extensional definition, 36

F distribution (*see* Statistics)
Factor analysis (*see* Statistics)
"Facts," 39
Filters:
  electronic, 115, 116
  role in systematic observation, 5, 6, 57
Finitude of relevant factors, 41, 42
Ford Foundation, 274
Friedman two-way analysis of variance (*see* Statistics)
Funding for research, 52, 54, 55, 274, 275

Galvanic skin response, 114, 122
Generality:
  of answers, 217, 220-222, 226
  as consideration when selecting a research design, 87
  differences between individual and typical subject designs, 69
  of nonrandom samples, 56, 221
  population concept, 201, 202
  of qualitative data, 94
  of quantitative data, 97
  relation to scientific method, 27
  in reporting research findings, 232
  use of inferential statistics for assessing, 201, 202
  "logical" basis for, 71, 72
  statistical basis for, 71

General Semantics formulations:
　abstraction, 89-91
　allness, 20
　identification, 24
　interrelatedness of events, 42
　levels of abstraction, 98
　map-territory analogy, 90, 91, 93, 94, 231
　space-time continuum, 250, 251
General Systems theory, 42
Group designs (see Research designs, typical subject)

Heart Association, 274
High-speed photography, 114
History of science, relationship to scientific method, 27, 28
　(see also Scientific method)
Hypernasality (see Examples)
Hypotheses:
　null, 204-207, 223, 224, 248, 249, 257, 258, 295, 297, 298, 300, 302, 304, 306, 307, 309, 311, 313
　research, 204, 248, 249
　tentative nature of, 15, 16
　"testable," 15

Iowa Scale for Rating Severity of Stuttering, 159
Index Medicus, 58
Individual subject designs (see Research designs)
Instrumentation schemes for measurement:
　calibration errors and validity, 222, 223
　components of, 114-122
　　amplification stage, 115
　　control stage, 116
　　data reduction and analysis stage, 121
　　detection stage, 114, 115
　　modification and shaping stage, 115, 116
　　recording and readout stage, 116-121
　　transmitting stage, 116
　illustration of function, 122
Interdisciplinary research, exploiting opportunities for, 18, 19
International Association of Logopedics and Phoniatrics, 241
Interquartile range (see Statistics)
Intersubjective testability, 43
Intraclass correlation coefficient (see Statistics)

Jewish Hospital in St. Louis, 16
Journal articles (see Reporting research findings)
Journal of Communication Disorders, 241
Journal of Speech and Hearing Disorders, 7, 8, 21, 22, 52, 53, 58, 91, 168, 171, 200, 217, 229, 236, 240
Journal of Speech and Hearing Research, 7, 8-11, 52, 132, 133, 171, 200, 217, 236, 239, 240

Kendall coefficient of concordance (see Statistics)
Kruskal-Wallis one-way analysis of variance (see Statistics)

Language and Language Behavior Abstracts, 58, 59, 235
Language and language disorders (see Examples)
Language, Speech, and Hearing Services in Schools, 21, 52, 171, 229, 240
Laryngectomy (see Examples)
Letters to the Editor (see Reporting research findings)
Levels of confidence (see Statistics)
Lingual strength measurement, 114
Literature search, 56-59
Loading effects, 126, 127

Mann-Whitney U test (see Statistics)
Marquette University, 110
Mayo Clinic, 16
Mean (see Statistics)
Measurement:
　definition, 36, 97, 98
　error:
　　line measuring illustration, 110
　　random, 110, 111, 223, 224
　　sources from readout devices, 125-128
　　systematic, 110-112, 223-226, 255-257
　instrumentation for, 114
　from magnetic tape recordings, 125
　psychological and educational instruments, for, 128-130
　of readouts from instrumentation schemes, 122-125
　　by distance measuring, 123
　　by frequency counting, 123-125
　role of the observer in the measurement process, 109-113
　scales of:
　　interval, 95, 96, 102-104, 132, 135-137, 140, 141, 172, 175, 176, 178-181, 188, 189, 192, 195, 200, 206, 207, 214
　　logarithmic, 96, 106, 107, 172, 200
　　nominal, 95, 98-101, 172, 176, 179, 186, 188-190, 206, 207
　　ordinal, 95, 100-102, 132, 134, 135, 140, 172, 175, 176, 178-181, 185, 186, 188-192, 195, 200, 206, 207, 214
　　ratio, 96, 104-106, 132, 137-139, 141, 172, 175, 176, 178-181, 188, 189, 192, 195, 200, 206, 207, 214
　scaling methods, 112, 113, 130-161
　schemes that utilize an instrument to supplement observer judgment, 113-130
　use of instrumentation for, 112
Measures, significance tests for (see Statistics)

Median (*see* Statistics)
Meters, 117, 122, 123, 126
Microphones, 115
Minneapolis Veterans' Administration Hospital, 16
Mode (*see* Statistics)
Multidimensional scaling (*see* Statistics)
Multiple correlation (*see* Statistics)
Multivariate statistical techniques, 42 (*see also* Statistics)

National Institute of Health, 274, 275
National Science Foundation, 274
Normal distribution (*see* Statistics)
Null hypothesis (*see* Hypotheses and Statistics)
Numerals:
  definition, 95, 98
  interval meaning of, 95, 96, 102-104
  logarithmic meaning of, 96, 106, 107
  nominal meaning of, 95, 98-101
  ordinal meaning of, 95, 100-102
  ratio meaning of, 96, 104-106

Oakland Schools, 16
Objective attitude toward research, 20-25
Office of Education, 274
Operational definition, 33, 63
Order effect, 69, 70, 144, 154
Organismic variables, 32

Paired comparisons (*see* Scaling methods)
Palatography, 114
Partial correlation coefficient (*see* Statistics)
Peabody Picture Vocabulary Test, 128
Pearson product-moment correlation coefficient (*see* Statistics)
Perceptual and Motor Skills, 241
Permutations:
  in constant sums scaling, 137, 138
  of numerals on a nominal scale, 99
  for paired comparisons and constant sums, 141
  in paired comparisons scaling, 134
Phi coefficient (*see* Statistics)
Philosophy of science, 27-44 (*see also* Scientific method)
Photoelectric cells, 115
Placebo effect, 32, 260, 261
Pneumotactographs, 115
Preamplifiers, 115
Prediction (*see also* Scientific method)
  principle of causality and, 40, 41
  of therapy outcome, 32
Prognosis, 32, 33
Psychological Abstracts, 58, 59, 235
Psychological scaling techniques (*see* Scaling methods)
Purdue pitch meter, 114
Pure research, 3

Questions:
  answerable from client folder data, 23
  of causality, 31, 32

Questions (*cont.*)
  that clinicians need to answer, 4, 5
  generating relevant, 51-62
  interpreting answers to, 216-226
  selecting, 56-62
  structuring to make answerable, 15, 28, 62-64

Radio telemetry, 114, 116
Random fluctuation, 68, 201-205, 257
Random numbers, 143, 144, 220, 226, 327-335
Random sampling, 57, 74, 77, 146, 153, 154, 201, 202, 220, 221, 226
Randomization, 73
Range (*see* Statistics)
Rank order (*see* Scaling methods)
Rank ordering, 100
Recorders (*see also* Instrumentation schemes for measurement)
  magnetic:
    audiotape, 119
    instrumentation, 119, 120
  oscillographic, 117, 118, 122-125
  oscilloscopes, 119
  strip chart, 117, 118, 122-125
  X-Y, 120-125
Regression analysis, 33 (*see also* Statistics and Scaling methods)
Relations pertaining to measurement scales (*see also* Measurement)
  concidence and precedence, 101
  equivalence, 99
Relevance of research to clinical process, 4, 5, 13-25
Relevance of research, need for belief in, 3, 4
Reliability:
  of answers, 217-220, 223-226
  of clinicians, 17
  as a consideration when selecting a research design, 87
  as a consideration when selecting research questions, 57
  difference between individual and typical subject designs, 68-71
  equal-appearing intervals vs. direct magnitude-estimation, 141
  in individual subject designs, 65, 75-78
  intraclass correlation coefficient, 158-159
  mean Q values, 159
  of qualitative data, 93, 94
  of quantitative data, 97, 172, 175
  of ratings, 147, 152, 159
  relation to scientific method, 27, 30, 34, 35, 43
  in reporting research findings, 232
  role of systematic observation, in, 6
  Spearman-Brown formula, 158
  split-half, 157, 158
  test-retest, 157
  in therapy outcome research, 252, 253
  in typical subject designs, 66

Reliability (cont.)
  use of inferential statistics for assessing, 201
Reporting research findings, 228-243
  audiotapes, 228, 230
  editorial processing of manuscripts, 241, 243
  locating outlets for research, 240, 241
  motion picture films, 228, 230, 231
  oral presentations, 228, 230, 231, 240
    convention papers, 228, 230, 240
    poster sessions, 228, 230
    scientific exhibits, 228, 230
  organization of written reports, 233-238
    abstract (or summary), 233-236
    acknowledgments, 233, 238
    appendices, 233, 238
    discussion, 58, 233, 237, 238
    introduction, 52, 233, 236
    methodology, 233, 236, 237
    references, 233, 238
    results, 233, 237
    title, 233, 234
  organization of oral presentations, 238, 239
  overall purpose of scientific communication, 231
  preparation of oral and written reports, 239
  specific objectives of scientific communication, 231-233
  videotapes, 228, 230
  written reports, 228-231
    articles, 229
    case reports, 229
    clinical exchange contributions, 229
    letters to the editor, 229, 230
    point-of-view papers, 229
    reports, 229
Research:
  considerations when identifying a problem area, 52-55
  defining a topic for, 55-62
  definition, 3, 44
  factors influencing completion of, 50, 51
  generating relevant questions for, 55-62
  needs, 11
  as process underlying asking and answering of questions, 3
  relevant questions for:
    generating, 51-62
    need for selecting, 51-52
Research designs:
  "before and after," 65, 75, 254, 255, 258
  combined individual subject and typical subject, 66
  differences between individual subject and typical subject, 67-72
  for generating qualitative data, 78
  individual subject:
    advantages and disadvantages, 72, 73
    for clinical case studies, 13, 15
    definition, 65
    increasing reliability of, 75-78
    variations, 75-78

Research designs (cont.)
  selecting appropriate, 65-87
  time series, 255-257
  typical subject (group):
    advantages and disadvantages, 73, 74
    definition, 66
    for detecting differences, 78-81
    for detecting relationships, 78, 81-87
    variations, 78-87
Research programs, clinical, 270-276
  achieving administrative support for, 270, 271
  preparing a research proposal, 271-274
  research funding, 51, 274, 275
  use of consultants in, 275, 276
Research reports (see Reporting research findings)
Review papers, 58
Rorschach test, 128

Samples:
  nonrandom, 56
  size of for testing null hypothesis, 223-226
Sampling:
  error, 57
  random (see Random sampling)
  sequential, 152, 154
Scales, 132, 134 (see also Measurement)
Scaling methods (see also Measurement)
  analyses of judges' ratings, 156-161
    computation of scale values, 156
    determining degree of interjudge agreement, 159, 160
    estimating reliability of scale values, 156-159
  anchoring scale points, 136, 137, 139, 144
  comparisons between scale values (table), 140
  considerations in the choice of, 139-143
    age and intelligence level of judges, 141
    computational ease, 141, 142
    duration of individual stimuli, 142, 143
    judges' reactions to task, 143
    maximum length of judging session, 142
    maximum number of judges available, 141
    minimum level of measurement required, 139-141
    number of stimuli to be rated, 141
    statistical sophistication of the intended audience, 142
    stimuli to be scaled at different times, need for, 142
  constant sums, 134, 137, 138, 140-143, 156
  constructing master scales, 159, 160
  definition, 131, 132
  direct magnitude-estimation, 105, 106, 134, 138, 139, 140-144, 147, 152, 156
  eliminating questionable ratings, 160
  end effect, 145

Scientific method (*cont.*)
  equal-appearing intervals, 95, 134-136, 140-142, 144, 145, 147, 152, 156, 159, 160
    Lewis-Sherman Scale of Stuttering Severity, 103
  as measuring instruments, 132, 134-139
  modes of stimulus presentation, 154-156
    headphones vs. speakers, 155
    individual vs. group presentation, 154
    loudness level of audiotape stimuli, 155
    number of judging sessions, 155, 156
    physical environment, 155
  multidimensional scaling, 199
  need for, 130-132
  paired (pair) comparisons, 134, 135, 140-143, 156
  preparation of stimuli, 143-147
    acquainting judges with range of attribute, 147
    duration of judging interval, 144
    equating for extraneous attributes, 146, 147
    methods of assembling tapes, 143
    number of presentations of each stimulus, 147
    numbering stimuli, 147
    ordering stimuli, 143, 144
    segmenting stimuli, 145, 146
    standard stimuli, 144, 145
  rank order (order of merit), 134, 135, 140-142, 156
  reliability of ratings, 219
  response sheets, 150, 151
  role of observer in, 110
  selection of a judging panel, 152-154
    defining population from which selected, 152, 153
    number of judges, 152
    sampling from population, 153, 154
  semantic differentials, 261-267
    administration, 265
    analyses of ratings, 265-267
    construction, 262, 264
    standard stimuli, 138, 139
  successive intervals (successive categories; graded dichotomies), 134, 136, 137, 140, 142, 144, 145, 147, 152, 156
  types of observer judgments, 113
  use of multiple regression with, 160, 161
  writing instructions to judges, 147-151
    for direct magnitude-estimation, 149, 150
    for equal-appearing intervals, 148-150
    for successive intervals, 150
Scattergrams, 82-87, 192, 199
Scientific justification, 52, 232, 236, 243
  (*see also* Reporting research findings)
Scientific method, 27-44
  assumptions (or presuppositions), 28
  characteristics, 33-40
    coherence or systematic structure, 36-38
    comprehensiveness, 38-40
    definiteness and precision, 35, 36
    intersubjective testability, 33, 34, 232
    reliability, 34, 35
  in clinical functioning, 14-16
  definition, 27
  historical perspective, 42, 43
  need for intuitive understanding of, 27-29
  objectives, 29-33
  role of in answering questions, 27-29
  role in description, 30
  role in explaining events, 30-32
  role in predicting events, 32, 33
  as a set of rules, 43, 44
  underlying assumptions, 40-42
    causality, 40, 41
    finitude of relevant factors, 41, 42
    uniformity, 41
  value of for clinicians, 28, 29
  viewed as a game, 28
Self-corrective aspect of science, 39
Semantic differential technique (*see* Scaling methods)
Semi-interquartile range (*see* Statistics)
Sequence effects, 70, 144, 154
Sign test (*see* Statistics)
Significance Tests (*see* Statistics)
Skinnerian operant conditioning, 29
Spearman rank-order coefficient (*see* Statistics)
Standard deviation (*see* Statistics)
Statistics (*see also* Measurement and Scaling methods)
  description of computational appendix, 170-172
  descriptive statistics, 172-200
    confidence interval estimates of, 202
    contingency coefficient, 185-189, 289, 290
    correlation coefficients, 184-195, 203, 289-294
    correlation coefficients for more than two sets of measures, 195
    correlation matrices, 196, 197
    definition of, 172
    discriminant function analysis, 33, 87, 197-199
    factor analysis, 195-197
    frequencies, 203
    geometric mean, 179
    harmonic mean, 179
    interquartile range, 160, 181, 182, 287, 288
    intraclass correlation coefficient, 158, 159, 195
    Kendall coefficient of concordance, 87, 195
    mean, 66-69, 73-76, 79, 80, 156, 174-177, 180, 182, 184, 201, 206-208, 214, 283, 285
    mean vs. median, 178, 179
    measures of association (*see under descriptive statistics* contingency coefficient, Kendall coefficient of concordance, multiple correlation coefficient, partial correlation

Statistics (*cont.*)
   coefficient, Pearson product-moment correlation coefficient, phi coefficient, Spearman rank-order coefficient)
   measures of central tendency (*see under* descriptive statistics geometric mean, harmonic mean, mean, median, mode)
   measures of variability (*see under* descriptive statistics interquartile range, range, semi-interquartile range, standard deviation)
   median, 66-69, 75, 76, 79, 80, 156, 177-181, 201-203, 206-208, 214, 284, 285
   mode, 67, 68, 179, 203, 285, 286
   multidimensional scaling, 199
   multiple correlation, 88, 160, 161, 194, 195
   nonlinear correlation coefficients, 194
   partial correlation coefficients, 194
   Pearson product-moment correlation coefficient, 157, 158, 185, 189, 191-194, 196, 293, 294
   percentages, 79, 203
   phi coefficient, 185, 189, 190, 290, 291
   proportions, 79, 203
   range, 160, 180, 181, 286, 287
   role of, 172-174
   semi-interquartile range, 159, 160, 181, 182
   Spearman rank-order coefficient, 185, 189-192, 292, 293
   standard deviation, 160, 182-184, 203, 288, 289
   two-dimensional graphical displays, 199, 200
   distributions of:
      binomial, 209, 211, 212, 320
      bivariate, 173, 174
      chi square, 209-211, 319
      definition of, 172
      multivariate, 173, 174
      normal, 183, 184, 209, 211, 212, 321
      t, 209-212, 322
      F, 209, 210, 212, 323-326
      univariate, 172, 173
   inferential statistics, 71, 201-215
      alpha level, 224
      analysis of variance, 81, 207, 208, 309-314
      Bayesian decision theory, 214, 215
      chance probability, 203, 204
      Chi square test, 207, 294-296
      confidence intervals, 202, 212-215, 314-318
      critical value of statistic, 210
      degrees of freedom (df), 210-212, 295, 302, 304, 306, 307, 309, 311, 313, 314
      estimation of population values, 212-215
      experiment-wise error rate, 206

Statistics (*cont.*)
      Friedman two-way analysis of variance, 207, 301, 302
      game theory, 215
      generality of conclusions from, 226
      identifying an appropriate significance test, 206-209
      Kruskal-Wallis one-way analysis of variance, 207, 302-304
      levels of confidence, 204, 209-212
      McNemar test for the significance of change, 208
      Mann-Whitney U test, 207, 298-301
      null hypothesis, 204-207, 211, 212, 248, 249, 295, 297, 298, 300, 302, 304, 306, 307, 309, 311, 312
      one-tailed vs. two-tailed tests, 209-212
      power of significance tests, 178, 179, 205, 207
      research hypothesis, 204
      sign test, 207, 208, 296-298
      significance tests, 201-212, 257, 258, 294-314
      t-test for related measures, 207, 304-306
      t-test for independent measures, 207, 306-308
      t-test for Pearson r, 308, 309
      Type I error, 205, 206, 249, 294, 296, 298, 301, 302, 304, 306, 308, 309, 312
      Type III error, 275, 276
      Type II error, 205, 207, 219, 220, 223, 224, 249, 253-255, 257
Strain gage transduction systems, 114, 115
Stuttering (*see* Examples)
Subject bias, 111, 112
Successive intervals (*see* Scaling methods)
Systematic observation:
   definition, 5, 6
   influence on reliability, 6
   influence on validity, 6
   relation to scientific method, 7
   satisfying need for, 7, 8

t distribution (*see* Statistics)
t-tests (*see* Statistics)
Tacit knowing, 60
Target attributes, 6, 128
Teacher-investigator, 14
Tentativeness of answers, 44
Therapist variables, 32
Therapy outcome research, 247-269
   choice of presumption in, 247-249
   designs for, 75-78
   experimenter bias in, 205, 206
   generality of, 201, 202
   identifying a problem area, 52-55
   impact of systematic measurement error on, 224-226
   need for organizing data, 165, 166
   principle of uniformity, 41
   questions to consider in, 250, 251
   relapse as a consideration in, 268, 269

Therapy outcome research (*cont.*)
  relation to clinical functioning, 15
  relevance of, 5, 8
  research design considerations in, 252-269
    choosing criterion measures, 252, 253
    controlling placebo effect contamination, 260, 261
    establishing baselines, 253, 254
    establishing measurement intervals, 254-257
    identifying alternatives to research hypotheses, 258
    identifying relevant organismic variables, 259
    identifying relevant therapist variables, 259, 260
    judging effectiveness, 257, 258
    measuring attitudes, 261-267
    reducing impact of experimenter bias, 258, 259
    statistics for, 252
  time required for, 23
  use of individual subject designs, 65
Transducers, 114, 115
Type I error (*see* Statistics)
Type II error (*see* Statistics)
Typical subject design (*see* Research designs)

Ultrasound, 114
"Unanswerable" questions, 62-64
Uniformity, principle of, 41
United Cerebral Palsy, 274
University of Iowa, 132
Unobjective attitudes toward research, 21-24

Validity:
  of answers, 217, 218, 222, 223
  as a consideration when selecting a research design, 87
  as a consideration when selecting research questions, 57
  face validity, 131, 132
  mean vs. median, 178
  of published findings, 62
  of qualitative data, 93
  of quantitative data, 96, 97
  of ratings, 147, 153
  relation to map-territory analogy, 91
  relation to scientific method, 27, 30
  in reporting research findings, 232
  role of systematic observation, 6
  in therapy outcome research, 253
  in therapy selection, 34
Variables:
  dependent, 59, 60, 161
  extraneous, 68, 73, 75, 146, 147, 255-258
  independent, 59, 60, 161
  organismic, 32, 152, 257, 259
  relationships between:
    cubic, 84, 85
    curvilinear, 84, 85
    linear, 81-86
    negative, 81, 84
    nonlinear, 81, 84, 85
    positive, 81, 82, 83
    strength of, 83-86
  therapist, 32, 259, 260
Velopharyngeal closure (*see* Examples)
Voice disorders (*see* Examples)

Wilson's disease, 51